CW01496983

Baillière's
CLINICAL ENDOCRINOLOGY AND METABOLISM
INTERNATIONAL PRACTICE AND RESEARCH

Baillière's

CLINICAL ENDOCRINOLOGY AND METABOLISM

INTERNATIONAL PRACTICE AND RESEARCH

Volume 7/Number 2
April 1993

Catecholamines

P.-M. G. BOULOUX
Guest Editor

Baillière Tindall
London Philadelphia Sydney Tokyo Toronto

This book is printed on acid-free paper.

Baillière Tindall   24–28 Oval Road
W.B. Saunders   London NW1 7DX, UK

The Curtis Center, Independence Square West,
Philadelphia, PA 19106–3399, USA

55 Horner Avenue
Toronto, Ontario M8Z 4X6, Canada

Harcourt Brace Jovanovich Group (Australia) Pty Ltd,
30–52 Smidmore Street, Marrickville, NSW 2204, Australia

Harcourt Brace Jovanovich Japan, Inc.
Ichibancho Central Building,
22–1 Ichibancho, Chiyoda-ku, Tokyo 102, Japan

ISSN 0950–351X

ISBN 0–7020–1698–5 (single copy)

Baillière's Clinical Endocrinology and Metabolism is published four times each year by Baillière Tindall. Prices for Volume 7 (1993) are:

TERRITORY	ANNUAL SUBSCRIPTION	SINGLE ISSUE
Europe including UK	£72.00 post free	£27.50 post free
All other countries	Consult your local Harcourt Brace Jovanovich office	

The editor of this publication is Catriona Byres, Baillière Tindall,
24–28 Oval Road, London NW1 7DX, UK.

Baillière's Clinical Endocrinology and Metabolism was published from 1972 to 1986 as *Clinics in Endocrinology and Metabolism*.

Typeset by Phoenix Photosetting, Chatham.
Printed and bound in Great Britain by Mackays of Chatham PLC, Chatham, Kent.

Contributors to this issue

SAAD AL-DAMLUJI BSc, MB, BS, MRCP, MD, Visiting Scientist, National Institute of Neurological Diseases, National Institute of Health, Building 10, Room 5N214, Bethesda, MD 20892, USA.

PIERRE-MARC BOULOUX MD, BSc, MRCP, Senior Lecturer of Endocrinology, Department of Endocrinology, Royal Free Hospital School of Medicine, Pond Street, London NW3 2QG, UK.

MURRAY DAVID ESLER B Med Sci, MB BS, PhD, FRACP, Head, Human Autonomic Function Laboratory; Associate Director, Alfred and Baker Medical Unit, Baker Medical Research Institute, Commercial Road, Prahran 3181, Melbourne, Australia.

VIVIAN FONSECA MRCP, Senior Registrar, Department of Endocrinology, Royal Free Hospital, Pond Street, London NW3 2QG, UK.

MICHAEL P. GILBEY BSc, PhD, Honorary Senior Lecturer, Senior Research Fellow, Department of Physiology, Royal Free Hospital School of Medicine, Rowland Hill Street, London NW3 2PF, UK.

PAUL HJEMDAHL MD, PhD, Associate Professor in Clinical Pharmacology, Karolinska Institute, Karolinska Hospital, S-10401 Stockholm, Sweden.

STEPHEN B. LIGGETT MD, Associate Professor of Medicine, Molecular Genetics and Pharmacology; Chief, Pulmonary and Critical Care Medicine, University of Cincinnati College of Medicine, 231 Bethesda Avenue, Room 7511, Cincinnati, OH 45267-0564, USA.

IAN ANDREW MACDONALD BSc, PhD, Professor of Metabolic Physiology, Department of Physiology and Pharmacology, Medical School, Queen's Medical Centre, Nottingham NG7 2UH, UK.

BARRY P. McGRATH MB, BS, MD (Sydney), FRACP, Associate Professor of Medicine, Monash University, Department of Medicine, Monash Medical Centre, Clayton, Victoria, Australia 3168.

CHRISTOPHER J. MATHIAS DPhil, FRCP, Professor of Neurovascular Medicine, The Cardiovascular Medicine Unit, Department of Medicine, St Mary's Hospital Medical School, Imperial College of Science, Technology and Medicine; the Autonomic Unit, University Department of Clinical Neurology, Institute of Neurology and National Hospital for Neurology and Neurosurgery, Queen Square, London WC1N 3BG, UK.

JOHN R. RAYMOND, Department of Medicine (Nephrology), Duke University Medical Center and the Veterans Administration Hospital, Durham, North Carolina, USA.

BRAHM SHAPIRO MB, ChB, PhD, Division of Nuclear Medicine, Department of Internal Medicine, University of Michigan Medical Center and the Department of Veteran's Affairs Medical Center, Ann Arbor, Michigan 48109-0028, USA.

KAZUMASA SHIMIZU MD, The Second Department of Internal Medicine, Tohoku University School of Medicine, Sendai, Japan 980.

K. MICHAEL SPYER BSc, PhD, DSc, MD (Hons) Lisbon, Chairman of Basic Medical Sciences, Professor and Chairman of Department of Physiology, Department of Physiology, Royal Free Hospital School of Medicine, Rowland Hill Street, London NW3 2PF, UK.

JONATHAN WEBBER BM, BCh, MRCP (UK), Clinical Research Fellow, Department of Physiology and Pharmacology, Medical School, Queen's Medical Centre, Nottingham NG7 2UH, UK.

Table of contents

Foreword

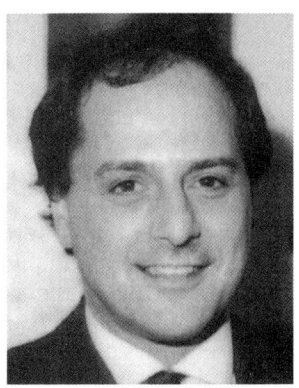

The last *Clinics in Endocrinology and Metabolism* to deal exclusively with catecholamines was in 1977. Since then, innumerable advances have occurred in catecholamine research, both at basic and clinical levels. In the present volume I have compiled contributions from basic scientists and clinical researchers covering a wide spectrum of interest. Within the space allocated it was not possible to be exhaustive; there are some notable omissions and I have had to be selective.

In the first chapter, Gilbey and Spyer describe the essential organization of the sympathetic nervous system, from a neuroanatomical and physiological standpoint. The central projections involved in cardiovascular regulation are discussed in detail, together with their complex interrelationships. The contribution of Stephen Liggett and John Raymond is a concise presentation of the pharmacology and molecular biology of adrenergic receptors. The modern classification of adrenergic receptors and the relationship between the molecular structure of these receptors and their various functions is described, as well as the important mechanisms of desensitization. Paul Hjemdahl then reviews critically the methodological approaches to quantifying the sub-nanomolar concentrations of circulating plasma catecholamines. Those who, like me, have been involved in catecholamine measurement over the past decade will welcome his critical assessment of methods which have been much used and abused.

Webber and MacDonald present a clear account of the role of the sympathoadrenal system in the control of metabolic function in the resting state, in altered nutritional states and obesity. Murray Esler reviews the issues governing the debate on the role of catecholamines in the pathogenesis of essential hypertension, and assesses the many methods used for assessment of sympathetic nervous system function in man. He further discusses the importance of the now well-documented sympathetic nervous system overactivity which characterizes the early developmental phases of essential hypertension. This logically leads on to a consideration of the circulatory pathophysiology of the congestive heart failure syndrome and the consequences of sympathetic dysfunction. This, and the effects of cardiac transplantation on sympathetic activity are further discussed by Shimizu and McGrath. The pathophysiology of autonomic nervous dysfunction is reviewed by Mathias, as well as recent data on dopamine beta hydroxylase deficiency. Al Damluji discusses the role of adrenoceptors in the regulation of hypothalamo–pituitary function, a complex and confusing area which his human experiments have done much to disentangle. Shapiro reviews the imaging of catecholamine-secreting tumours, focusing on the uses of MIBG (metaiodobenzylguanidine) in both diagnosis and treatment of these tumours. Finally, Fonseca and Bouloux review recent advances in the biology, diagnosis and treatment of phaeochromocytomas and para-gangliomas.

Editing the manuscripts has been a most stimulating exercise. This volume highlights in a selective manner some of what has been achieved in the past decade, and alludes to the future direction of catecholamine research at the physiological, cellular and subcellular levels.

P.-M. G. BOULOUX

1

Essential organization of the sympathetic nervous system

MICHAEL P. GILBEY
K. MICHAEL SPYER

The sympathetic nervous system consists of efferent neurones supplying the viscera. Sympathetic preganglionic neurones, which form the final common pathway out of the central nervous system involved in sympathetic control, arise from the thoracic and upper lumbar segments of the spinal cord and project to ganglia or innervate adrenal chromaffin cells. Sympathetic postganglionic neurones originating in these ganglia then innervate the end organs (Loewy, 1990b).

The axons of the sympathetic preganglionic neurones exit the spinal cord at their segment of origin via the ventral roots. They then project through the white rami communicantes by way of the segmental nerve and join the sympathetic chain. They may then synapse in chain ganglia (paravertebral). The axons of postganglionic neurones may then project back into a segmental nerve or, alternatively, the postganglionic axons may emerge from the paravertebral chain as a postganglionic nerve trunk. Other preganglionic axons pass through the sympathetic chain to synapse in peripheral ganglia (prevertebral) which are located in the abdominal cavity or chromaffin cells of the adrenal medulla (Langley, 1921).

Within the last 20 years technological innovations in methods of track tracing and the cellular localization of putative neurotransmitter substances, or the enzymes associated with their synthesis, have led to a rapid growth of information concerning the location of sympathetic preganglionic neurones and the central pathways, and the nature of the neurotransmitters involved in regulating their activity. Tracing methods have involved the use of anterograde tracers such as radiolabelled excitatory amino acids (Ross et al, 1984) and phaseolus vulgaris leukoagglutinin (Li et al, 1992a), retrograde tracers such as horseradish peroxidase (Ross et al, 1984) and rhodamine latex microspheres (Hirsch and Helke, 1988), and transneuronal retrograde tracers such as pseudorabies virus (Strack et al, 1989b). Immunohistochemical techniques have provided the major means of identifying the cellular localization of putative neurotransmitters or their synthesizing enzymes (Hancock, 1982). Modern neurophysiology and neuropharmacology techniques have been used to investigate the function of these central

Baillière's Clinical Endocrinology and Metabolism—
Vol. 7, No. 2, April 1993
ISBN 0–7020–1698–5

259

neurones and putative neurotransmitters in the central nervous control of sympathetic activity (Coote, 1988; Gebber, 1990; Guyenet, 1990).

The essence of this chapter is to describe the central neural networks and neurotransmitters involved in the control of sympathetic activity, including those involved in the afferent and efferent loops of cardiovascular reflexes and tonic and phasic sympathetic responses. The data and ideas presented in this chapter are drawn from animal studies (mainly on rat, cat and rabbit); however, we believe that the essential features of the central nervous control of the sympathetic nervous system are likely to be similar across species. For detailed accounts we refer the reader to a number of recent reviews in this area (Jordan and Spyer, 1986; Coote, 1988; Cabot, 1990; Cervero and Foreman, 1990; Gebber, 1990; Guyenet, 1990; Kumada et al, 1990; Loewy, 1990a,b, 1991; Spyer, 1990).

NEUROANATOMY OF THE CENTRAL REGULATORY AREAS OF SYMPATHETIC FUNCTION

The locations of sympathetic preganglionic neurones within the thoracic and lumbar spinal cord

Petras and Cummings (1972) mapped the distribution of sympathetic preganglionic neurones within the spinal cord of the rhesus monkey. This

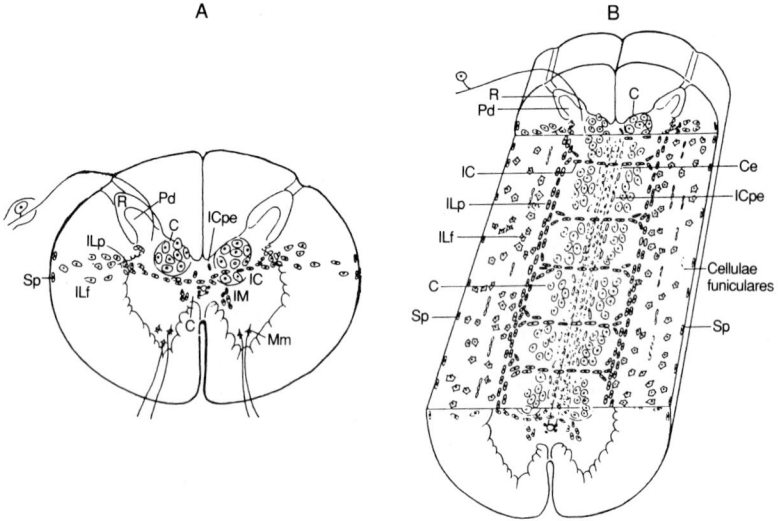

Figure 1. Schematic diagram of the location of autonomic nuclei (ILp, ILf, IC and ICpe) in the spinal cord. (a) Transverse section. (b) Horizontal plane. ILp = nucleus intermediolateralis thoracolumbalis pars principalis; ILf = nucleus intermediolateralis thoracolumbalis pars funicularis; IC = nucleus intercalatus spinalis; ICpe = nucleus pars paraependymalis. Adapted from Petras and Cummings (1972). Sp = subpial neurones; R = substantia gelatinosa of Rolando; Pd = nucleus proprius cornus dorsalis; C = Clarke's column; IM = nucleus intermediomedialis; Mm = motor neurone; Ce = cells of central grey substance. Adapted from Petras and Cummings (1972) with permission.

distribution has subsequently been confirmed in a number of species (Cabot, 1990).

Sympathetic preganglionic neurones are found in four main nuclei within the intermediate spinal grey matter. The nomenclature used varies; that employed by Petras and Cummings (1972) is given in parentheses in the following description. Figure 1 shows the location of the four sympathetic nuclei. The bulk of sympathetic preganglionic neurones are found within the intermediolateral cell column (IML) (in the nucleus intermediolateralis thoracolumbalis pars principalis; ILp), which is located in the lateral horn of the grey matter. Another group is found extending from the IML into the lateral funiculus (the nucleus intermediolateralis thoracolumbalis pars funicularis; ILf). The intercalated cell group (the nucleus intercalatus spinalis; IC) is found medial to the IML, and a fourth group dorsolateral to the central canal is known as the central autonomic nucleus (the nucleus intercalatus pars paraependymalis; ICpe). The cell bodies of sympathetic preganglionic neurones form a ladder-like arrangement when viewed in horizontal section (see Figure 4).

It has only recently become feasible to attempt to investigate the locations of sympathetic preganglionic neurones influencing specific target organs using retrograde transneuronal labelling techniques (see below), as conventional retrograde tracers do not travel trans-synaptically and sympathetic preganglionic neurones synapse in ganglia remote from the end organs they innervate (see above). Most of the information available at present describes the rostrocaudal and intrasegmental distribution of sympathetic preganglionic neurones projecting into specific nerves or synapsing in particular ganglia (Chung et al, 1979; Kuo et al, 1980; Deuschl and Illert, 1981; Oldfield and McLachlan, 1981; Janig and McLachlan, 1986; Morgan et al, 1986; Strack et al, 1988), the exception being with regard to the location of sympathetic preganglionic neurones innervating the chromaffin cells of the adrenal medulla (Holets and Elde, 1983; Bacon and Smith, 1988; Strack et al, 1988; Vera et al, 1990). Strack et al (1988) examined the segmental distribution of sympathetic preganglionic neurones projecting to a number of sympathetic ganglia and the adrenal gland of rats. Preganglionic neurones projecting to a particular ganglia were found to arise from a number of segments, but with one segment making the predominant contribution (Figure 2). They also found that, although the main source of sympathetic preganglionic neurones was primarily the IML, those projecting to the inferior mesenteric ganglion were located mainly in the central autonomic nucleus. In addition, in the upper thoracic cord the lateral funiculus contained a significant number of sympathetic preganglionic neurones, whereas in the lumbar cord the central autonomic nucleus was prominent. Recently studies using retrograde transneuronal labelling techniques involving viral infections have examined the locations of sympathetic preganglionic neurones innervating postganglionic sympathetic neurones projecting into the renal nerve, where in rat and rabbit they are found in the IML of segments T7–T13 and T7–L2, respectively (Schramm et al, 1991; Li et al, 1992a), and the medial gastrocnemius muscle in the rat, where they are found in the IML of T11–L2 (Rotto-Percelay et al, 1992).

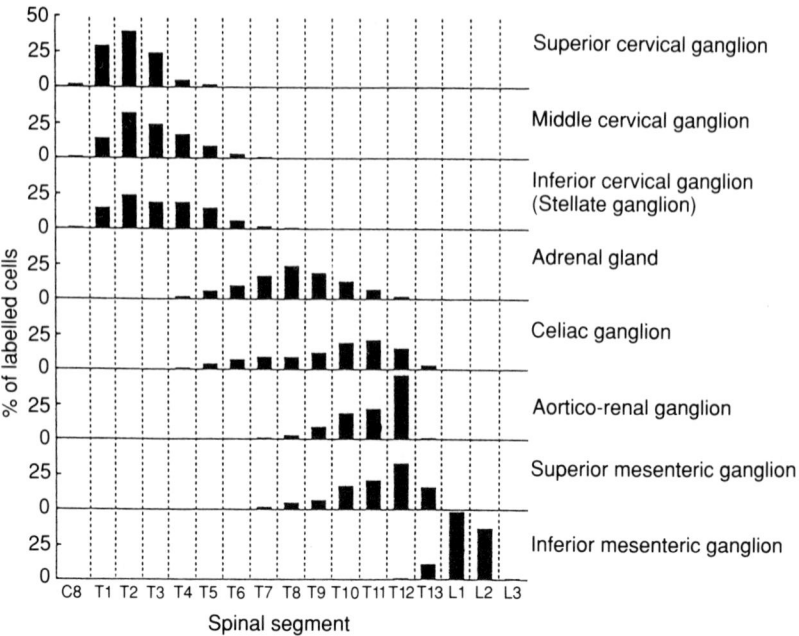

Figure 2. A series of histograms showing the segmental distribution of labelled sympathetic preganglionic neurones after fluoro-gold injections into the major sympathetic ganglia and adrenal gland of rats. From Strack et al (1988) with permission.

Supraspinal neurones projecting to spinal sympathetic nuclei

The above description of the topography of sympathetic preganglionic neurones reveals considerable overlap, with respect to the intrasegmental and the rostrocaudal segments of origin, of sympathetic preganglionic neurones projecting into different nerves or ganglia. Therefore sympathetic preganglionic neurones with different functions are likely to be intermixed, at least to a degree. Such an arrangement of sympathetic preganglionic neurones raises a number of technical problems concerning the identification of supraspinal pathways regulating the activity of sympathetic preganglionic neurones with known function or identified projections. For example, retrograde tracing methods involving the injection of substances into the IML label supraspinal cell bodies with axons projecting to, or through, this nucleus and therefore demonstrate that such cell bodies are probably involved in the control of sympathetic activity without indicating which specific sympathetic function they are regulating. Similarly, most anterograde tracing studies have only shown that particular cell groups project to sympathetic nuclei in the spinal cord.

In an early study in the cat, Amendt et al (1979), following unilateral injection of horseradish peroxidase into the IML, examined the brain stem for labelled perikarya between the first cervical segment and the inferior colliculi. Labelled neurones were found within the nucleus tractus solitarius, the ventrolateral reticular formation from the obex to 8 mm rostral, and in the caudal raphe nuclei (pallidus, obscurus and magnus) 2–9 mm rostral to the obex. Other studies using conventional retrograde and anterograde tracing methods have confirmed and extended the above findings (Saper et al, 1976; Loewy and Burton, 1978; Loewy et al, 1979a,b; Saper and Loewy, 1980; Blessing et al, 1981; Loewy, 1981, 1982; Ross et al, 1984; Tucker and Saper, 1985; Hirsch and Helke, 1988; Hosoya et al, 1991). These studies, whilst demonstrating the location of cell groups projecting to the region of the IML, failed to discern whether these cells make direct contact with sympathetic preganglionic neurones. Injection of an anterograde tracer, phaseolus vulgaris leucoagglutinin (PHA-L), centred on the raphe nuclei pallidus and magnus or the rostral ventrolateral medulla has led to the demonstration of labelled terminals making synaptic contact with retro-gradely labelled adrenal sympathetic neurones (Bacon et al, 1990; Zagon and Smith, 1990).

Recently, transneuronal labelling techniques have been developed and utilized in an attempt to locate the cell bodies of neurones with axons terminating in the immediate vicinity of sympathetic preganglionic neurones. Pseudorabies virus has been injected into either the adrenal gland or the superior cervical, stellate, coeliac or sympathetic ganglia of rats (Strack et al, 1989a,b). From its retrograde transsynaptic transport, it appears that five brain regions innervate sympathetic outflow at all thoracolumbar levels: the ventromedial and rostral ventrolateral medulla, the area encompassing the caudal raphe nuclei, the A5 noradrenergic cell group, and the paraventricular nucleus of the hypothalamus. In addition, numerous small interneurones in Rexed laminae VII and X of the spinal cord were labelled. Other cell groups were only infected following the injection of some ganglia. After superior cervical and stellate ganglia injections, labelled cell bodies were found in the periaqueductal grey matter of the midbrain and the lateral hypothalamic area. The zona incerta was labelled solely from the stellate ganglion. The experiments also indicated a topographical organization of neurones within the paraventricular nucleus of the hypothalamus; those regulating the upper thoracic sympathetic outflow were found medially, whilst those projecting to the mid and lower thoracic levels were located dorsolaterally. Schramm et al (1991), in similar experiments, also observed labelling of neurones in the rostral ventrolateral medulla, the A5 cell group and the paraventricular nucleus following renal injections of pseudorabies virus. However, not all neurones appear to be susceptible to pseudorabies virus infection and therefore not all neurones projecting to sympathetic preganglionic neurones may be identified using this technique. Figure 3 summarizes the locations of supraspinal regions with major projections to the IML.

Obviously not all supraspinal neurones projecting to the spinal cord necessarily influence sympathetic preganglionic neurones directly; they may synapse on propriospinal or segmental interneurones that themselves influence sympathetic preganglionic neurones (Strack et al, 1989a; Cabot et al, 1991). The brain nuclei involved in this kind of circuitry remain to be identified.

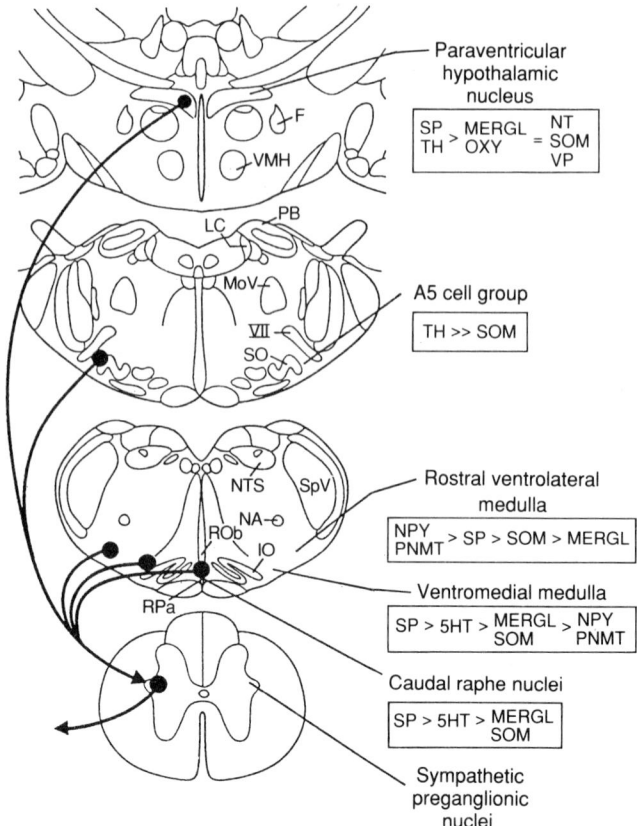

Figure 3. Summary diagram illustrating brain regions with major projections to sympathetic preganglionic neurones. Also shown are some of the neurotransmitters colocalized in neurones retrogradely labelled from the adrenal gland using pseudorabies virus. A5 = noradrenergic cell group; F = fornix; 5HT = 5-hydroxytryptamine; IO = inferior olivary nucleus; LC = locus coeruleus; MERGL = metenkephalin-arg-gly-leu; MoV = motor trigeminal nucleus; NA = nucleus ambiguus; NPY = neuropeptide Y; NT = neurotensin; NTS = nucleus tractus solitarius; OXY = oxytocin; PB = parabrachial nucleus; PNMT = phenylethanolamine-N-methyltransferase (enzyme marker for adrenaline); ROb = raphe obscurus; RPa = raphe pallidus; SO = superior olivary nucleus; SOM = somatostatin; SP = substance P; SpV = spinal trigeminal nucleus; TH = tyrosine hydroxylase (enzyme marker for noradrenaline); TRH = thyrotropin-releasing hormone; VII = facial nerve; VIP = vasoactive intestinal polypeptide; VMH = ventromedial hypothalamic nucleus; VP = vasopressin. Adapted from Strack et al (1989b) with permission.

Supraspinal networks influencing descending pathways regulating sympathetic activity

There is evidence that supraspinal neurones projecting to autonomic areas of the spinal cord receive inputs from many neuronal cell groups which are reciprocally connected. This network of interconnecting neurones has been studied using the anatomical tracing techniques described above. The areas and nuclei of the brain included in this matrix are the rostral and caudal ventrolateral medulla (including A1 and C1), the raphe nuclei, the A5 cell group, the periaqueductal grey matter, the parabrachial nuclei, the Kölliker–Fuse nucleus, the locus coeruleus, the paraventricular nucleus of the hypothalamus, the lateral hypothalamic area, the zona incerta, the perifornical area of the hypothalamus and the bed nucleus of the stria terminalis (Cedarbaum and Aghajanian, 1978; Sapar and Loewy, 1980; McKellar and Loewy, 1981, 1982; Blessing et al, 1982; Lovick, 1985; Byrum and Guyenet, 1987; Tucker et al, 1987; Van Bockstaele et al, 1989; Li et al, 1992b; Loewy, 1991). Although these neuroanatomical studies demonstrate projections from one nucleus or area to another, they do not demonstrate connectivity or that the circuitry is necessarily involved in sympathetic control; for the latter to be demonstrated unequivocally requires the application of neurophysiological techniques (see below).

Recently, the combination of transneuronal retrograde tracing (using herpes simplex virus) with anterograde tracing (using PHA-L) from the caudal medulla has provided strong evidence for connections between the caudal medulla and 'premotor sympathetic neurones' of the rostral ventrolateral medulla and A5 region labelled from the adrenal medulla (Li et al, 1992a). Future studies employing the similar application of anterograde and retrograde tracing techniques promise to provide important information on the detailed connections of cell groups rather than general areas of projection (see above).

BRAIN STEM NUCLEI INVOLVED IN TONIC AND PHASIC SYMPATHETIC RESPONSES

Sympathetic nerves demonstrate ongoing (tonic) activity under resting conditions. Various perturbations or changes in behavioural state elicit phasic changes in sympathetic activity which can involve the generation of differential patterns of sympathetic activity (see Gebber, 1990). The central neural circuitry and mechanisms of generation of these types of sympathetic activity have been the subject of extensive investigation. Neuronal circuits within the spinal cord are capable of generating sympathetic activity (Schramm, 1986), yet the role of supraspinal mechanisms appears to be of particular importance. The supraspinal aspects will be considered here.

Modern neuronal tracing methods have been used to identify cell groups which may be involved in central 'sympathetic' circuitry (see above). The cells in these areas have then been investigated for characteristics congruent with 'sympathetic' function, such as a firing pattern correlated to sympathetic efferent nerve discharge and/or axonal projections to the IML. Such neurones, if they have a cardiovascular function, can then be tentatively identified as being sympatho-inhibitory or excitatory by determining whether they are activated or inhibited by baroreceptor activation. Neurones with some of these properties have been found in the rostral ventrolateral medulla, the caudal raphe nuclei, the lateral tegmental field and the hypothalamus (Morrison and Geber, 1984, 1985; Barman and

Gebber, 1985, 1989a,b; Morrison et al, 1988; Guyenet et al, 1989; McCall and Clement, 1989; Barman, 1990; Huangfu et al, 1991). It is likely that these neurones are involved in the generation of phasic and tonic sympathetic activities.

For many years the 'Holy Grail' has been the search for the source of tonic sympathetic activity. In the latter part of the last century lesions of the rostral ventrolateral medulla (RVLM) were found to reduce blood pressure to levels seen in the spinal animal (see Gebber, 1990). This area was 'rediscovered' just over a decade ago, when it was realized that it provided a major source of innervation to the IML (see above). It has since been the focus of extensive investigation and is now implicated as being of great importance in cardiovascular control. This area has also been referred to as the C1 region, the nucleus reticularis rostroventralis, the nucleus paragigantocellularis and the subretrofacial nucleus (Ross et al, 1984; Dampney et al, 1987; Sun et al, 1988; Reis et al, 1989).

Much has been learned about neurones within this area with respect to: (a) the sympathetic responses evoked by influencing their activity using electrical or chemical methods; (b) the physiological characteristics of the spinally projecting neurones; and (c) their neurochemical content. Electrical lesions of this area have been observed to decrease blood pressure in anaesthetized animals, as does the application of inhibitory chemicals to the overlying ventral surface of the medulla or their microinjection into the area (Reis et al, 1984; Benarroch et al, 1986). All these procedures can reduce blood pressure to that seen in the spinal animal, indicating that the neurones of the RVLM are tonically active and responsible for resting tone. Conversely, stimulation of neurones within the RVLM either electrically or by the microinjection of excitatory amino acids (which activate cell bodies but not fibres of passage) produces pressor responses and a tachycardia (Reis et al, 1984). In the cat, there is evidence that the RVLM regulates sympathetic drive to the heart, vasculature and adrenal medulla, but not that involved with pupillomotor, sudomotor and gut function (McAllen, 1986). The physiological characteristics of spinally projecting neurones in this area are also consistent with cardiovascular function (see above).

Work from Guyenet's laboratory (Guyenet et al, 1989) has indicated that some neurones within the RVLM have pacemaker properties, and Guyenet has suggested that the 'pacemaker neurones' may contribute to tonic sympathetic activity. However, Gebber's laboratory contests this view, suggesting that sympathetic activity is generated by neurones antecedent to those found in the RVLM (Barman and Gebber, 1989a). Gebber (1990) suggests that the lateral tegmental field neurones may form part of a sympathetic rhythm generator.

It is clear that the RVLM is an important supraspinal site involved in the relay of excitatory drive to sympathetic preganglionic neurones involved in cardiovascular control—a 'vasomotor centre'. However, the relative compactness of 'cardiovascular' IML-projecting neurones in this region has made studies (e.g. ablation) possible which cannot be done on dispersed cell populations, and consequently it is possible that the functional significance of this region has been exaggerated. Recent studies give some credence to this view. Following bilateral lesions of the RVLM, conscious rats maintain normal blood pressure and baroreceptor reflexes are functional. Similarly lesions, although producing maintained hypotension in rats anaesthetized with urethane, only produced a transient hypotension in rats anaesthetized with α-chloralose or pentobarbitone sodium (pentobarbital sodium *USP*) (Cochrane et al, 1988; Cochrane and Nathan, 1989). The RVLM may therefore not be '*the* vasomotor centre'.

The involvement of the RVLM in the mediation of phasic sympathetic responses has been the subject of intense investigation. It has been implicated in the mediation of responses to stimulation of a number of nerves: superior laryngeal, vagus and numerous somatosensory afferents (Brown and Guyenet, 1985; Sun and Guyenet, 1987; Morrison and Reis, 1989; Stornetta et al, 1989; Sun and Spyer, 1991a). A baroreceptor reflex pathway appears to relay through this area (see below), as do afferents from the area postrema (Sun and Spyer, 1991b). The spinal projecting neurones of this area also have their activity modulated by central respiratory drive (McAllen, 1987; Haselton and Guyenet, 1989a) and therefore are one site of origin of the respiratory-related modulation of sympathetic activity (Gilbey et al, 1986).

NEUROANATOMICAL CONNECTIONS AND TRANSMITTERS INVOLVED IN THE CARDIOVASCULAR REFLEXES

Central projections of afferents

Both visceral and somatic afferents can influence the sympathetic nerve activity supplying the cardiovascular system (Janig, 1985; Janig and McLachlan, 1987; Coote, 1988). The afferents enter the central nervous system by way of spinal and cranial nerves. Cranial visceral afferents enter the brain where they synapse in brain stem nuclei, whereas spinal visceral afferents pass via the sympathetic or parasympathetic nerves into the spinal cord. Spinal visceral afferents terminate either in the dorsal horn or project rostrally to the dorsomedial medulla, including the commissural nucleus of the nucleus tractus solitarius (NTS) (Simon and Schramm, 1984; Willis, 1986; Knuepfer et al, 1988). Most organs receive a dual afferent innervation via fibres which travel in sympathetic and parasympathetic nerves (Cervero and Foreman, 1990).

The focus here is on visceral afferents that arise within the cardiovascular system and terminate within the NTS. These project into the brain via the vagal and glossopharyngeal nerves. The central projections of cardiovascular afferents have been studied for decades using many methods (see Jordan and Spyer, 1986), but again the major advances have been made within the last 20 years.

Modern anterograde and retrograde tracing techniques have provided a detailed picture of the central projections of these nerves. Visceral afferents entering the NTS project in an organ-specific manner to subnuclei (the NTS has a viscerotopic organization) and also to the commissural nucleus of the

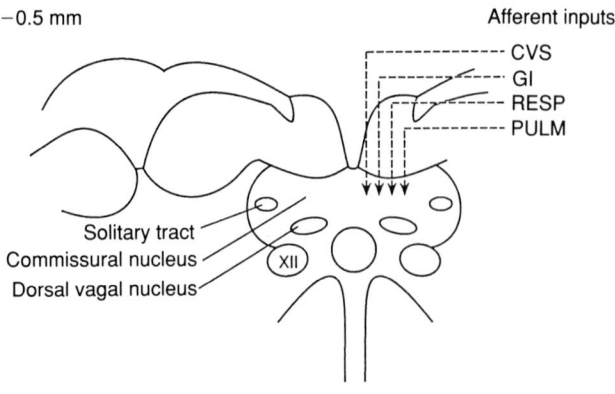

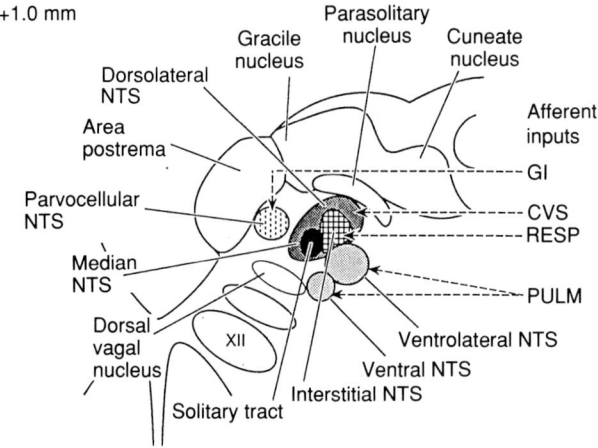

Figure 4. Projections of various afferents in the NTS of the cat shown in transverse plane. The upper diagram illustrates a common site of projection for various afferents 0.5 mm caudal to the obex. The lower diagram shows the viscerotopic pattern of innervation 1.0 mm rostral to the obex. CVS = cardiovascular system; GI = gastrointestinal; RESP = respiratory tract; PULM = pulmonary; XII = hypoglossal nucleus. Adapted from Loewy (1990a).

NTS, where afferents converge (Figure 4). The carotid sinus and aortic depressor nerves (branches of the glossopharyngeal and vagal nerves, respectively) which carry information from the arterial baroreceptors and chemoreceptors project to the dorsolateral and medial NTS and the commissural nucleus (Loewy, 1990a).

Mapping of afferent projections using neurophysiological techniques has identified arterial baroreceptor afferents innervating chiefly the dorsolateral and dorsomedial regions of the NTS rostral to the obex, and to a lesser extent lateral and ventrolateral subdivisions (Jordan and Spyer, 1986). Neurophysiological studies have demonstrated both presynaptic and post-synaptic interactions between afferents within the NTS (Jordan and Spyer,

1986; Spyer, 1990). Although lung stretch and superior laryngeal afferents appear to interact presynaptically, such is not the case for aortic and sinus nerve afferents (Jordan and Spyer, 1986). Many NTS neurones receive a postsynaptic convergent input from a number of afferents such as those contained within the sinus, aortic, vagus and superior laryngeal nerves (Spyer, 1990). Thus the NTS may be one site for the integration of afferent inputs.

Neurotransmitters in cardiovascular afferents

A number of neurochemicals have been found to be associated with the ninth and tenth cranial nerves, including neuropeptides such as substance P, calcitonin gene-related peptide, vasoactive intestinal polypeptide, cholecystokinin, neuropeptide Y and neurokinin A (Helke and Hill, 1988; Cryzyk-Krzeska et al, 1991), and 5-hydroxytryptamine (5-HT) (Gaudin-Chazal et al, 1982). Subnuclei of the NTS (dorsal, medial and commissural) which receive afferents from the carotid sinus nerve contain high levels of glutamate which are greatly reduced following sectioning of the ninth and tenth cranial nerves (Dietrich et al, 1982).

An excitatory amino acid, perhaps glutamate, is most favoured as the neurotransmitter released by baroreceptor afferents. The evidence, however, is quite tentative. Amino acid receptor agonists microinjected into the nucleus decrease blood pressure and heart rate, and endogenous glutamate and aspartate are released in response to perfusion with high potassium levels (see Kumada et al, 1990). Importantly, a number of excitatory amino acid antagonists applied to the NTS have been observed to reduce or block the excitation of single NTS units produced by stimulation of the solitary tracts (Miller and Felder, 1988), the depressor reflex evoked by aortic nerve stimulation (Leone and Gordon, 1989), and the baroreceptor reflex (Guyenet et al, 1987).

Supraspinal interneurones involved in the transmission of cardiovascular reflexes

Neurones of the NTS send projections to a number of areas or nuclei within the supraspinal matrix (see above) thought to be involved in regulating the activity of bulbospinal neurones controlling the activity of sympathetic preganglionic neurones, such as the parabrachial nucleus, the Kölliker–Fuse nucleus, the central nucleus of the amygdala and bed nucleus of the stria terminalis (Loewy, 1990a). The NTS is also connected reciprocally to a number of cell groups that probably provide direct inputs to sympathetic preganglionic neurones; these include the caudal raphe nuclei, the RVLM, the central grey matter, the lateral hypothalamic area and the paraventricular nucleus of the hypothalamus. The NTS also sends projections to the spinal cord. This labyrinth of projections from the NTS supports the contention that the baroreceptor reflex is mediated by a number of parallel pathways.

There are two mechanisms by which sympathetic preganglionic neuronal activity may be decreased by baroreceptor activity: sympathetic preganglionic neuronal activity may be inhibited, in the true sense of the word, or baroreceptor activation may lead to the diminution of excitatory drive to these neurones (disfacilitation). The balance of neurophysiological evidence also indicates that baroreceptor control of sympathetic activity occurs over a number of parallel pathways: spinally projecting 'sympatho-excitatory' neurones located in the caudal raphe nuclei and RVLM have their activity decreased by baroreceptor activity, and spinally projecting 'sympatho-inhibitory' neurones in these same areas are activated by baroreceptor activation (McCall and Clement, 1989; Barman, 1990; Gebber, 1990; Guyenet, 1990; Li et al, 1991).

The RVLM is considered to be a major relay station in a baroreceptor reflex pathway which functions by decreasing the activity of RVLM sympatho-excitatory neurones. Recent intracellular studies demonstrated that the decrease in activity is mediated by disfacilitation in one population of neurones and direct inhibition in another (Granata and Kitai, 1992). The baroreceptor-mediated inhibition appears to involve γ-aminobutyric acid (GABA) as it is blocked by bicuculline, a selective $GABA_A$ antagonist (Sun and Guyenet, 1985). There is evidence that this inhibitory input is relayed to the RVLM via interneurones located in the caudal ventrolateral medulla (CVLM), an area which also receives a heavy projection from the NTS. For example, injection of excitatory amino acid antagonists into the CVLM blocked the aortic baroreceptor reflex and caused a rise in blood pressure (Somogyi et al, 1989). However, other observations indicate that, although the aortic baroreceptor reflex is blocked under these circumstances, renal sympathetic nerve activity is still influenced by changes in arterial blood pressure (Blessing, 1989). Recent observations indicate that it is the rostral portion of the CVLM that is responsible for mediating the baroreceptor reflex (Cravo et al, 1991). Although experiments in anaesthetized animals, where tonic sympathetic activity is maintained, have indicated that the RVLM has to be intact for the baroreceptor reflex to remain functional (see Kumada et al, 1990), conscious rats were normotensive following bilateral lesions of the RVLM and had normal baroreceptor sensitivity to an increase in blood pressure (Cochrane and Nathan, 1989).

Baroreceptor stimulation causes an increase in the discharge rate of some bulbospinal neurones originating in the RVLM and caudal raphe nuclei. These observations indicate that baroreceptor inhibition also occurs at a spinal site (see Coote, 1988).

Neurotransmitters influencing sympathetic preganglionic neurones

Numerous putative neurotransmitters or enzymes involved in their synthesis have been found within neurones identified as projecting to the IML (see Figure 3) or within terminals within the IML, sometimes identified as being contiguous with, or making synaptic contacts with, sympathetic preganglionic neurones. The neurochemicals implicated in the direct control of sympathetic preganglionic neuronal activity include: (a) the monoamines—

adrenaline, noradrenaline and 5-HT; (b) peptides—substance P, thyrotropin-releasing hormone (TRH), metenkephalin, vasopressin, oxytocin and neuropeptide Y; (c) amino acids—glutamate, GABA and glycine (see Cabot, 1990). Many of these substances have been found to influence the excitability and/or the firing pattern of sympathetic preganglionic neurones (Coote, 1988; Marks et al, 1990; Gilbey and Stein, 1991). In some cases a putative neurotransmitter may have more than one action on sympathetic preganglionic neuronal activity. This diversity of action of a transmitter (e.g. the catecholamines) is due to the presence of receptor subtypes on the preganglionic neurones (Nishi, 1990; Gilbey and Stein, 1991). Because of the problems involved in identifying sympathetic preganglionic neurones functionally, it is not clear which of these transmitters are involved in determining the activity of sympathetic preganglionic neurones with a particular cardiovascular function (Gilbey and Stein, 1991). However, it has been shown that nerve terminals containing 5-HT, GABA, substance P and phenylethanolamine-N-methyltransferase (PNMT; the enzyme involved in the synthesis of adrenaline) make synaptic contact with adrenal sympathetic preganglionic neurones (Bacon and Smith, 1988; Milner et al, 1988) and that these neurones are excited by the local application of substance P, TRH, glutamate and 5-HT (Backman et al, 1990).

The neurochemical content of neurones in the RVLM is heterogeneous; there is now evidence that glutamate, neuropeptide Y, enkephalin, 5-HT and adrenaline are present either singly or in combination (Strack et al, 1989b; Minson et al, 1991). However, until recently attention was focused on the coincidence of the C1 (adrenergic) cell group (Reis et al, 1989). Although there is strong circumstantial evidence that some of the baroreceptor-sensitive neurones are adrenergic (Haselton and Guyenet, 1989b), some baroreceptor-sensitive cells in this region do not stain positively for PNMT (Granata and Kitai, 1992), as is the case for 'pacemaker' cells (Sun et al, 1991). Indeed, evidence is now accumulating that glutamate is the most important excitatory transmitter released by these sympathetic 'premotor' neurones, with adrenaline and other monoamines and peptides probably serving an important modulatory role (Morrison et al, 1989).

Neurotransmitters in sympathetic efferents

It is well established that sympathetic preganglionic neurones utilize acetylcholine as a neurotransmitter and that the postganglionic neurones release principally noradrenaline, with those innervating the sweat glands employing acetylcholine. However, in the last decade it has become apparent that many neurochemicals may be involved.

Sympathetic preganglionic neurones have been shown to contain several neuroactive peptides, and different peptides have been shown to coexist within the same neurone (e.g. substance P, neurotensin, somatostatin, enkephalin, corticotrophin-releasing factor and vasoactive intestinal polypeptide) (Krukoff, 1987). Neurotransmission between sympathetic postganglionic neurones and vascular smooth muscle is thought to involve at least three neurotransmitters—adenosine triphosphate (ATP), noradrenaline and neuropeptide Y—which are thought to mediate fast depolarizations, slow depolarizations and very slow contractions, respectively (Morris and Gibbins, 1992).

CONCLUDING REMARKS

The various anatomical and neurophysiological studies that have been reviewed have indicated that the activity of sympathetic preganglionic neurones is determined by the actions of a complex series of parallel, and often reciprocal, pathways that descend from several levels of the neuraxis. The actions of the sympathetic nervous system in homeostasis, and in the expression of behaviour, are thus dependent on the balance of influences that are exerted through this integrative matrix. Whilst the chemical content of the neurones involved in these pathways and the receptors present on sympathetic preganglionic neurones and the various interneurones are being identified, the challenge is now the physiological issue of understanding the mechanisms of action and interaction of these pathways. Following the acquisition of these new physiological insights, it may be possible to understand the pathological consequences of lesions (developmental, chemical and structural) on autonomic function and so be in a position to offer rational clinical approaches to several disease states.

SUMMARY

The sympathetic nervous system consists of efferent neurones supplying the viscera. The cell bodies of preganglionic neurones are located in four areas in the thoracolumbar cord; however, the majority are found in the IML. Various tracing techniques have provided information concerning the location of the cell bodies of sympathetic preganglionic neurones projecting into various nerves and ganglia and regulating the adrenal gland, the kidney and the sympathetic supply to skeletal muscle. Numerous supraspinal neurones project to the neuropil surrounding sympathetic preganglionic neurones and may form synaptic contacts with these neurones. The areas of the brain that project to the IML appear to be part of a network of reciprocally connected supraspinal cell groups. Although much emphasis has been placed on the importance of the RVLM in the mediation of tonic and phasic inputs to sympathetic preganglionic neurones, it appears that other areas are of significant import; the RVLM should not be considered to be 'the vasomotor centre'. Spinal and cranial afferents influence the sympathetic nervous system. Baroreceptor afferents terminate in the NTS and may utilize an excitatory amino acid as their neurotransmitter. However, a number of neuropeptides are also associated with these afferents. Neurones within the NTS project to a number of brain stem areas thought to be involved in the regulation of sympathetic activity; consequently the baroreceptor reflex may be mediated over a number of parallel pathways involving both supraspinal and spinal sites of inhibition. Many neurotransmitters are thought to regulate the activity of sympathetic preganglionic neurones: monoamines, peptides and amino acids. Matching the chemical content of the cell bodies of neurones within a particular cell group with physiological characteristics is a challenging task; some barosensitive neurones of the RVLM do not appear to be adrenergic although they are in the midst of the C1 adrenergic cell group. Besides acetylcholine and noradrenaline, neurotransmission in the periphery appears to involve numerous peptides and ATP.

Acknowledgements

The authors thank the British Heart Foundation and Medical Research Council for supporting the studies from their laboratories.

REFERENCES

Amendt K, Czachurski J, Dembowsky K et al (1979) Bulbospinal projections to the intermediolateral cell column: a neuroanatomical study. *Journal of the Autonomic Nervous System* 1: 103–107.

Backman SB, Sequeira Martinho H & Henry JL (1990) Adrenal versus nonadrenal sympathetic preganglionic neurones in the lower thoracic intermediolateral nucleus of the cat: effects of serotonin, substance P, and thyrotropin-releasing hormone. *Canadian Journal of Physiology and Pharmacology* 68: 1108–1118.

Bacon SJ & Smith AD (1988) Preganglionic sympathetic neurones innervating the rat adrenal medulla: immunocytochemical evidence of synaptic input from nerve terminals containing substance P, GABA or 5-hydroxytryptamine. *Journal of the Autonomic Nervous System* 24: 97–122.

Bacon SJ, Zagon A & Smith AD (1990) Electron microscopic evidence of a monosynaptic pathway between cells in the caudal raphe nuclei and sympathetic preganglionic neurons in the rat spinal cord. *Experimental Brain Research* 79: 589–602.

Barman SM (1990) Descending projections of hypothalamic neurons with sympathetic nerve-related activity. *Journal of Neurophysiology* 64: 1019–1032.

Barman SM & Gebber GL (1985) Axonal projection patterns of ventrolateral medullospinal sympathoexcitatory neurons. *Journal of Neurophysiology* 53: 1551–1566.

Barman SM & Gebber GL (1989a) Basis for the naturally occurring activity of rostral ventrolateral medullary sympathoexcitatory neurons. *Progress in Brain Research* 81: 117–129.

Barman SM & Gebber GL (1989b) Lateral tegmental field neurons of cat medulla: a source of basal activity of raphespinal sympathoinhibitory neurons. *Journal of Neurophysiology* 61: 1011–1024.

Benarroch EE, Granata AR, Ruggiero DA et al (1986) Neurons of C1 area mediate cardiovascular responses initiated from ventral medullary surface. *American Journal of Physiology* 250: R932–R945.

Blessing WW (1989) Baroreceptor-vasomotor reflex after N-methyl-D-aspartate receptor blockade in rabbit caudal ventrolateral medulla. *Journal of Physiology* 416: 67–78.

Blessing WW, Goodchild AK, Dampney RA et al (1981) Cell groups in the lower brain stem of the rabbit projecting to the spinal cord, with special reference to catecholamine-containing neurons. *Brain Research* 221: 35–55.

Blessing WW, Jaeger CB, Ruggiero DA et al (1982) Hypothalamic projections of medullary catecholamine neurons in the rabbit: a combined catecholamine fluorescence and HRP transport study. *Brain Research Bulletin* 9: 279–286.

Brown DL & Guyenet PG (1985) Electrophysiological study of cardiovascular neurons in the rostral ventrolateral medulla in rats. *Circulation Research* 56: 359–369.

Byrum CE & Guyenet PG (1987) Afferent and efferent connections of the A5 noradrenergic cell group in the rat. *Journal of Comparative Neurology* 261: 529–542.

Cabot JB (1990) Sympathetic preganglionic neurons: cytoarchitecture, ultrastructure, and biophysical properties. In Loewy AD & Spyer KM (eds) *Central Regulation of Autonomic Functions*, pp 44–67. New York: Oxford University Press.

Cabot JB, Mennone A, Bogan N et al (1991) Retrograde, trans-synaptic and transneuronal transport of fragment C of tetanus toxin by sympathetic preganglionic neurons. *Neuroscience* **40:** 805–823.

Cedarbaum JM & Aghajanian GK (1978) Afferent projections to the rat locus coeruleus as determined by a retrograde tracing technique. *Journal of Comparative Neurology* **178:** 1–16.

Cervero F & Foreman RD (1990) Sensory innervation of the viscera. In Loewy AD & Spyer KM (eds) *Central Regulation of Autonomic Functions*, pp 104–125. New York: Oxford University Press.

Chung K, Chung JM, Lavelle FW et al (1979) Sympathetic neurons in the cat spinal cord projecting to the stellate ganglion. *Journal of Comparative Neurology* **185:** 23–29.

Cochrane KL & Nathan MA (1989) Normotension in conscious rats after placement of bilateral electrolytic lesions in the rostral ventrolateral medulla. *Journal of the Autonomic Nervous System* **26:** 199–211.

Cochrane KL, Buchholz RA, Hubbard JW et al (1988) Hypotensive effect of lesions in the rostral ventrolateral medulla in rats are anesthetic-dependent. *Journal of the Autonomic Nervous System* **22:** 181–187.

Coote JH (1988) The organisation of cardiovascular neurons in the spinal cord. *Reviews of Physiology, Biochemistry and Pharmacology* **110:** 147–285.

Cravo SL, Morrison SF & Reis DJ (1991) Differentiation of two cardiovascular regions within caudal ventrolateral medulla. *American Journal of Physiology* **261:** R985–R994.

Cryzyk-Krzeska MF, Bayliss DA, Seroogy KB et al (1991) Gene expression for peptides in neurons of the petrosal and nodose ganglia in rat. *Experimental Brain Research* **83:** 411–418.

Dampney RA, Goodchild AK & McAllen RM (1987) Vasomotor control by subretrofacial neurones in the rostral ventrolateral medulla. *Canadian Journal of Physiology and Pharmacology* **65:** 1572–1579.

Deuschl G & Illert M (1981) Cytoarchitectonic organization of lumbar preganglionic sympathetic neurons in the cat. *Journal of the Autonomic Nervous System* **3:** 193–213.

Dietrich WD, Lowry OH & Loewy AD (1982) The distribution of glutamate, GABA and aspartate in the nucleus tractus solitarius of the cat. *Brain Research* **237:** 254–260.

Gaudin-Chazal G, Seyfritz N, Araneda S et al (1982) Selective retrograde transport of ^{3}H-serotonin vagal afferents. *Brain Research Bulletin* **8:** 503–509.

Gebber GL (1990) Central determinants of sympathetic nerve discharge. In Loewy AD & Spyer KM (eds) *Central Regulation of Autonomic Functions*, pp 126–144. New York: Oxford University Press.

Gilbey MP & Stein RD (1991) Characteristics of sympathetic preganglionic neurones in the lumbar spinal cord of the cat. *Journal of Physiology* **432:** 427–443.

Gilbey MP, Numao Y & Spyer KM (1986) Discharge patterns of cervical sympathetic preganglionic neurones related to central respiratory drive in the rat. *Journal of Physiology* **378:** 253–265.

Granata AR & Kitai ST (1992) Intracellular analysis in vivo of different barosensitive bulbospinal neurons in the rat rostral ventrolateral medulla. *Journal of Neuroscience* **12:** 1–20.

Guyenet PG (1990) Role of ventral medulla oblongata in blood pressure regulation. In Loewy AD & Spyer KM (eds) *Central Regulation of Autonomic Functions*, pp 145–167. New York: Oxford University Press.

Guyenet PG, Filtz TM & Donaldson SR (1987) Role of excitatory amino acids in rat vagal and sympathetic baroreflexes. *Brain Research* **407:** 272–284.

Guyenet PG, Haselton JR & Sun MK (1989) Sympathoexcitatory neurons of the rostroventrolateral medulla and the origin of the sympathetic vasomotor tone. *Progress in Brain Research* **81:** 105–116.

Hancock MB (1982) Leu-enkephalin, substance P, and somatostatin immunohistochemistry combined with the retrograde transport of horseradish peroxidase in sympathetic preganglionic neurons. *Journal of the Autonomic Nervous System* **6:** 263–272.

Haselton JR & Guyenet PG (1989a) Central respiratory modulation of medullary sympathoexcitatory neurons in rat. *American Journal of Physiology* **256:** R739–R750.

Haselton JR & Guyenet PG (1989b) Electrophysiological characterization of putative C1 adrenergic neurons in the rat. *Neuroscience* **30:** 199–214.

Helke CJ & Hill KM (1988) Immunohistochemical study of neuropeptides in vagal and glossopharyngeal afferent neurons in the rat. *Neuroscience* **26:** 539–551.

Hirsch MD & Helke CJ (1988) Bulbospinal thyrotropin-releasing hormone projections to the intermediolateral cell column: a double fluorescence immunohistochemical-retrograde tracing study in the rat. *Neuroscience* **25:** 625–637.

Holets V & Elde R (1983) Sympathoadrenal preganglionic neurons: their distribution and relationship to chemically-coded fibers in the kitten intermediolateral cell column. *Journal of the Autonomic Nervous System* **7:** 149–163.

Hosoya Y, Sugiura Y, Okado N et al (1991) Descending input from the hypothalamic paraventricular nucleus to sympathetic preganglionic neurons in the rat. *Experimental Brain Research* **85:** 10–20.

Huangfu D, Koshiya N & Guyenet PG (1991) A5 noradrenergic unit activity and sympathetic nerve discharge in rats. *American Journal of Physiology* **261:** R393–R402.

Janig W (1985) Organization of the lumbar sympathetic outflow to skeletal muscle and skin of the cat hindlimb and tail. *Reviews of Physiology, Biochemistry and Pharmacology* **102:** 119–213.

Janig W & McLachlan EM (1986) Identification of distinct topographical distributions of lumbar sympathetic and sensory neurons projecting to end organs with different functions in the cat. *Journal of Comparative Neurology* **246:** 104–112.

Janig W & McLachlan EM (1987) Organization of lumbar spinal outflow to distal colon and pelvic organs. *Physiological Review* **67:** 1332–1404.

Jordan D & Spyer KM (1986) Brainstem integration of cardiovascular and pulmonary afferent activity. *Progress in Brain Research* **67:** 295–314.

Knuepfer MM, Akeyson EW & Schramm LP (1988) Spinal projections of renal afferent nerves in the rat. *Brain Research* **446:** 17–25.

Krukoff TL (1987) Coexistence of neuropeptides in sympathetic preganglionic neurons of the cat. *Peptides* **8:** 109–112.

Kumada M, Terui N & Kuwaki T (1990) Arterial baroreceptor reflex: its central and peripheral neural mechanisms. *Progress in Neurobiology* **35:** 331–361.

Kuo DC, Yamasaki DS & Krauthamer GM (1980) Segmental organization of sympathetic preganglionic neurons of the splanchnic nerve as revealed by retrograde transport of horseradish peroxidase. *Neuroscience Letters* **17:** 11–16.

Langley JN (1921) *The Autonomic Nervous System.* Cambridge: W Heffer and Sons.

Leone C & Gordon FJ (1989) Is L-glutamate a neurotransmitter of baroreceptor information in the nucleus of the tractus solitarius? *Journal of Pharmacology and Experimental Therapeutics* **250:** 953–962.

Li Y-W, Gieroba ZJ, McAllen RM et al (1991) Neurons in the rabbit caudal ventrolateral medulla inhibit bulbospinal barosensitive neurons in rostral medulla. *American Journal of Physiology* **261:** R44–R51.

Li YW, Ding ZQ, Wesselingh SL et al (1992a) Renal and adrenal sympathetic preganglionic neurons in rabbit spinal cord—tracing with herpes simplex virus. *Brain Research* **573:** 147–152.

Li YW, Wesselingh SL & Blessing WW (1992b) Projections from rabbit caudal medulla to C1 and A5 sympathetic premotor neurons, demonstrated with phaseolus leucoagglutinin and herpes simplex virus. *Journal of Comparative Neurology* **317:** 317–379.

Loewy AD (1981) Raphe pallidus and raphe obscurus projections to the intermediolateral cell column in the rat. *Brain Research* **222:** 129–133.

Loewy AD (1982) Descending pathways to the sympathetic preganglionic neurons. *Progress in Brain Research* **57:** 267–277.

Loewy AD (1990a) Central autonomic pathways. In Loewy AD & Spyer KM (eds) *Central Regulation of Autonomic Functions*, pp 88–103. New York: Oxford University Press.

Loewy AD (1990b) Anatomy of the autonomic nervous system: an overview, In Loewy AD & Spyer KM (eds) *Central Regulation of Autonomic Functions*, pp 3–16. New York: Oxford University Press.

Loewy AD (1991) Forebrain nuclei involved in autonomic control. *Progress in Brain Research* **87:** 253–268.

Loewy AD & Burton H (1978) Nuclei of the solitary tract: efferent projections to the lower brain stem and spinal cord of the cat. *Journal of Comparative Neurology* **181:** 421–449.

Loewy AD, McKellar S & Saper CB (1979a) Direct projections from the A5 catecholamine cell group to the intermediolateral cell column. *Brain Research* **174:** 309–314.

Loewy AD, Saper CB & Baker RP (1979b) Descending projections from the pontine micturition center. *Brain Research* **172:** 533–538.

Lovick TA (1985) Projections from the diencephalon and mesencephalon to nucleus paragigantocellularis lateralis in the cat. *Neuroscience* **14:** 853–861.

Marks SA, Stein RD, Dashwood MR et al (1990) [³H]Prazosin binding in the intermediolateral cell column and the effects of iontophoresed methoxamine on sympathetic preganglionic neuronal activity in the anaesthetized cat and rat. *Brain Research* **530:** 321–324.

McAllen RM (1986) Action and specificity of ventral medullary vasopressor neurones in the cat. *Neuroscience* **18:** 51–59.

McAllen RM (1987) Central respiratory modulation of subretrofacial bulbospinal neurones in the cat. *Journal of Physiology* **388:** 533–545.

McCall RB & Clement ME (1989) Identification of serotonergic and sympathetic neurons in medullary raphe nuclei. *Brain Research* **477:** 172–182.

McKellar S & Loewy AD (1981) Organization of some brain stem afferents to the paraventricular nucleus of the hypothalamus in the rat. *Brain Research* **217:** 351–357.

McKellar S & Loewy AD (1982) Efferent projections of the A1 catecholamine cell group in the rat: an autoradiographic study. *Brain Research* **241:** 11–29.

Miller BD & Felder RB (1988) Excitatory amino acid receptors intrinsic to synaptic transmission in nucleus tractus solitarii. *Brain Research* **456:** 333–343.

Milner TA, Morrison SF, Abate C et al (1988) Phenylethanolamine N-methyltransferase-containing terminals synapse directly on sympathetic preganglionic neurons in the rat. *Brain Research* **448:** 205–222.

Minson J, Pilowsky P, Llewellyn-Smith I et al (1991) Glutamate in spinally projecting neurones of the rostral ventral medulla. *Brain Research* **555:** 326–331.

Morgan C, de Groat WC & Nadelhaft I (1986) The spinal distribution of sympathetic preganglionic and visceral primary afferent neurons that send axons into the hypogastric nerves of the cat. *Journal of Comparative Neurology* **243:** 23–40.

Morris JL & Gibbins IL (1992) Co-transmission and neuromodulation. In Burnstock G & Hoyle CHV (eds) *Autonomic Neuroeffector Mechanisms*, pp 33–120. Chur: Harwood Academic.

Morrison SF & Gebber GL (1984) Raphe neurons with sympathetic-related activity: baroreceptor responses and spinal connections. *American Journal of Physiology* **246:** R338–R348.

Morrison SF & Gebber GL (1985) Axonal branching patterns and funicular trajectories of raphespinal sympathoinhibitory neurons. *Journal of Neurophysiology* **53:** 759–772.

Morrison SF & Reis DJ (1989) Reticulospinal vasomotor neurons in the RVL mediate the somatosympathetic reflex. *American Journal of Physiology* **256:** R1084–R1097.

Morrison SF, Milner TA & Reis DJ (1988) Reticulospinal vasomotor neurons of the rat rostral ventrolateral medulla: relationship to sympathetic nerve activity and the C1 adrenergic cell group. *Journal of Neuroscience* **8:** 1286–1301.

Morrison SF, Ernsberger P, Milner TA et al (1989) A glutamate mechanism in the intermediolateral nucleus mediates sympathoexcitatory responses to stimulation of the rostral ventrolateral medulla. *Progress in Brain Research* **81:** 159–169.

Morrison SF, Callaway J, Milner TA et al (1991) Rostral ventrolateral medulla—a source of the glutamatergic innervation of the sympathetic intermediolateral nucleus. *Brain Research* **562:** 126–135.

Nishi S (1990) Catecholaminergic modulation and transmission in sympathetic preganglionic neurons. *Japanese Journal of Physiology* **40:** 775–787.

Oldfield BJ & McLachlan EM (1981) An analysis of the sympathetic preganglionic neurons projecting from the upper thoracic spinal roots of the cat. *Journal of Comparative Neurology* **196:** 329–345.

Petras JM & Cummings JF (1972) Autonomic neurons in the spinal cord of the rhesus monkey: a correlation of the findings of cytoarchitectonics and sympathectomy with fiber degeneration following dorsal rhizotomy. *Journal of Comparative Neurology* **146:** 189–218.

Reis DJ, Ross CA, Ruggiero DA et al (1984) Role of adrenaline neurons of ventrolateral medulla (the C1 group) in the tonic and phasic control of arterial pressure. *Clinical and Experimental Hypertension, Part A: Theory and Practice* **6:** 221–241.

Reis DJ, Ruggiero DA & Morrison SF (1989) The C1 area of the rostral ventrolateral medulla oblongata. A critical brainstem region for control of resting and reflex integration of arterial pressure. *American Journal of Hypertension* **2**: 363S–374S.

Ross CA, Ruggiero DA, Joh TH et al (1984) Rostral ventrolateral medulla: selective projections to the thoracic autonomic cell column from the region containing C1 adrenaline neurons. *Journal of Comparative Neurology* **228**: 168–185.

Rotto-Percelay DM, Wheeler JG, Osorio FA et al (1992) Transneuronal labelling of spinal interneurons and sympathetic preganglionic neurons after pseudorabies virus injections in the rat medial gastrocnemius muscle. *Brain Research* **574**: 291–306.

Saper CB & Loewy AD (1980) Efferent connections of the parabrachial nucleus in the rat. *Brain Research* **197**: 291–317.

Saper CB, Loewy AD, Swanson LW et al (1976) Direct hypothalamo-autonomic connections. *Brain Research* **117**: 305–312.

Schramm LP (1986) Spinal factors in sympathetic regulation. In Magro A, Osswald W, Reis D & Vanhoutte P (eds) *Central and Peripheral Mechanisms of Cardiovascular Regulation*, pp 303–352. New York: Plenum.

Schramm LP, Strack AM, Platt KB et al (1991) CNS neurones infected by renal injection of pseudorabies virus. *Society for Neuroscience Abstracts* **17**: 245.6 (abstract).

Simon OR & Schramm LP (1984) The spinal course and medullary termination of myelinated renal afferents in the rat. *Brain Research* **290**: 239–247.

Somogyi P, Minson JB, Morilak D et al (1989) Evidence for an excitatory amino acid pathway in the brainstem and for its involvement in cardiovascular control. *Brain Research* **496**: 401–407.

Spyer KM (1990) The central nervous organization of reflex circulatory control. In Loewy AD & Spyer KM (eds) *Central Regulation of Autonomic Functions*, pp 168–188. New York: Oxford University Press.

Stornetta RL, Morrison SF, Ruggiero DA et al (1989) Neurons of rostral ventrolateral medulla mediate somatic pressor reflex. *American Journal of Physiology* **256**: R448–R462.

Strack AM, Sawyer WB, Marubio LM et al (1988) Spinal origin of sympathetic preganglionic neurons in the rat. *Brain Research* **455**: 187–191.

Strack AM, Sawyer WB, Hughes JH et al (1989a) A general pattern of CNS innervation of the sympathetic outflow demonstrated by transneuronal pseudorabies viral infections. *Brain Research* **491**: 156–162.

Strack AM, Sawyer WB, Platt KB et al (1989b) CNS cell groups regulating the sympathetic outflow to adrenal gland as revealed by transneuronal cell body labelling with pseudorabies virus. *Brain Research* **491**: 274–296.

Sun MK & Guyenet PG (1985) GABA-mediated baroreceptor inhibition of reticulospinal neurons. *American Journal of Physiology* **249**: R672–R680.

Sun MK & Guyenet PG (1987) Arterial baroreceptor and vagal inputs to sympathoexcitatory neurons in rat medulla. *American Journal of Physiology* **252**: R699–R709.

Sun MK & Spyer KM (1991a) Nociceptive inputs into rostral ventrolateral medulla spinal vasomotor neurones in rats. *Journal of Physiology* **436**: 685–700.

Sun MK & Spyer KM (1991b) GABA-mediated inhibition of medullary vasomotor neurones by area postrema stimulation in rats. *Journal of Physiology* **436**: 669–684.

Sun MK, Hackett JT & Guyenet PG (1988) Sympathoexcitatory neurons of rostral ventrolateral medulla exhibit pacemaker properties in the presence of a glutamate-receptor antagonist. *Brain Research* **438**: 23–40.

Sun MK, Stornetta RL & Guyenet PG (1991) Morphology of rostral medullary neurons with intrinsic pacemaker activity in the rat. *Brain Research* **556**: 61–70.

Tucker DC & Saper CB (1985) Specificity of spinal projections from hypothalamic and brainstem areas which innervate sympathetic preganglionic neurons. *Brain Research* **360**: 159–164.

Tucker DC, Saper CB, Ruggiero DA et al (1987) Organization of central adrenergic pathways: I. Relationships of ventrolateral medullary projections to the hypothalamus and spinal cord. *Journal of Comparative Neurology* **259**: 591–603.

Van Bockstaele EJ, Pieribone VA & Aston Jones G (1989) Diverse afferents converge on the nucleus paragigantocellularis in the rat ventrolateral medulla: retrograde and anterograde tracing studies. *Journal of Comparative Neurology* **290**: 561–584.

Vera PL, Hurwitz BE & Schneiderman N (1990) Sympathoadrenal preganglionic neurons in the adult rabbit send their dendrites into the contralateral hemicord. *Journal of the Autonomic Nervous System* **30:** 193–198.

Willis Jr, WD (1986) Visceral inputs to sensory pathways in the spinal cord. *Progress in Brain Research* **67:** 207–226.

Zagon A & Smith AD (1990) Projections from the rostral ventrolateral medulla to identified spinal sympathetic neurons and serotinergic medullary raphe neurons in rat. *Society for Neuroscience Abstracts* **16:** 97.6 (abstract).

2

Pharmacology and molecular biology of
adrenergic receptors

STEPHEN B. LIGGETT
JOHN R. RAYMOND

Catecholamines exert their physiological effects via binding to cell surface
receptors, which are collectively known as adrenergic receptors. First
classified as either α or β based on the physiological effects of various
agonists, the family of adrenergic receptors now has many members which
have been cloned and the deduced primary amino acid sequence established. In this chapter we will review the current classification of adrenergic
receptors, and the relationship between the molecular structure of these
receptors and their various functions.

CLASSIFICATION OF ADRENERGIC RECEPTORS

The first adrenergic receptor to be cloned and sequenced was the hamster
β_2-adrenergic receptor (β_2AR) (Dixon et al, 1986). This was accomplished
by purification of the receptor to homogeneity, amino acid analysis of
cyanogen bromide (CNBR) cleaved products, and the probing of hamster
genomic DNA with degenerate oligonucleotide probes based on the amino
acid sequences. The subsequent cloning of the full-length complementary
DNA (cDNA) enabled an amino acid sequence to be deduced that revealed
several key components that have become hallmarks of not only the
adrenergic receptor family, but the G protein coupled receptor superfamily
as a whole. Shown in Figure 1 is the human β_2AR presented in a manner that
conceptually illustrates some of these hallmarks. All adrenergic receptors
are proteins with extracellular amino termini, which often contain sites for
asparagine-linked glycosylation. Within each receptor are seven clusters of
hydrophobic-rich amino acids which are thought to represent transmembrane segments. Each is connected by extracellular and intracellular loops.
The carboxy terminus is intracellular. The third intracellular loop and
cytoplasmic tails can be highly variable in length and amino acid composition between different adrenergic receptors, as can be appreciated by
comparing the β_2AR with the α_2AR of Figure 2. While the seven hydrophobic segments are commonly depicted in two dimensions as in Figures 1

Baillière's Clinical Endocrinology and Metabolism—
Vol. 7, No. 2, April 1993
ISBN 0–7020–1698–5

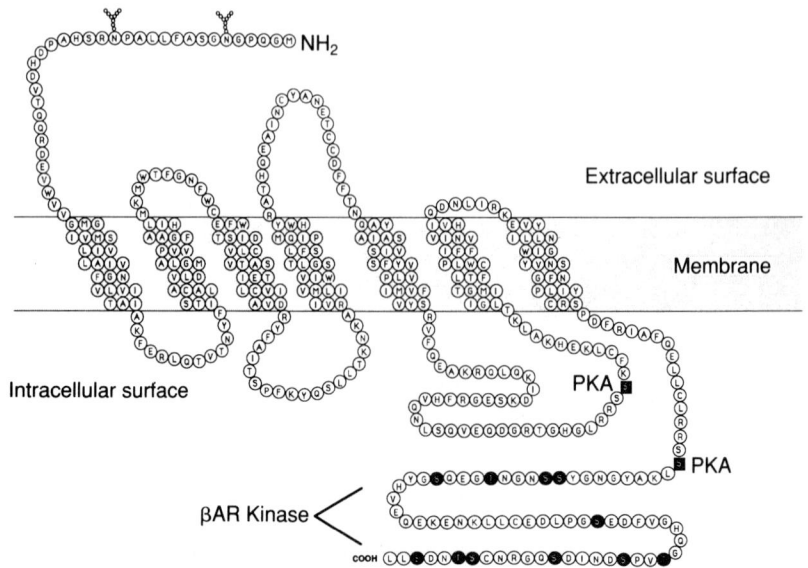

Figure 1. Primary amino acid sequence and proposed membrane topography of the human β_2AR. The locations of potential phosphorylation sites and the residues which were mutated, as discussed in the text, are indicated. PKA = protein kinase A.

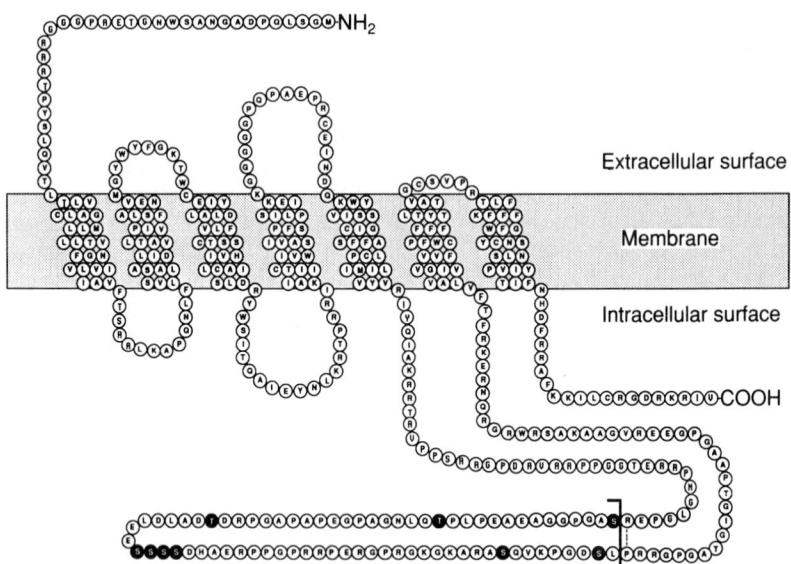

Figure 2. Primary amino acid sequence and proposed membrane topography of the human α_2AR α_2C10. The locations of potential phosphorylation sites in a deletion mutation, as discussed in the text, are indicated.

and 2, the bulk of evidence based on site-directed mutagenesis and crystallographic data suggests that these are arranged in clusters such that the side chains of various amino acids in one segment interact with those of other segments to which they are not necessarily adjacent in the two dimensional depiction of Figures 1 and 2.

The similarities between amino acid sequences in adrenergic receptors are greatest in the transmembrane segments which, as discussed below, are the regions that comprise the agonist binding domains. Based on the transmembrane spanning homology alone, the adrenergic receptors segregate into three major groups α_1, α_2 and β, which are identical to the groups in the classification scheme developed pharmacologically prior to the cloning of the adrenergic receptors. Each type of adrenergic receptor has three, or in some cases possibly more, subtypes, giving rise to subtype designations such as α_{1A}, α_{1B}, etc. Some authors suggest the use of the term subsubtype to describe these receptors, but in this chapter we prefer the term subtype to refer to a specific adrenergic receptor within a major group. The classification scheme along with some molecular and pharmacological properties of adrenergic receptor subtypes are shown in Table 1.

In a manner similar to that which occurred with the muscarinic receptors, some differences in nomenclature have developed between receptors classified originally pharmacologically and those classified by molecular cloning. In some cases, cloning has given rise to new adrenergic receptor subtypes which were not previously well-defined pharmacologically. The major problems in nomenclature have been with α_1AR and α_2AR. The cloned α_2AR subtypes have been frequently designated according to their human chromosomal location, i.e. α_2C10, α_2C4, α_2C2 (for chromosomes 10, 4 and 2, respectively), but this convention has not been uniformly applied, resulting in considerable confusion and debate (Lomasney et al, 1991). Pharmacological characterization of the α_2AR in various cell lines and tissues has led to other classifications (Harrison et al, 1991b). At the time of writing, it is clear that the human α_2AR of platelets (α_2C10) (Kobilka et al, 1987b) is the same as that of HT29 cells and is designated α_{2A}. A closely related rat clone has been isolated and tentatively assigned a distinct designation as an α_{2D} receptor due to some pharmacological differences from α_{2A} (Lanier et al, 1991). The human α_2C4 (Regan et al, 1988) is most likely homologous to the rat cerebral cortex receptor previously designated α_{2B} and the α_2AR from OK cells previously designated as α_{2C}. It is also closely related to the rat clones RG10 (Lanier et al, 1991) and RBα_{2D} (Harrison et al, 1991a). In keeping with the recommendations of Lomasney et al (1990, 1991), we will designate α_2C4 as α_{2C}. Finally, apparent homologues to the rat lung α_{2B} receptor have been cloned and designated RNGα_2 (Zeng et al, 1990) and clone 5A (Weinshank et al, 1990). This classification scheme does not rectify all known pharmacological and genetic subtypes of α_2AR. Moreover, even within groups of putative species homologues, large functional differences have been reported, such as the preference of the putative rat α_{2C} (RG20) for G_o rather than G_i (Coupry et al, 1992) while the closely related human putative α_{2C} (α_2C4) couples to G_i species with a higher affinity than to G_o (Kurose et al, 1991). A

Table 1. Pharmacologic and molecular properties of the cloned adrenergic receptors.

Subtype	Number of amino acids*	Human chromosome	TMS identity†	Primary G protein‡	Third loop size (Number of amino acids)	Tail size (Number of amino acids)	Agonist potency§
βAR:							
β_1AR	477 (h)	10		G_s	~80	~97	Iso > A = NA
β_2AR	413 (h)	5	71	G_s	~54	~84	Iso > A ≥ NA
β_3AR	402 (h)	8	65	G_s	~66	~55	BRL ≥ Iso > NA > A
α_1AR:							
α_{1A}AR	560 (r)	5		G_q	~70	~160	NA > A > Phenyl > Oxy
α_{1B}AR	515 (ham)	5	72	G_q	~71	~164	Oxy > A ≥ NA > Phenyl
α_{1C}AR	466 (b)	8	77	G_q	~70	~139	Oxy ≫ A ≥ NA > Phenyl
α_2AR¶:							
α_2C10	450 (h)	10		G_i	~158	~21	Oxy ≫ A ≥ NA
α_2C4	450 (h)	4	75	G_i	~158	~21	Oxy = A ≥ NA
α_2C2	461 (h)	2	74	G_i	~180	~22	Oxy = A ≥ NA

* The number of amino acids in the receptor is based on the species of the cloned receptor as listed: h = human; r = rat; b = bovine; ham = hamster.
† The amino acid identity within the transmembrane spanning portions (TMS) of a given adrenergic receptor is listed as a percentage of the first member of each group.
‡ Listed is the primary G protein to which the receptor is known to couple. The α_2AR is also known to couple to G_s. In addition, there are some subtype differences in the coupling of the α_2AR to the various $G_{i\alpha}$ subunits, and to G_o. See text for discussion.
§ Agonist abbreviations are: Iso = isoprenaline; A = adrenaline; NA = noradrenaline; BRL = BRL 33744; Phenyl = phenylephrine; Oxy = oxymetazoline.
¶ Several additional α_2AR subtypes have been cloned and are not easily classified. These include the α_{2B} from rat and human, the rat α_{2D} which may be the homologue of α_{2A}, RG10, RNGα_2 and RBα_{2B}. See text for discussion.

very recent direct comparison of the pharmacological properties of three cloned human α_2ARs and the α_2ARs of HT29 cells, rat neonatal lung cells and OK cells has convincingly established these relationships: α_2C10 is equivalent to HT29, α_2C2 is a homologue of α_2B from rat neonatal lung, and α_2C4 is a homologue of α_2C from opposum OK cells (Bylund et al, 1992). Nevertheless, a more definitive scheme that integrates chromosomal location, pharmacology, species differences, second messenger and G protein coupling characteristics is clearly needed.

A consistent feature of the amino acids of the transmembrane spanning regions is the degree of identity between different subtypes within a given adrenergic receptor group. For example, the transmembrane spanning identity between α_2AR subtypes is approximately 70%. However, this falls to less than 45% when an α_2AR is compared with a βAR or an α_1AR. Despite the high degree of identity in these ligand binding transmembrane spanning segments between subtypes, clear differences in agonist (and antagonist) binding affinities have been demonstrated (Table 1).

STRUCTURAL REQUIREMENTS FOR RECEPTOR BINDING OF CATECHOLAMINES AND OTHER LIGANDS

When the structural and functional similarities of the adrenergic receptors to rhodopsin became apparent, it was hypothesized that the adrenergic receptor binding pocket would reside within the transmembrane clusters of hydrophobic residues. Previous studies with rhodopsin strongly suggested that the chromophore retinal is covalently attached to lysine 296 within transmembrane domain 7 (TM7) (Ovchinikov, 1982; Thomas and Stryer 1982). Biochemical studies with avian βARs (Rubenstein et al, 1987), β_2ARs (Dohlman et al, 1988) and α_2ARs (Matsui et al, 1989) showed that photoaffinity labels were covalently attached to transmembrane domains of these receptors. Site-directed mutagenesis studies further confirmed the importance of the hydrophobic regions in ligand binding. Structural determinants important for distinguishing agonist and antagonists between β_1 and β_2 adrenergic receptors are localized primarily within TM6 and TM7 (Frielle et al, 1988). In contrast, TM7 is the most important determinant of antagonist specificity between α_2AR and β_2AR. Elegant mutagenesis studies demonstrated that a uniquely conserved asparagine residue within TM7 conferred high affinity for classical β antagonists amongst βARs. Substitution of asparagine for the analogous phenylalanine 412 of α_2C10 conferred an ability to bind to βAR antagonists (Suryanaryana et al, 1991). Interestingly, the serotonin (5-hydroxytryptamine; 5HT) 1A receptor (5HT$_{1A}$) shares the conserved asparagine 385 with the βAR and has a high affinity for βAR antagonists. Mutation of the asparagine 385 to valine ablates the ability of the 5HT$_{1A}$ receptor to recognize βAR antagonists (Guan et al, 1992).

Insight regarding specific residues involved in agonist binding has also been derived from site-directed mutagenesis studies (Strader et al, 1989a; Tota et al, 1991). The positively charged catecholamine putatively interacts with the negatively charged carboxy group of the aspartic acid 113 in TM3 of β_2AR (Strader et al, 1988). Hydroxyl groups in the meta and para positions of the catechol ring may form hydrogen bonds with side chains of serine 204 and 207 within TM 5 (Strader et al, 1989b). Therefore, these residues are thought to interact directly with the catecholamines. Other residues appear to be important for ligand binding to adrenergic receptors in a less direct manner. For example, four extracellular cysteine residues of the β_2AR (at locations 106, 184, 190 and 191) appear to participate in disulphate bonds that stabilize the β_2AR in a conformation favourable to agonist binding. Reduction of those residues or substitution by site-directed mutagenesis (Dohlman et al, 1990) lowers ligand binding and alters binding specificity. Interestingly, in one instance a mutation of an extracellular cysteine evidently altered the β_2AR tertiary structure in such a way that agonist-promoted desensitization and phosphorylation were enhanced (Liggett et al, 1989b). In contrast, substitution of four transmembrane cysteines does not alter ligand binding. Studies with rhodopsin examined the role of the analogous cysteine residues and yielded similar results (Karnik et al, 1988). Because these cysteine residues are well conserved amongst members of the G protein coupled receptor superfamily, they may be assumed to play at least some role for all of the adrenergic and other receptors.

Clearly the determinants of the ligand binding specificity of adrenergic receptors are complex. They reside primarily within the transmembrane domains, but can be affected by other extracellular residues. Therefore, the ligand binding properties of adrenergic receptors represent the convergence of numerous structural characteristics.

Domains responsible for G-protein coupling

As shown in Table 1, the adrenergic receptors couple primarily to G_s, G_i or G_q. All βARs couple to G_s, thus stimulating adenylyl cyclase and resulting in increased intracellular concentrations of the second messenger cyclic adenosine monophosphate (cAMP). All α_2ARs couple to G_i, inhibiting adenylyl cyclase and lowering cellular cAMP. Presumably, all α_1ARs couple to the less well characterized pathway that activates phospholipase C, probably via G_q, and increasing phosphoinositide turnover. Adrenergic receptors also couple to ion channels, primarily via the above mentioned G proteins, although these pathways have been less well delineated. The regions of these receptors which are responsible for the coupling of the agonist-bound receptor to G proteins and thus initiation of the signal transduction cascade have been elucidated primarily by site-directed mutagenesis. The first global evaluation of regions of α_2ARs and β_2ARs and their G protein coupling domains was reported by Kobilka and colleagues (1988) using chimeric α_2/β_2ARs. These investigators were able to delineate not only the regions that are responsible for agonist binding, but also those involved in G protein coupling. A chimeric α_2/β_2AR which contains primarily the α_2AR up to the fifth transmembrane spanning segment, but having the sixth and seventh transmembrane spanning regions as well as the third intracellular loop and third extracellular loop of the β_2AR, stimulated adenylyl cyclase in response to an α_2AR agonist. This suggested that the regions responsible for agonist binding were still present and identified this as an α_2AR; however G protein coupling had been switched from G_i to G_s. That the third intracellular loop of the β_2AR is the key region for G protein coupling has been shown by more specific mutations in a number of different studies (O'Dowd et al, 1988). Of the residues in the third intracellular loop, it appears that those adjacent to the transmembrane spanning regions are the most critical for the β_2AR to couple to G_s. Removal of 12 residues on the carboxy terminal portion of the third intracellular loop causes an impairment in the functional coupling of the β_2AR to G_s as demonstrated by agonist-stimulated adenylyl cyclase activity (Hausdorff et al, 1990b). Interestingly, the physical coupling (as identified by agonist competition studies) showed no impairment of formation of the agonist-receptor-G protein complex. In a group of mutated β_2ARs we recently have shown that the regions responsible for G protein coupling probably comprise a concerted cooperation of multiple segments of the intracellular domains (Liggett et al, 1991). We constructed five mutated β_2ARs (Figure 3), three which had regions in the N-terminal (denoted S1) and C-terminal (denoted S2) portions of the third intracellular loop and proximal portion of the cytoplasmic tail (denoted S3) substituted with analogous portions of the α_2AR, and two combination mutations (denoted S2, 3 and S1, 2, 3). We then studied the physical and functional coupling properties of each mutated receptor. We found that G_s coupling was virtually abolished with any

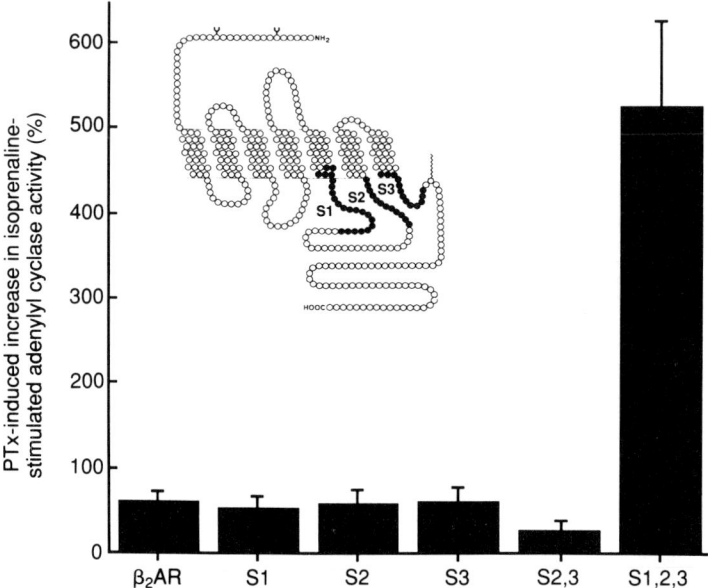

Figure 3. Effects of ablating G_i coupling with pertussis toxin (PTX) on agonist-promoted adenylyl cyclase activities of wild type and mutant β_2AR.

mutation containing the S2 substitution. Addition of more substitutions at the aforementioned regions did not further depress G_s coupling. When all of the substitutions were made, a frank inhibition of adenylyl cyclase could still not be demonstrated. We considered whether, in fact, these mutated receptors containing pieces of the α_2AR might be coupling simultaneously to G_s and G_i. In order to assess this possibility, we incubated cells expressing these mutated receptors in vivo to pertussis toxin, thereby releasing any functional receptor-G_i interaction. When each of these mutations was assessed in this manner, we were able to show that the S1, 2, 3 mutation underwent a dramatic increase in agonist-stimulated adenylyl cyclase activity after pertussis toxin treatment (Figure 3), suggesting that in fact this receptor was coupling to both G_i and G_s. Such an increase was not seen with any other mutant receptors containing smaller pieces of the α_2AR, thus suggesting that for coupling to G_i a concerted effort of at least three sub-segments of the receptor is required. Such a scheme is supported by a recent study with α_2AR and peptides used for blocking coupling (Dalman and Neubig, 1991). Peptides from the second and third intracellular loops of the $\alpha_{2A}AR$ were found to decrease high affinity binding of agonists to both α_{2A}- and $\alpha_{2B}AR$.

While some information is known about the structural requirements of adrenergic receptors coupling to their respective G proteins, little is known about subtle differences in G protein coupling that may occur between adrenergic receptor subtypes. Recently we have examined this in detail with

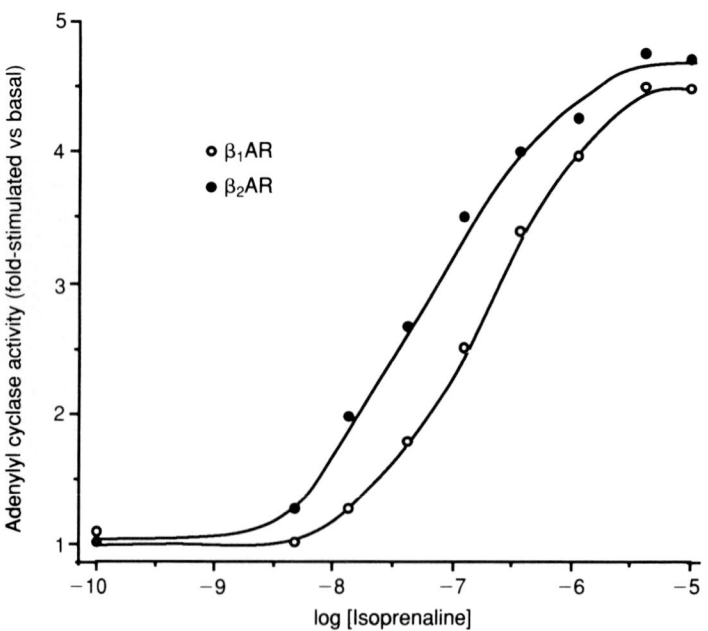

Figure 4. Differences in functional coupling between human recombinant β_1AR and β_2AR expressed in CHW cells.

the β_1AR and β_2AR, which have classically been thought to couple with equal efficacies to G_s (Greene et al, 1992). We transfected Chinese hamster fibroblast (CHW) cells with human β_1AR (Frielle et al, 1987) and β_2AR (Kobilka et al, 1987a) cDNAs in the mammalian expression vector pBC12BI, and selected clones expressing equal receptor densities (~ 350 fmol/mg) for further study. As shown in Figure 4, there was a clear difference in the EC_{50} (concentration at which 50% of a response is obtained) for isoprenaline (isoproterenol *USP*) in stimulating adenylyl cyclase between β_1AR and β_2AR. This approximately five-fold higher EC_{50} for the β_1AR was not due to a difference in the binding affinity of isoprenaline for these two receptor subtypes. In competition studies in the presence of guanosine triphosphate (GTP), we showed that isoprenaline has an equal affinity of binding to β_1AR and β_2AR. However, when competition studies were performed in the absence of GTP, where high (K_H) and low (K_L) binding states could be assessed, we found that there was a clear difference between them. The β_2AR had an approximately five-fold lower K_H and a higher K_L/K_H ratio compared with the β_1AR, thus revealing a greater tendency to form the high affinity ternary complex for the β_2AR. We therefore showed for the first time that β_1AR and β_2AR couple in a subtype-selective manner to G_s. (The β_3AR was not assessed in these studies, because it appears to have a low affinity for all catecholamines, as assessed both by radioligand binding and agonist-stimulated adenylyl cyclase studies.) The molecular basis of such subtype-selective coupling to G_s is currently under investigation. The most likely region of the β_1AR that confers such specificity is a long string of prolines which is present in the β_1AR third intracellular loop and which is not present in the β_2AR.

Recently some of the determinants of α_2AR coupling to G proteins have been delineated. We have shown that such coupling to G_i must reside primarily in the N-terminal and C-terminal portions of the third intracellular loop (which is considerably larger in the α_2AR compared with the β_2AR), as a mutation deleting the middle portion of the $\alpha_{2A}AR$ third intracellular loop still couples normally to G_i (Liggett et al, 1992b). As discussed below, this region is rich in serines and threonines and has been found to be the key determinant of phosphorylation of the α_2AR during agonist-promoted desensitization. We have also had the opportunity to assess the subtype-selective nature of α_2ARs in coupling to G_i (Eason et al, 1992). We expressed α_2C10, α_2C4 and α_2C2 independently in Chinese hamster ovary (CHO) cells and studied adenylyl cyclase activation by agonists in washed membranes. Unexpectedly, we found a biphasic adenylyl cyclase dose-response curve for the agonist UK 14304 in cells expressing 5 pmol/mg of α_2C10 (Figure 5). This finding suggested that α_2AR may couple to both G_i and G_s. In order to evaluate this we selectively ablated either receptor-G_s or receptor-G_i coupling using in vivo incubations of cells with cholera toxin or pertussis toxin. Membranes were then prepared and agonist-stimulated adenylyl cyclase activities determined. Such treatments resulted in monophasic curves revealing either stimulation or inhibition of adenylyl cyclase (Figure 5). To further evaluate whether physical coupling of α_2AR to G_s does occur, we developed a system utilizing highly specific antibodies to

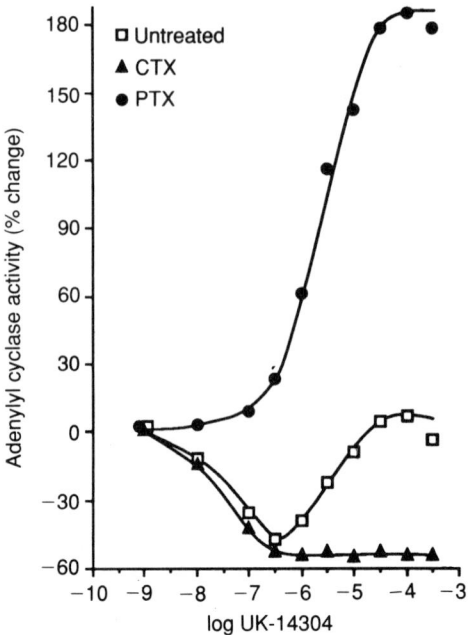

Figure 5. Effects of selective ablation of G_s and G_i coupling on the function of the α_2C10 adrenergic receptor. CTX = cholera toxin; PTX = pertussis toxin.

both the α_{2A}AR and the α subunit of G_s. Membranes were exposed to agonist for 15 min, then the α_2C10 was purified by immunoprecipitation and probed for the presence of an agonist-receptor-G_s complex by Western blotting with G_s antibody or cholera toxin-mediated adenosine diphosphate (ADP) ribosylation. As shown in Figure 6, there was no physical coupling of the α_{2A}AR to G_s in the absence of agonist. However, after exposure to agonist, G_s co-purified with α_2AR in the above mentioned techniques. This effect was blocked by co-incubation with the α_2AR antagonist yohimbine. When the extent of inhibition or stimulation was assessed in each of the three α_2AR subtypes, clear differences in receptor-G_s, but not receptor-G_i, coupling were noted. As shown in Figure 7, there was no difference in the coupling of these α_2AR subtypes to G_i, with an approximately 50% decrease in adenylyl cyclase induced by agonist after treatment with cholera toxin (to ablate G_s coupling) being found in each case. On the other hand, a clear rank order for coupling to G_s was observed.

This rank order for G_s coupling was α_2C10 > α_2C4 > α_2C2. (It should be noted that these studies were performed with only one agonist, UK 14304, and that it is conceivable that the rank order may be different with other agonists.) Thus, it appears that, within the group of α_2ARs, several receptor subtypes may demonstrate selective coupling to a common G protein. In this case, it appears that all human α_2AR subtypes couple equally well to their primary G protein, G_i, but show differing tendencies to couple to a

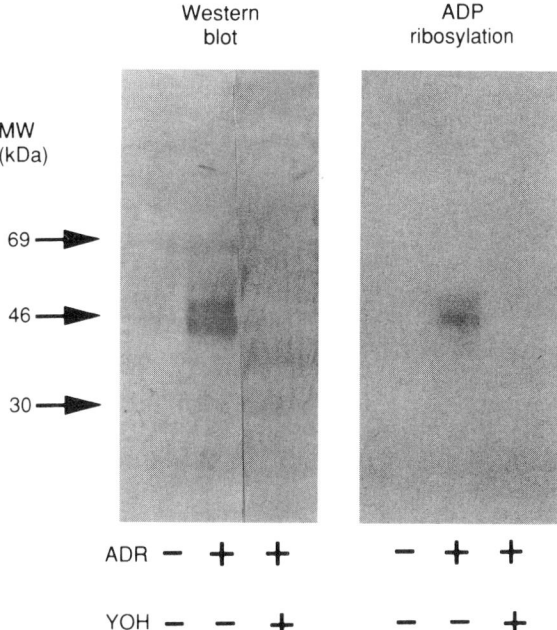

Figure 6. Direct functional coupling of α_2C10 to G_s. Membranes were treated with buffer alone, agonist, or agonist with antagonist, the α_2AR purified, and receptor-G_s complexes probed by cholera toxin-mediated ADP ribosylation or Western blots using G_s antibody. ADR = adrenaline; YOH = yohimbine.

secondary G protein, G_s. We are currently studying the molecular basis of subtype selectivity using site-directed mutagenesis. The most likely region which imparts such selectivity is again the third intracellular loop, which shows regions of low homology between the α_2AR subtypes.

Another important consideration is that of which G_i subtype the respective α_2ARs couple. Several groups have addressed the issue of specificity of coupling of the various α_2ARs to $G_{i\alpha}$ subunits. Kurose et al (1991) used purified G proteins and α_2ARs to establish a rank order of coupling preference of $G_{i3} > G_{i2} > Gi_{i1} > G_o$ for both the α_2C10 and α_2C4 receptors, although the α_2C10 appeared to couple more efficiently to all of the G proteins. Other groups have used transfected mammalian cells to establish physical and functional coupling between the α_2C10 receptor and G_{i3} and G_{i2} (McClue and Milligan, 1990; Milligan et al, 1991). Another group used a similar approach to show that α_{2B}ARs and α_{2D}ARs inhibit adenylyl cyclase in NIH3T3 fibroblasts primarily through $G_{i\alpha2}$ (Duzic et al, 1992). They also showed that the α_{2C}AR could couple to G_{i2} and/or G_{i3}, but this coupling was much less effective than that of α_{2B}AR or α_{2D}AR. In contrast, α_{2C}AR (but not α_{2B} or α_{2D}) were very efficiently coupled to G_o (Duzic et al, 1992). These studies provided further evidence for the heterogeneous nature of the coupling of the α_2AR subtypes to multiple G proteins.

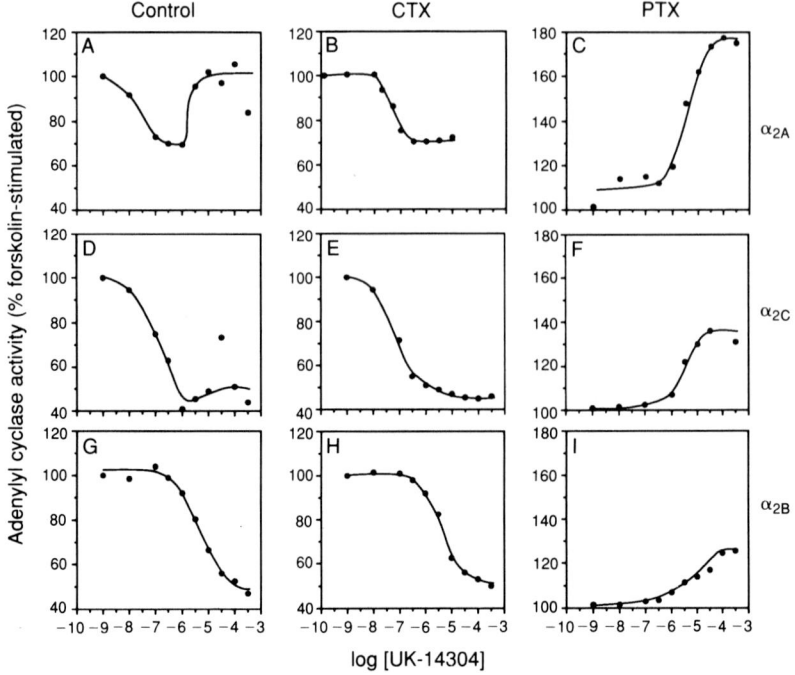

Figure 7. Subtype-selective coupling of the α_2AR subtypes to G_s and G_i. Adenylyl cyclase activities determined in membranes from transfected CHO cells treated with pertussis toxin (PTX) represent G_s coupling, and from cells treated with cholera toxin (CTX) represent G_i coupling.

CATECHOLAMINE-PROMOTED DESENSITIZATION OF ADRENERGIC RECEPTORS

Desensitization is defined as a waning of a response despite the continuous presence of a stimulus of constant intensity. Desensitization is a common phenomenon, being found in a diverse number of biological systems such as slime mould, yeast mating behaviour and light adaptation (Dohlman et al, 1991). Desensitization has been observed in many G protein coupled receptor systems. Amongst the adrenergic receptors, desensitization has been studied most extensively with the βARs (Hausdorff et al, 1990a; Dohlman et al, 1991; Liggett, 1991). Recently, some of the mechanisms of α_2AR desensitization have also been elucidated (Liggett et al, 1992b,c). Three general mechanisms have been invoked during desensitization of the adrenergic receptors, and these are defined here to minimize ambiguity. Perhaps the earliest event that occurs in agonist-induced desensitization of some adrenergic receptors is an *uncoupling* of the receptor from its G protein. While there may be several components to the uncoupling process, it is clear from the studies of the β_2AR and the α_2AR that rapid uncoupling is due to phosphorylation of the receptor by various kinases. Another process which may occur later in the course of agonist-promoted desensitization is receptor *sequestration*, also known as internalization or compartmentalization. Affected receptors are presumably not available to interact with G proteins, and in some model systems as many as 70% of the cell surface receptors may undergo sequestration after exposure to agonists. After a more prolonged agonist exposure, the total receptor complement (regardless of localization) is decreased in some adrenergic receptor systems. This process, which requires several hours of agonist exposure, has been termed receptor *downregulation*. Downregulation has, unfortunately, also been used synonymously with desensitization. For purposes of this review, however, desensitization is defined functionally. It may involve some or all of the above general mechanisms. Whenever possible we will utilize expressions such as 'decrease in receptor expression' for the term 'downregulation'. Other terms which require definition are 'homologous' and 'heterologous' desensitization. Homologous desensitization is said to occur when a subsequent blunted response is found only to the desensitizing stimulus, but not with other stimuli which may terminate in common pathways (for example, stimulation of adenylyl cyclase). Heterologous desensitization occurs when not only is the response to the desensitization agent subsequently reduced, but responses to other stimuli also undergo desensitization. As is implied by the above definition, receptor desensitization may occur by agonist- or non-agonist-promoted mechanisms.

Mechanism of short-term βAR desensitization

Of the adrenergic receptors, desensitization of the β_2AR has been studied most extensively. Studies in a number of systems including intact animals, cultured cells and reconstituted systems, have shown desensitization of the β_2AR. The hallmark of short-term agonist-promoted desensitization of the β_2AR is an uncoupling of the receptor from G_s. For example, within minutes of agonist exposure to β_2AR expressed on S49 lymphoma cells, receptor-mediated stimulation of adenylyl cyclase activity in subsequently prepared membranes is reduced (Shear et al, 1976). Concomitant with this reduced activity is a decrease in the ability of the receptor to form the high affinity agonist-receptor-G_s ternary complex. In systems involving membranes prepared from cells or tissues, this is assessed in agonist competition curves performed in the absence of guanine nucleotides. These curves are shallow and can be resolved by fitting techniques into high and low affinity forms of the receptor.

Direct evidence that the βAR was in fact directly modified during desensitization was first demonstrated by Lefkowitz and colleagues (Strulovici et al, 1984). They showed that purified βARs derived from desensitized cells were functionally impaired in their ability to couple to purified G_s in a reconstituted phospholipid vesicle system. That such alterations were in fact covalent modifications of the βAR by phosphorylation was demonstrated in numerous subsequent studies (Sibley et al, 1987; Bouvier et al, 1988; Lohse et al, 1990). Thus, βARs of cells exposed to agonists undergo rapid, stoichiometric phosphorylation which is temporally related to desensitization. A key finding in these early studies, which were performed prior to the cloning of any adrenergic receptor, was that cAMP analogues, or agents that increase intracellular cAMP such as forskolin or prostaglandin E_1, also induced β_2AR phosphorylation and desensitization. This strongly suggested that the cAMP-dependent protein kinase, also known as protein kinase A (PKA), played a role in β_2AR desensitization. As will be further discussed below, subsequent cloning of the β_2AR has indeed revealed two consensus sequences for PKA phosphorylation in the deduced amino acid sequence of this receptor. Another series of studies revealed that yet another kinase was involved in agonist-promoted desensitization of the βAR. Agonists were found to invoke phosphorylation of β_2ARs in cells which were incapable of increasing cAMP (such as the S49 lymphoma cell variant cyc- which lacks functional G_s), and also in cells which lack PKA activity (the kin- variant) (Sibley et al, 1987). The phosphorylation induced in these cells, then, was dependent *only* on receptor occupancy by agonists. Reconstitution of these receptors with purified G_s and phospholipid vesicles also revealed an impaired agonist-promoted coupling of the receptor to G_s. Monumental efforts culminated in the discovery of the kinase involved in this agonist-specific phosphorylation of the β_2AR (Benovic et al, 1987a,b), which has been termed the βAR kinase, or βARK.

Recent studies utilizing the cloned human β_2AR expressed in CHW cells and site-directed mutagenesis have identified the molecular determinants of desensitization and their relationship to receptor phosphorylation (Bouvier et al, 1988; Hausdorff et al, 1989; Liggett et al, 1989a). We mutated the

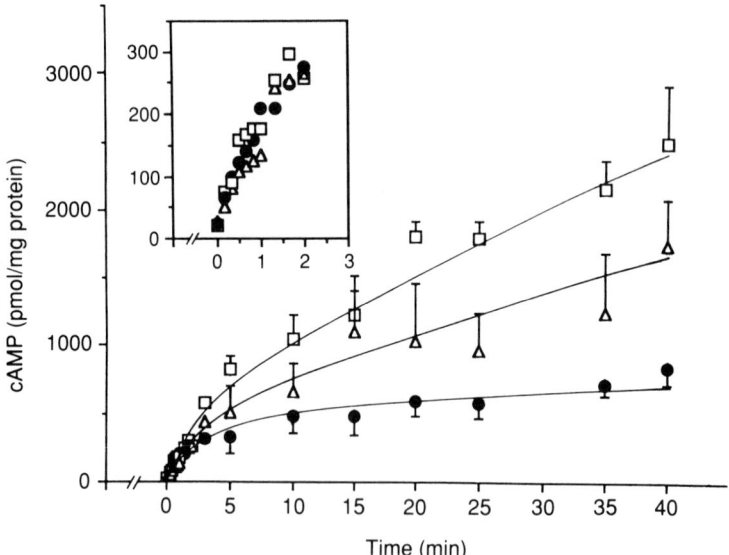

Figure 8. Altered agonist-promoted desensitization of mutant β_2AR lacking phosphorylation sites. ● = wild type β_2AR; □ = mutated β_2AR lacking βARK phosphorylation sites; △ = mutated β_2AR lacking PKA phosphorylation sites.

β_2AR by substituting alanines for the serines in the PKA consensus sequences (R-R-X-S) in the third intracellular loop and the proximal cytoplasmic tail (Figure 1). A second mutated β_2AR had serines and threonines in the carboxy terminal tail substituted with alanines or glycines, thus removing potential βARK phosphorylation sites (Figure 1). The mutated cDNA was inserted into the mammalian expression vector pBC12BI, and CHW cells were transfected by the calcium phosphate precipitation method, thus establishing stable cell lines expressing wild type and mutated receptors. In preliminary studies, the mutated receptors displayed normal coupling to G_s as assessed by high affinity binding and agonist-stimulated adenylyl cyclase activities. Several models of desensitization were then assessed. In one approach (Liggett et al, 1989a), we found that intracellular cAMP production in CHW cells expressing the wild type β_2AR became markedly dampened during continuous exposure to 2 μmol/litre isoprenaline (Figure 8). The initial rates of cAMP production during the first 2 min were reduced by 75% during subsequent time periods up to 40 min. In marked contrast, cAMP production rates did not undergo extensive dampening in cells expressing either $\beta_2(PKA-)$ receptors or $\beta_2(\beta ARK-)$ receptors, thus revealing critical roles in desensitization for the regions mutated. In these same cells, Hausdorff et al (1989) showed that in vivo phosphorylation of both mutated receptors was depressed in response to micromolar concentrations of the agonist (Figure 9). These studies also show that desensitization, as assessed by agonist-stimulated adenylyl cyclase assays, was perturbed by these mutations. An important finding of this study was that desensitization and phosphorylation of the β_2AR were highly dependent on agonist concentrations, as was predicted by the biochemical properties of βARK and PKA. During high agonist concentrations, phosphorylation of the β_2AR occurred by two mechanisms: each occupied receptor became phosphorylated by βARK and, since intracellular cAMP is elevated, by PKA as well.

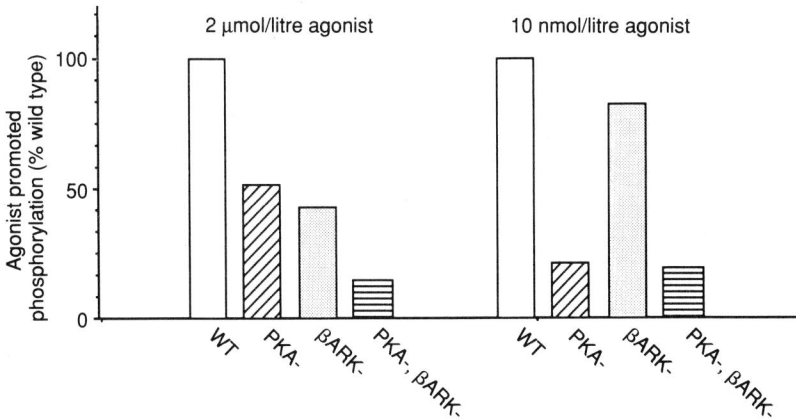

Figure 9. Phosphorylation of wild type and mutant β_2AR by low (10 nmol/litre) and high (2 μmol/litre) concentrations of agonist. Adapted from Hausdorff et al, 1989. WT = wild type; PKA− = mutated β_2AR lacking PKA sites; βARK− = mutated β_2AR lacking βARK sites; PKA−, βARK− = mutated β_2AR lacking sites for both PKA and βARK.

On the other hand, during low agonist concentration exposure (nanomolar), the majority of receptors are not occupied by agonist and thus βARK phosphorylation was found to play no significant role. However, since even at this concentration of agonist a rise in intracellular cAMP occurs, PKA is then activated and phosphorylates all βARs (regardless of occupancy by agonist) present in a cell.

Clinical implications of high and low dose catecholamine-promoted mechanisms of βAR desensitization

It seems that β_2ARs (and most probably β_1ARs) undergo desensitization by two different mechanisms depending on agonist concentrations. Clinically, this is potentially manifested in several different scenarios. High agonist concentrations (in the micromolar range) are present in the synaptic terminal, in the lung during inhalation of aerosolized βAR agonist, in the heart during cardiopulmonary bypass, and in the systemic circulation during administration of agonist for the treatment of cardiovascular arrest. Under these circumstances, both βARK and PKA phosphorylation mechanisms are in play. The rapid onset of βARK phosphorylation (Roth et al, 1991) is particularly suited to the rapid changes in agonist concentrations that may occur in the synapse. On the other hand, PKA plays the dominant role during desensitization with low agonist concentrations. Nanomolar concentrations of agonist are present during intense exercise, during a number of clinical states such as myocardial infarction and diabetic ketoacidosis, during intravenous administration of standard doses of βAR agonist for the treatment of heart failure and shock, and during the oral administration of βAR agonists such as terbutaline and xamoterol.

We have recently examined (Liggett et al, 1992a) the potential for desensitization of the β_3AR (Emorine et al, 1989). Unlike the β_2AR, which contains 11 serines and threonines in its cytoplasmic tail, or the β_1AR, which contains ten serines or threonines in an analogous position, the β_3AR contains only three such residues. In addition, while both β_1AR and β_2AR contain sites for PKA-mediated phosphorylation, no such consensus sequences are found within the β_3AR. This suggested to us that perhaps the β_3AR would undergo little or no agonist-promoted desensitization. We therefore cloned the β_3AR from a leukocyte genomic library (Liggett and Schwinn, 1991), and expressed it in CHO cells and compared the desensitization patterns of the β_2AR and the β_3AR. Cells were exposed to 100 μmol/litre isoprenaline for 15 min, scraped, membranes prepared and agonist-stimulated adenylyl cyclase activities determined. We found that, unlike the β_2AR (top panel, Figure 10), the β_3AR undergoes no agonist-promoted desensitization (middle panel, Figure 10). The β_2AR desensitization pattern was characterized by both a shift in the EC_{50} to the right, and a decrease in the maximal stimulation of adenylyl cyclase. To determine the molecular basis of this lack of desensitization of the β_3AR, we constructed a chimeric β_3/β_2AR (Liggett et al, 1992a). This receptor contained all the amino acids in the transmembrane regions and intracellular and extracellular loops, but contained the β_2AR C-terminal tail starting at amino acid 364 of the β_3AR.

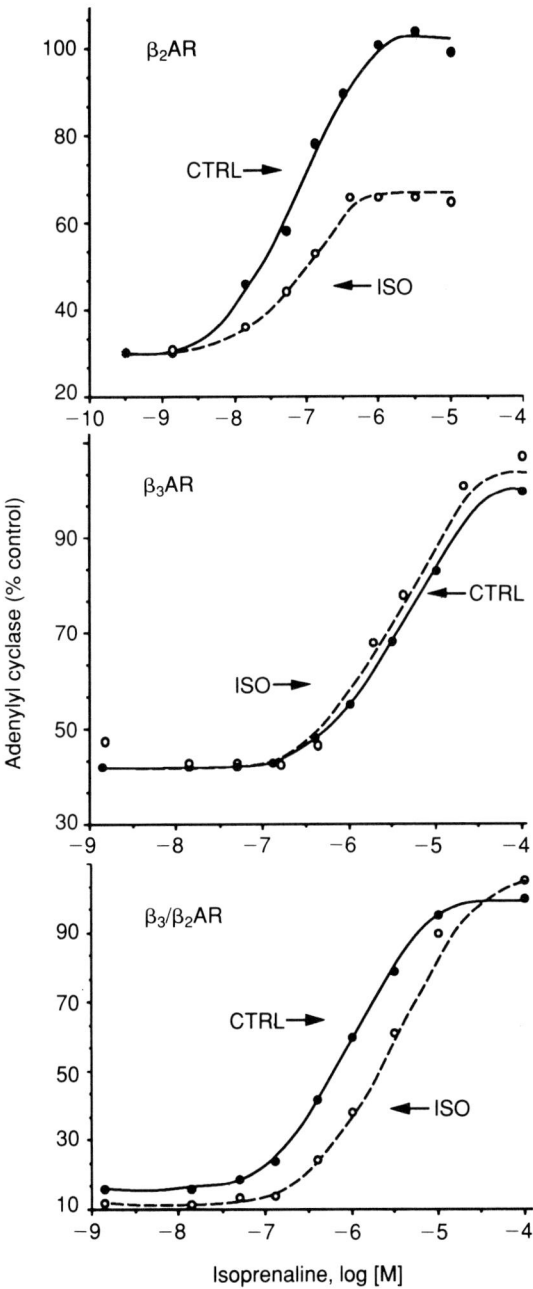

Figure 10. Agonist-promoted desensitization of the β_2AR, the β_3AR and a chimeric β_3/β_2AR. CTRL = control; ISO = isoprenaline.

Thus, this chimeric receptor contained all the possible βARK phosphorylation sites found in the β_2AR. It was then expressed in CHW cells and found to undergo a clear agonist-promoted desensitization. As shown in Figure 10 (bottom panel), a five-fold shift of the EC_{50} for stimulation of adenylyl cyclase was indeed observed in this chimeric receptor. This is indicative of approximately 40% desensitization when examining the adenylyl cyclase activities of a submaximal concentration of isoprenaline (e.g. 1 μmol/litre). Thus, desensitization of the βAR subtypes appears to be clearly subtype specific. We have not examined the β_1AR in detail, but it is clear the β_2AR and the β_3AR have markedly different patterns of short-term desensitization. We found virtually no desensitization with the β_3AR compared with a marked desensitization of the β_2AR after 15 min of agonist exposure. The lack of β_3AR desensitization may serve to permit continued production of energy substrates from fat cells or skeletal muscle during continuous exposure to catecholamines in states of increased sympathetic activity.

Mechanisms of long-term agonist-promoted desensitization of β_2AR

While the events required for phosphorylation of the β_2AR occur over a time frame of seconds to minutes, after a more prolonged exposure several additional events occur. Beginning several minutes after agonist exposure and continuing for up to a few hours, a sequestration or internalization of the β_2AR occurs. The nature and importance of such sequestration of the β_2AR remains controversial (Perkins et al, 1991). Only recently has sequestration been examined extensively using light microscopic (Von Zastrow and Kobilka, 1992) and ultrastructural electron microscopic (Saffitz and Liggett, 1992) approaches. It has been thought for a number of years that such sequestration is the beginning of a cycle of receptor internalization which then leads to degradation and ultimately results in a decrease in the total number of cellular receptors (downregulation). However, several lines of evidence suggest that the appearance of sequestration is not required for downregulation to occur (Perkins et al, 1991). For example, a mutated receptor which lacks four serines in the cytoplasmic tail of the β_2AR (Figure 1) undergoes no agonist-promoted sequestration, yet undergoes a normal pattern of a long-term agonist-promoted decrease in receptor expression (Hausdorff et al, 1991). Similarly, treatment of cells with concanavalin A, which blocks sequestration, has no effect on agonist-promoted downregulation. The molecular determinants of sequestration are also controversial. One group has shown that normal receptor G_s coupling is required for agonist-promoted sequestration (Cheung et al, 1989), whilst another group has shown that sequestration is unaffected by mutations that affect agonist-G_s coupling, but that downregulation is depressed by such mutations (Campbell et al, 1991).

We therefore consider downregulation to be a separate component of agonist-promoted desensitization. The disappearance of receptors during prolonged agonist exposure is thought to be due to several different processes. These include a decrease in the transcription of β_2AR messenger

RNA (mRNA), a decrease in the stability of β_2AR mRNA, and an increase in degradation of β_2AR expressed at the cell surface. Several interesting observations have recently been made regarding transcriptional control. Collins et al (1989) have shown that during agonist exposure β_2AR mRNA initially increases during the first 1–3 h and then undergoes a marked decrease, so that at 24 h less than 20% of the basal level of mRNA is present. The increase in β_2AR mRNA suggested the possibility that a cAMP response element (CRE) may be present in the 5′ flanking region of the β_2AR coding block which initially increases the rate of β_2AR mRNA transcription. Such a CRE is indeed present in the β_2AR (Kobilka et al, 1987a) and has been shown to increase transcription in response to agents that increase cAMP (Collins et al, 1990). This mechanism, however, does not appear to play a critical role in alterations in receptor expression, as downregulation of β_2AR occurs nevertheless. Indeed, downregulation of β_2AR occurs even in transfected cell lines in which transcription is controlled by viral and other promoters (Campbell et al, 1991). This suggests that it is not transcriptional control that is the key factor in the processes involved in agonist-promoted decreases in receptor expression, but pathways distal to the transcriptional process. Malbon and colleagues have shown that agonist-promoted decreases in β_2AR mRNA and receptor expression are paralleled by enhanced degradation of β_2AR mRNA (Hadcock et al, 1989). Thus it appears that processes involved in degradation of β_2AR mRNA are critical to the receptor downregulation process. It has also been shown that the PKA phosphorylation sites of the β_2AR enhance receptor downregulation (Bouvier et al, 1989); a mutant β_2AR which lacks the third intracellular PKA site underwent less of a decrease in β_2AR mRNA and receptor expression. Finally, two tyrosine residues in the carboxy tail of the β_2AR appear to be required for full agonist-promoted downregulation (Valiquette et al, 1990).

The pattern of agonist-promoted downregulation of the β_1AR and the β_2AR does not appear to occur with the β_3AR. This receptor has no PKA phosphorylation sites, and has a number of potential transcriptional control elements in the 5′ flanking region (Liggett and Schwinn, 1991). We have recently shown that there are at least three active CREs in this region (Thomas et al, 1992). These elements—TGACTCCA, TGAGGTCT and CGAGGTCA—are located 518, 622 and 1125 bases upstream of the β_3AR coding block. Each was inserted upstream of the promoter sequence in the vector pA_{10} CAT_2, which has a chloramphenicol acetyltransferase (CAT) reporter gene downstream. VERO cells were transfected with these constructs, and the synthesis of CAT assessed under conditions of increased cAMP. As shown in Figure 11, these three elements caused increased transcription of the CAT reporter gene in response to cAMP (Thomas et al, 1992). 3T3F442A cells express β_3ARs after undergoing a change in phenotype from fibroblast to adipocyte-like during insulin exposure (Thomas et al, 1992). We therefore examined the effects of agonist exposure on β_3AR mRNA and expression in these cells.

In contrast to what occurs with the β_2AR, β_3AR mRNA was found to undergo no decrease even after 30 h of agonist exposure. Indeed, a mild

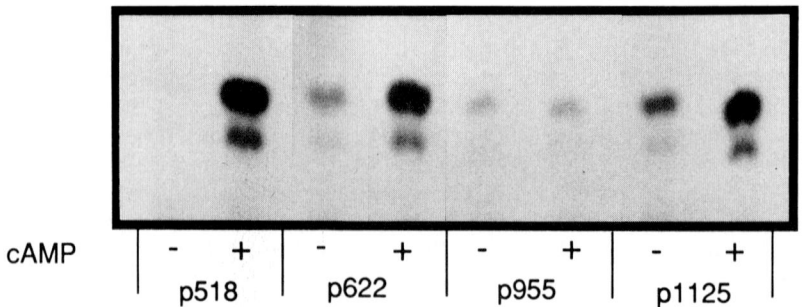

Figure 11. Effects of potential CREs of the 5′ flanking region of the β_3AR on transcription of the CAT reporter gene. The elements p518, p622 and p1125 (named according to the number of nucleotides upstream of the β_3AR initiator methionine) were responsive to cAMP.

increase, up to 165% of basal levels, was detected (Thomas et al, 1992). β_3AR expression was also found to be increased by agonist exposure, as shown in Figure 12. In contrast, β_1AR expression in undifferentiated 3T3F442A cells underwent a classic downregulation of receptor expression in response to agonist. Thus, downregulation of βARs appears to be subtype selective. The β_1AR and the β_2AR undergo marked agonist-promoted downregulation, while the β_3AR appears to be resistant to this process. We have shown that one mechanism which contributes to the lack of downregulation is an agonist-promoted increase in β_3AR mRNA. The β_3AR thus undergoes a paradoxical increase in expression mediated by the end product of the signal transduction cascade, cAMP.

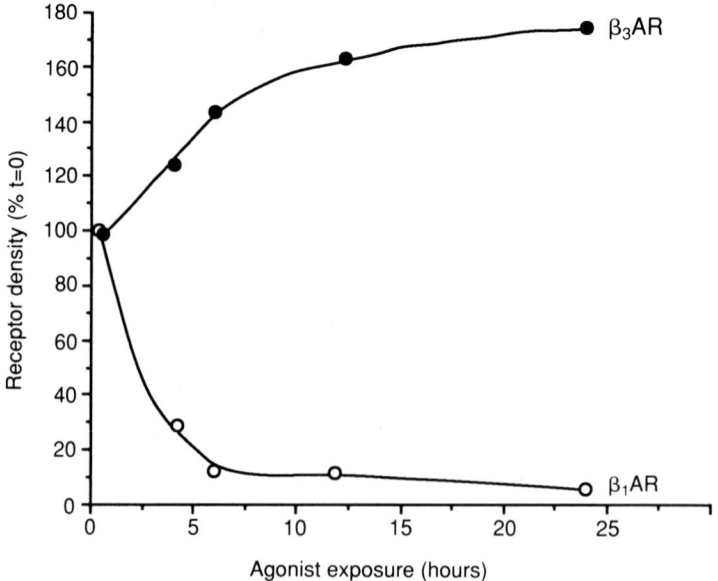

Figure 12. Effects of long-term agonist exposure on β_1AR and β_3AR expression.

Mechanism of short-term agonist-promoted αAR desensitization

Compared with the $\beta_2 AR$, little is known about $\alpha_2 AR$ desensitization. For a number of years there was no consensus as to whether the $\alpha_2 AR$ undergoes any agonist-promoted desensitization or downregulation (reviewed in Liggett et al, 1992b,c). Contributing to the varying results of previous studies may have been the use of tissue preparations containing more than one subtype of $\alpha_2 AR$, the use of cell lines expressing undefined $\alpha_2 ARs$, the use of cell lines expressing low receptor numbers with low radioligand binding or adenylyl cyclase signals, and the use of platelets for 'intact cells' studies. To circumvent these potential problems, we recently undertook studies of recombinant $\alpha_2 ARs$ expressed in CHW cells (Liggett et al, 1992b). The advantage of this system is that it provides a pure population of well-defined $\alpha_2 ARs$ and varying levels of expression depending on which clonal cell line is studied, and permits the use of mutagenesis of the receptor as a method of investigating regions which may be involved in specific mechanisms of desensitization. When the $\alpha_2 AR$ was expressed in CHW cells at a level of 1 pmol/mg, two patterns of agonist-promoted desensitization were observed (Figure 13, upper panel). After 30 min of agonist exposure, a rightward shift in the EC_{50} for adrenaline (epinephrine *USP*) mediated inhibition of adenylyl cyclase was noted. This resulted in an approximately 80% desensitization of this inhibitory capacity as observed at a submaximal concentration of 1 μmol/litre adrenaline (Figure 13, upper panel). After 24 h of agonist exposure, a further rightward shift in the EC_{50} was found, and a decrease in the maximal inhibitory capacity was observed (Figure 13). We thus considered that perhaps two different processes were occurring. To assign a molecular basis for this desensitization, we compared the amino acid sequences of the $\alpha_{2A} AR$ with the $\beta_2 AR$. This latter receptor contains multiple serines and threonines in a long cytoplasmic tail which are substrates for βARK phosphorylation, and two PKA consensus sequences located in the third intracellular loop and the proximal cytoplasmic tail. In contrast, the $\alpha_{2A} AR$ has a small intracellular tail (Table 1), and contains a much larger third intracellular loop (Figure 2). Within this third intracellular loop, there are multiple serines and threonines which we considered to be potential βARK phosphorylation sites. No PKA consensus sequences are located in the $\alpha_{2A} AR$. In a reconstituted phospholipid system, the purified $\alpha_2 AR$ has been shown to be a substrate for βARK phosphorylation (Benovic et al, 1987c). We then considered the possibility that the $\alpha_2 AR$ may undergo short-term desensitization via a βARK or similar kinase-mediated mechanism. Within the third intracellular loop of the $\alpha_{2A} AR$, one particularly interesting sequence of amino acids (EESSS, Figure 2) has been recently shown to be an excellent substrate for βARK phosphorylation in vitro (Onorato et al, 1991). We therefore constructed a mutated $\alpha_{2A} AR$ which had this sequence, as well as other serines and threonines, deleted, as shown in Figure 2. When this mutated receptor was expressed in CHW cells, it displayed no agonist-promoted short-term desensitization (Figure 13, lower panel). It did, however, undergo a long-term desensitization pattern similar to the wild type. Thus at least one mechanism of desensitization which was involved in the short-term phenomenon seemed to be localized to the third intracellular loop which had been deleted and that this was most likely mediated by phosphorylation. In order to test this, we studied in vivo phosphorylation of the α_2AR in response to agonist exposure. Cells were incubated with phosphorus-32 for 2.5 h and then treated with agonist,

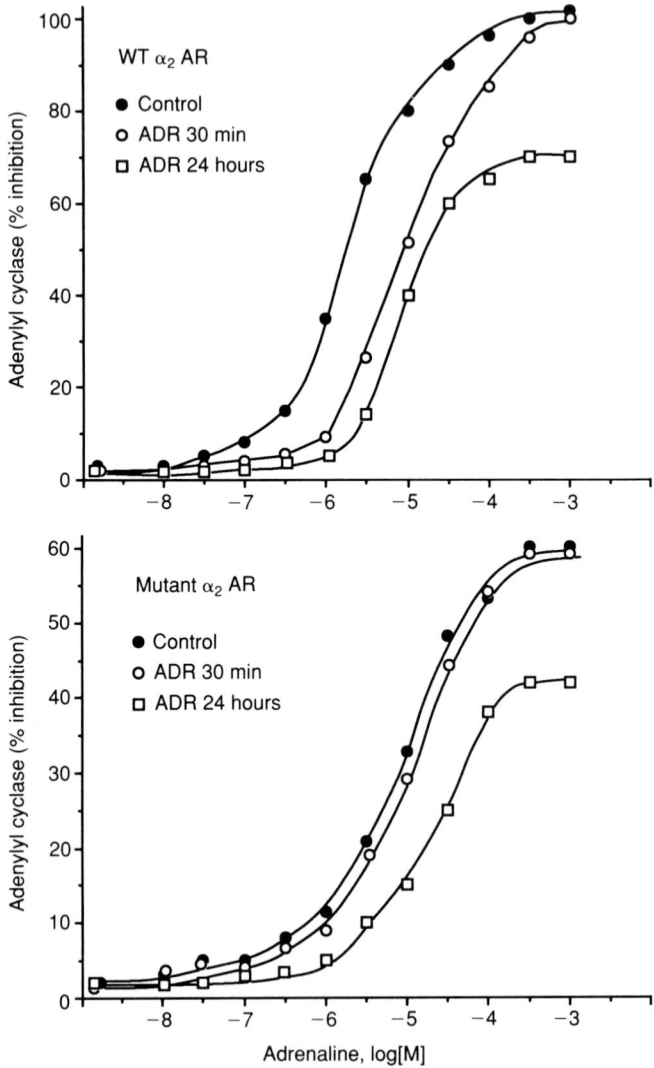

Figure 13. Desensitization of wild type (upper panel) α_2AR and a mutated (lower panel) receptor lacking a portion of the third intracellular loop. Short-term agonist exposure caused desensitization of the wild type α_2AR, as depicted by a shift in the EC_{50} for adrenaline-mediated inhibition of adenylyl cyclase. This effect was ablated when phosphorylation sites in the third loop were deleted (bottom panel, 30 min). Desensitization due to long-term agonist exposure (24 h) was unaffected by the mutation.

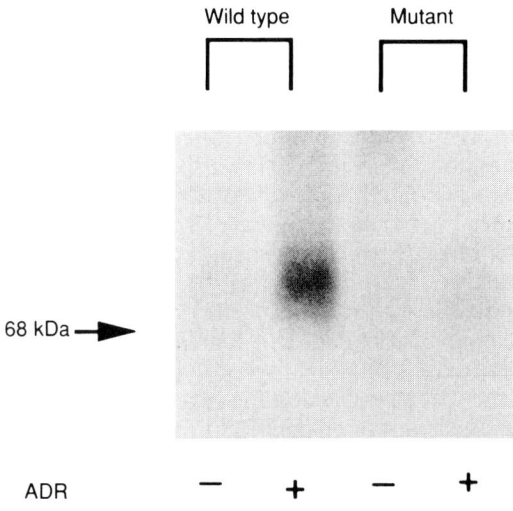

Figure 14. Agonist-promoted phosphorylation of the wild type α_2AR and a mutated α_2AR receptor lacking a portion of the third intracellular loop. ADR = adrenaline.

purified by immunoprecipitation with an α_2AR-specific antibody, and then electrophoresed through 10% polyacrylamide gels. As shown in Figure 14, an intense phosphorylation of the wild type α_2AR occurred after in vivo exposure to adrenaline for 15 min. In marked contrast, negligible phosphorylation was observed with the mutated α_{2A}AR which lacked potential βARK phosphorylation sites. We also assessed whether this mutation altered agonist-promoted sequestration of the α_{2A}AR. A mild degree ($\sim 30\%$) of sequestration of the α_2AR wild type was found to occur after agonist exposure, but this was not altered in the mutated receptor, which displayed the same time course and extent of sequestration. These series of experiments, therefore, showed unequivocally that the α_{2A}AR does indeed undergo a short-term agonist-promoted desensitization which is due to phosphorylation of the receptor at sites localized to the middle portion of the third intracellular loop.

Mechanisms of long-term desensitization of α_2AR

As discussed above, after 24 h of agonist exposure the α_{2A}AR underwent a different pattern of desensitization compared with that seen after 30 min. After this prolonged agonist exposure, there was both a rightward shift in the EC_{50} for adrenaline-mediated inhibition of adenylyl cyclase, as well as a decrease in the maximal inhibition of adenylyl cyclase. We considered several mechanisms that may be involved in long-term desensitization of α_2AR. One potential mechanism is a decrease in α_2AR expression after long-term agonist exposure. Such downregulation is commonly observed with the β_1AR and the β_2AR. In CHW cells expressing human α_{2A}ARs, we found that there was no decrease in receptor expression after prolonged agonist exposure of up to 48 h (Liggett et al, 1992b). We therefore considered that downregulation of receptor number was not an important factor in α_{2A}AR long-term desensitization. However, we do recognize that downregulation may be, to a certain extent, cell-type specific, and thus downregulation may occur in other cell types. Instead of a decrease in receptor expression, we found that the amount of G_i present in the cell was markedly decreased after agonist exposure. This was found using both detection of G_i by pertussis toxin-mediated ADP ribosylation and Western blots using G_i specific antibodies. Although it appeared that a clear reduction in G_i did occur after long-term agonist exposure, we wondered whether this was sufficient to cause reduced function of the α_{2A}AR (Figure 13, 24 h time points). To assess this we incubated cells expressing the α_{2A}AR with low concentrations of pertussis toxin, which ablated approximately 50% of the pertussis toxin-mediated ADP ribosylation in membranes. Thus, approximately 50% of the receptor-G_i coupling was ablated. These cells were then studied using agonist-promoted inhibition of adenylyl cyclase assays, and indeed it was found that the 50% decrease in G_i in these cells caused a rightward shift in the EC_{50} for adrenaline as well as a decrease in the maximal inhibitory capacity (Liggett et al, 1992b). Thus, the decrease of G_i by another mechanism (pertussis toxin incubation) also caused a pattern of depressed α_2AR function which was very similar to that induced by long-term agonist exposure. As further support that changes in G_i may be more important for long-term agonist desensitization of the α_2AR rather than a decrease in receptor expression, it has recently been shown that there is a CRE located in the 5' flanking region of the α_{2A}AR (Sakve and Hoffman, 1991). When cells were exposed to cAMP analogues these investigators showed that there was a marked increase in both receptor expression and α_{2A}AR mRNA. When α_2ARs are exposed to agonist for long periods of time and G_i is decreased, intracellular cAMP begins to increase. Thus it appears that there is a tendency during long-term agonist exposure in cells which naturally express the receptor and have the endogenous promoter to actually undergo an increase in receptor expression. Clearly, there is not the major impetus for a decrease in receptor expression which has been frequently described for the β_2AR. Further studies on the molecular mechanisms of this decrease in G_i as well as whether downregulation of α_2AR expression occurs in other cell types is underway.

SUMMARY

The recent cloning of multiple adrenergic receptors has moved our understanding of these receptors from a conceptual one (Alquist, 1948) to one based on well-defined unique cellular proteins. The biochemical and pharmacological properties of these receptors can now be studied in detail by expression of a single subtype in cells normally devoid of adrenergic receptors. By site-directed mutagenesis, the relationship between the structures of these receptors and their function is now being elucidated for each adrenergic receptor subtype. These functions include the binding of catecholamines and other ligands, G protein coupling and functional regulation.

Acknowledgements

The authors wish to thank Shirley McLean and Sabrina Campbell for typing the manuscript and Gerygraphics for the photography.

The authors are supported, in part, by the National Institutes of Health grants HL45967 (SBL) and NS30927 (JRR).

REFERENCES

Alquist RP (1948) A study of the adrenotropic receptors. *American Journal of Physiology* **153:** 586–600.

Benovic JL, Mayor F Jr, Staniszewski C, Lefkowitz RJ & Caron MG (1987a) Purification and characterization of the β-adrenergic receptor kinase. *Journal of Biological Chemistry* **262:** 9026–9032.

Benovic JL, Kuhn H, Weyand I, Codina J, Caron MG & Lefkowitz RJ (1987b) Functional desensitization of the isolated β-adrenergic receptor by the β-adrenergic receptor kinase: potential role of an analog for the retinal protein arrestin (48-kDa protein). *Proceedings of the National Academy of Sciences of the USA* **84:** 8879–8882.

Benovic JL, Regan JW, Matsui H et al (1987c) Agonist-dependent phosphorylation of the α_2-adrenergic receptor by the β-adrenergic kinase. *Journal of Biological Chemistry* **262:** 17251–17253.

Bouvier M, Hausdorff WP, DeBlasi A et al (1988) Removal of phosphorylation sites from the β_2-adrenergic receptor delays onset of agonist-promoted desensitization. *Nature* **333:** 370–373.

Bouvier M, Collins S, O'Dowd BF et al (1989) Two distinct pathways for cAMP-mediated down-regulation of the β_2-adrenergic receptor. *Journal of Biological Chemistry* **264:** 16786–16792.

Bylund DB, Blaxall HS, Iversen LJ, Caron MG, Lefkowitz RJ & Lomasney JL (1992) Pharmacological characteristics of alpha-2 adrenergic receptors: Comparison of pharmacologically defined subtypes with subtypes identified by molecular cloning. *Molecular Pharmacology* **42:** 1–5.

Campbell PT, Hnatowich M, O'Dowd BF, Caron MG, Lefkowitz RJ & Hausdorff WP (1991) Mutations of the human β_2-adrenergic receptor that impair coupling to G_s interfere with receptor down-regulation but not sequestration. *Molecular Pharmacology* **39:** 192–198.

Cheung AH, Sigal IS, Dixon RAF & Strader CD (1989) Agonist-promoted sequestration of the β_2-adrenergic receptor requires regions involved in functional coupling with G_s. *Molecular Pharmacology* **34:** 132–138.

Collins S, Bouvier M, Bolanowski MA, Caron MG & Lefkowitz RJ (1989) cAMP stimulates transcription of the β_2-adrenergic receptor gene in response to short-term agonist exposure. *Proceedings of the National Academy of Sciences of the USA* **86:** 4853–4857.

Collins S, Altschmied J, Herbsman O, Caron MG, Mellon PL & Lefkowitz RJ (1990) A cAMP response element in the β_2-adrenergic receptor gene confers transcriptional autoregulation by cAMP. *Journal of Biological Chemistry* **265:** 19330–19335.

Coupry I, Duzic E & Lanier SM (1992) Factors determining the specificity of signal transduction by guanine nucleotide-binding protein coupled receptors II. *Journal of Biological Chemistry* **267:** 9852–9857.

Dalman HM & Neubig RR (1991) Two peptides from the α_{2A}-adrenergic receptor alter receptor G protein coupling by distinct mechanisms. *Journal of Biological Chemistry* **266:** 11025–11029.

Dixon RAF, Kobilka BK, Strader DJ et al (1986) Cloning of the gene and cDNA for mammalian β-adrenergic receptor and homology with rhodopsin. *Nature* **32:** 75–79.

Dohlman HG, Bouvier M, Benovic JL, Caron MG & Lefkowitz RJ (1987) The multiple membrane spanning topography of the β_2-adrenergic receptor. *Journal of Biological Chemistry* **262:** 14282–14288.

Dohlman HG, Caron MG, Strader CD, Amlaiky N & Lefkowitz RJ (1988) Identification and sequence of a binding site peptide of the β_2-adrenergic receptor. *Biochemistry* **27:** 1813–1817.

Dohlman HG, Caron MG, DeBlasi A, Frielle T & Lefkowitz RJ (1990) A role of extracellular disulfide bonded cysteines in the ligand binding function of the β_2-adrenergic receptor. *Biochemistry* **29:** 2335–2342.

Dohlman HG, Thorner J, Caron MG & Lefkowitz RJ (1991) Model systems for the study of seven-transmembrane-segment receptors. *Annual Review of Biochemistry* **60:** 653–688.

Duzic E, Coupry I, Downing S & Lanier SM (1992) Factors determining the specificity of signal transduction by guanine nucleotide-binding protein-coupled receptors I. *Journal of Biological Chemistry* **267:** 9844–9851.

Eason MG, Kurose H, Holt BD, Raymond JR & Liggett SB (1992) Simultaneous coupling of α_2-adrenergic receptors to two G-proteins with opposing effects: subtype-selective coupling of α_2C10, α_2C4 and α_2C2 adrenergic receptors to G_i and G_s. *Journal of Biological Chemistry* **267:** 15795–15801.

Emorine LJ, Marullo S, Briend-Sutren MM et al (1989) Molecular characterization of the human β_3-adrenergic receptor. *Science* **245:** 1118–1121.

Frielle T, Collins S, Daniel KW, Caron MG, Lefkowitz RJ & Kobilka BK (1987) Cloning of the cDNA for the β_1-adrenergic receptor. *Proceedings of the National Academy of Sciences of the USA* **84:** 7920–7924.

Frielle Y, Daniel KW, Caron MG & Lefkowitz RJ (1988) Structural basis of β-adrenergic receptor subtype specificity studied with chimeric β_1/β_2-adrenergic receptors. *Proceedings of the National Academy of Sciences of the USA* **85:** 9494–9498.

Gerhardt MA & Neubig RR (1991) Multiple G_i protein subtypes regulate a single effector mechanism. *Molecular Pharmacology* **40:** 707–711.

Greene S, Holt B & Liggett SB (1992) β_1- and β_2-adrenergic receptors display subtype specific coupling to G_s. *Molecular Pharmacology* **41:** 889–893.

Guan XM, Peroutka SJ & Kobilka BK (1992) Identification of a single amino acid residue responsible for the binding of a class of β-adrenergic receptor antagonists to 5-hydroxytryptamine receptors. *Molecular Pharmacology* **41:** 695–698.

Hadcock JR, Wang H & Malbon CC (1989) Agonist-induced de-stabilization of β-adrenergic receptor mRNA. *Journal of Biological Chemistry* **264:** 19928–19933.

Harrison JK, D'Angelo DD, Zeng DW & Lynch KR (1991a) Pharmacological characterization of rat α_2-adrenergic receptors. *Molecular Pharmacology* **40:** 407–412.

Harrison JK, Pearson WR & Lynch KR (1991b) Molecular characterization of α_1 and α_2-adrenoceptors. *Trends in Pharmacological Sciences* **12:** 62–67.

Hausdorff WP, Bouvier M, O'Dowd BF, Irons GP, Caron MG & Lefkowitz RJ (1989) Phosphorylation sites on two domains of the β_2-adrenergic receptor are involved in distinct pathways of receptor desensitization. *Journal of Biological Chemistry* **264:** 12657–12665.

Hausdorff WP, Caron MG & Lefkowitz RJ (1990a) Turning off the signal: Desensitization of β-adrenergic receptor function. *FASEB Journal* **4:** 2881–2889.

Hausdorff WP, Hnatowich M, O'Dowd BF, Caron MG & Lefkowitz RJ (1990b) A mutation of the β_2-adrenergic receptor impairs agonist activation of adenylyl cyclase without affecting high affinity agonist binding. *Journal of Biological Chemistry* **265:** 1388–1393.

Hausdorff WP, Campbell PT, Ostrowski J, Yu SS, Caron MG & Lefkowitz RJ (1991) A small region of the β-adrenergic receptor is selectively involved in its rapid regulation. *Proceedings of the National Academy of Sciences of the USA* **88:** 2979–2983.

Karnik SS, Sukmar TP, Chen HB & Khorana HG (1988) Cysteine 110 and 187 are essential for the formation of correct structure of bovine rhodopsin. *Proceedings of the National Academy of Sciences of the USA* **85:** 75–84.

Kobilka BK, Frielle T, Dohlman HG et al (1987a) Delineation of the intronless nature of the human and hamster β_2-adrenergic receptor genes and their putative promoter regions. *Journal of Biological Chemistry* **262:** 7321–7327.

Kobilka BK, Matsui H, Kobilka TS et al (1987b) Cloning, sequencing, and expression of the gene coding for the human platelet α_2-adrenergic receptor. *Science* **238:** 650–656.

Kobilka BK, Kobilka TS, Daniel K, Regan JW, Caron MG & Lefkowitz RJ (1988) Chimeric α_2/β_2-receptors: Delineation of domains involved in effector coupling and ligand binding specificity. *Science* **240:** 1310–1316.

Kurose H, Regan JW, Caron MG et al (1991) Functional interactions of recombinant α_2 adrenergic receptor subtypes and G proteins in reconstituted phospholipid vesicles. *Biochemistry* **30:** 3335–3341.

Lanier SM, Downing S, Duzic E & Homcy CJ (1991) Isolation of rat genomic clones encoding subtypes of the α_2-adrenergic receptor. Identification of a unique receptor subtype. *Journal of Biological Chemistry* **266:** 10470–10478.

Liggett SB (1991) Desensitization of the β-adrenergic receptor: Distinct molecular determinants of phosphorylation by specific kinases. *Pharmacological Research* **24:** 29–41.

Liggett SB & Schwinn DA (1991) Multiple potential regulatory elements in the 5' flanking region of the human β_3-adrenergic receptor. *DNA Sequence* **2:** 61–63.

Liggett SB, Bouvier M, Hausdorff WP, O'Dowd BF, Caron MG & Lefkowitz RJ (1989a) Altered patterns of agonist-stimulated cAMP accumulation in cells expressing mutant β_2-adrenergic receptors lacking phosphorylation sites. *Molecular Pharmacology* **36:** 641–646.

Liggett SB, Bouvier M, O'Dowd BF et al (1989b) Substitution of an extracellular cysteine in the β_2-adrenergic receptor enhances receptor phosphorylation and desensitization. *Biochemical and Biophysical Research Communications* **165:** 257–263.

Liggett SB, Caron MG, Lefkowitz RJ & Hnatowich MR (1991) Coupling of a mutated form of the human β_2-adrenergic receptor to G_i and G_s: requirements for multiple cytoplasmic domains in the coupling process. *Journal of Biological Chemistry* **266:** 4816–4821.

Liggett SB, Schwinn DA & Lefkowitz RJ (1992a) A chimeric β_3/β_2 adrenergic receptor delineates the nature of subtype selective desensitization. *Clinical Research* **42:** 117.

Liggett SB, Ostrowski J, Chesnut LC et al (1992b) Sites in the third intracellular loop of the α_{2A}-adrenergic receptor confer short term agonist-promoted desensitization. Evidence for a receptor kinase-mediated mechanism. *Journal of Biological Chemistry* **267:** 4740–4746.

Liggett SB, Ostrowski J, Chesnut LC, Caron MG & Lefkowitz RJ (1992c) Role of the β-adrenergic receptor kinase in desensitization of the α_2-adrenergic receptor. *Transactions of the Association of American Physicians* **104:** 40–47.

Lohse MJ, Benovic JL, Caron MG & Lefkowitz RJ (1990) Multiple pathways of rapid β_2-adrenergic receptor desensitization: delineation with specific inhibitors. *Journal of Biological Chemistry* **265:** 3202–3209.

Lomasney JW, Cotecchia S, Lefkowitz RJ & Caron MG (1991) Molecular biology of α-adrenergic receptors: implications for receptor classification and for structure-function relationships. *Biochimica et Biophysica Acta* **1095:** 127–139.

Lomasney JW, Lorenz W, Allen LF et al (1990) Expansion of the alpha 2-adrenergic receptor family: cloning and characterization of a human alpha 2-adrenergic receptor subtype, the gene for which is located on chromosome 2. *Proceedings of the National Academy of Sciences of the USA* **87:** 5094–5098.

Matsui H, Lefkowitz RJ, Caron MG & Regan JW (1989) Localization of the fourth membrane spanning domain as a ligand binding site in the human platelet α_2-adrenergic receptor. *Biochemistry* **28:** 4125–4130.

McClue ST & Milligan G (1990) Molecular interaction of the human α_2-C10-adrenergic receptor, when expressed in RAT-1 fibroblasts, with multiple pertussis toxin-sensitive guanine nucleotide-binding proteins: studies with site-directed antisera. *Molecular Pharmacology* **40:** 627–632.

Milligan G, Carr C, Gould GW, Mullaney I & Lawan BE (1991) Agonist-dependent, cholera toxin-catalyzed ADP-mobilization of pertussis toxin-sensitive G-protein following transfections of the human α_{2D}-adrenergic receptor into rat-1 fibroblasts. *Journal of Biological Chemistry* **266:** 6447–6455.

O'Dowd BF, Hnatowich M, Regan JW, Leader WM, Caron MG & Lefkowitz RJ (1988) Site-directed mutagenesis of the cytoplasmic domains of the human β_2-adrenergic receptor: Localization of regions involved in G protein-receptor coupling. *Journal of Biological Chemistry* **263:** 15985–15992.

Onorato JJ, Palczewski K, Regan JW, Caron MG, Lefkowitz RJ & Benovic JL (1991) The role of acidic amino acids in peptide substrates of the β-adrenergic receptor kinase and rhodopsin kinase. *Biochemistry* **30:** 5118–5125.

Ovchinikov KY (1982) Rhodopsin and bacteriorhodopsin: structure-function relationships. *FEBS Letters* **148:** 179–191.

Perkins JP, Hausdorff WP & Lefkowitz RJ (1991) Mechanisms of ligand-induced desensitization of β-adrenergic receptors. In Perkins JP (ed) *The β-Adrenergic Receptor*, pp 125–180. Clifton, New Jersey: Humana Press.

Regan JW, Kobilka TS, Yang-Feng TL, Caron MG & Lefkowitz RJ (1988) Cloning and expression of a human kidney cDNA for a novel α_2-adrenergic receptor. *Proceedings of the National Academy of Sciences of the USA* **85:** 6301–6305.

Roth N, Campbell P, Caron MG, Lefkowitz RJ & Lohse MJ (1991) Comparative rates of desensitization of β-adrenergic receptor kinase and the cyclic AMP dependent protein kinase. *Proceedings of the National Academy of Sciences of the USA* **88:** 6201–6204.

Rubenstein RC, Wong SK-F & Ross EM (1987) The hydrophobic tryptic core of the β-adrenergic receptor retains G_s regulatory activity in response to agonists and thiols. *Journal of Biological Chemistry* **34:** 1655–1666.

Saffitz J & Liggett SB (1992) Subcellular distribution of β_2-adrenergic receptors delineated with quantitative ultrastructural autoradiography of radioligand binding sites. *Circulation Research* **70:** 1320–1325.

Sakue M & Hoffman BB (1991) cAMP regulates transcription of the α_{2A}-adrenergic receptor gene in HT-29 cells. *Journal of Biological Chemistry* **266:** 5743–5749.

Shear M, Insel PA, Melmon KL & Coffino P (1976) Agonist-specific refractoriness induced by isoproterenol. *Journal of Biological Chemistry* **251:** 7572–7576.

Sibley DR, Benovic JL, Caron MG & Lefkowitz RJ (1987) Regulation of transmembrane signalling by receptor phosphorylation. *Cell* **48:** 913–922.

Strader CD, Sigal IS, Calendor MR, Rands E, Hill WS & Dixon RA (1988) Conserved aspartic acid residues 70 and 113 of the β-adrenergic receptor have different roles in receptor function. *Journal of Biological Chemistry* **263:** 10267–10271.

Strader CD, Sigal IS & Dixon RA (1989a) Mapping the functional domains of the β-adrenergic receptor. *American Journal of Respiratory Cell and Molecular Biology* **1:** 81–86.

Strader CD, Calendore MR, Hill WS, Sigal IS & Dixon RA (1989b) Identification of two serine residues involved in agonist activation of β-adrenergic receptor function. *Journal of Biological Chemistry* **264:** 13572–13578.

Strulovici B, Cerione RA, Kilpatrick BF, Caron MG & Lefkowitz RJ (1984) Direct demonstration of impaired functionality of a purified desensitization β-adrenergic receptor in a reconstitution system. *Science* **225:** 837–840.

Suryanaryana S, Daunt DA, Von Zastrow M & Kobilka BK (1991) A point mutation in the seventh hydrophobic domain of the α_2-adrenergic receptor increases its affinity for a family of β-receptor antagonists. *Journal of Biological Chemistry* **266:** 15488–15492.

Thomas DD & Stryer L (1982) Transverse location of retinal chromophore of rhodopsin in rod outer segment disc membranes. *Journal of Molecular Biology* **154:** 145–157.

Thomas RF, Holt BD, Schwinn DA & Liggett SB (1992) Long term agonist exposure induces up regulation of β_3-adrenergic receptor expression via multiple cAMP response elements. *Proceedings of the National Academy of Sciences of the USA* **89:** 4490–4494.

Tota MR, Calendor MR, Dixon RA & Strader CD (1991) Biophysical and genetic analysis of the ligand-binding site of the β-adrenoceptor. *Trends in Pharmacological Sciences* **12:** 4–6.

Valiquette M, Bonin H, Hnatowich M, Caron MG, Lefkowitz RJ & Bouvier M (1990) Involvement of tyrosine residues located in the carboxyl tail of the human β_2-adrenergic receptor in agonist-induced down-regulation of the receptor. *Proceedings of the National Academy of Sciences of the USA* **87:** 5089–5093.

Voight MM, McCure SK, Kunterman RY et al (1991) The rat α_2-C4 adrenergic receptor gene encodes a novel pharmacological subtype. *FEBS Letters* **278:** 45–50.

Von Zastrow M & Kobilka BK (1992) Ligand regulated internalization of human β_2 adrenergic receptors between plasma membranes and endosomes containing transferrin receptors. *Journal of Biological Chemistry* **267:** 3530–3538.

Weinshank RL, Zgombick JM, Macchi M et al (1990) Cloning, expression and pharmacological characterization of a human α_{2B}-adrenergic receptor. *Molecular Pharmacology* **38:** 681–688.

Zeng D, Harrison JK, D'Angelo DD et al (1990) Molecular characterization of a rat α_{2B}-adrenergic receptor. *Proceedings of the National Academy of Sciences of the USA* **87:** 3102–3106.

3

Plasma catecholamines—analytical challenges
and physiological limitations

PAUL HJEMDAHL

Cardiovascular and metabolic adaptation to stress and disease states is often mediated by the autonomic nervous system. A comprehensive evaluation of autonomic function includes studies of sympathoadrenal activity, i.e. sympathetic nerve activity and the levels of the circulating 'stress hormone' adrenaline (ADR), parasympathetic (mainly vagal) nerve activity, and the various receptors mediating the effects of autonomic activation. Sympathetic nerves release noradrenaline (NA) as their primary transmitter. NA may also reach levels in plasma compatible with actions as a circulating hormone. This chapter will focus on the analytical problems of catecholamine measurement (mainly in plasma) and the information that can or cannot be derived from plasma catecholamine measurements.

Sympathetic nerve activity can be evaluated by axonal nerve activity recordings (in humans only in muscle and skin), by measuring NA in various ways, reflecting its release from sympathetic nerves, and/or by studying the effects of drugs influencing sympathetic function. These approaches will all be commented on in an attempt to provide a framework into which plasma catecholamine data can be fitted. Relationships between plasma NA and sympathetic nerve activity is a key topic, as 'plasma NA' is a frequently used and often misunderstood tool when assessing sympathetic nerve activity in humans.

The importance of ADR as a circulating 'stress hormone' or as a cotransmitter will also be discussed, in order to illustrate problems encountered when evaluating the physiological importance of a catecholamine. Methodological limitations are not always appreciated. Assessments of pre- and post-junctional receptor function will be commented on, as plasma catecholamine determinations may be used in this context, but not as indiscriminately as is sometimes the case. Examples of plasma catecholamine response patterns to physiological stimuli will be taken mainly from studies of autonomic mechanisms during mental stress, as this illustrates how differentiated the patterns of activity of the autonomic nervous system may be; other stimuli will be briefly commented upon.

The comments given here on sympathoadrenal mechanisms in humans will, by necessity, be brief in relation to the immense literature in the field. Taking examples mainly from our own studies may give a limited outlook on

Baillière's Clinical Endocrinology and Metabolism—
Vol. 7, No. 2, April 1993
ISBN 0–7020–1698–5

the literature, but has the advantages that the studies have been performed under similar conditions and the catecholamines have been determined with the same assay, which facilitates comparisons—analytical techniques and experimental design are important aspects when comparing studies.

ANALYTICAL CHALLENGES IN CATECHOLAMINE MEASUREMENT

There is an extremely large number of methods for measuring catecholamines in plasma and other biological matrices which have generated over 2000 references since 1980 (Candito et al, 1990). The seemingly never-ending publication of new methods or modifications of old ones clearly points towards problems with regard to precision, speed and economy with catecholamine assays (in addition to the eagerness to have 'one's own' methods referenced). It would not be appropriate to describe all the bio-chemical assays for catecholamines and their variations in detail in this context; I will therefore restrict my comments to more general descriptions of assay methodology and some opinions on problems with accuracy of the assays, as well as on how the assays should be validated. I will also give some practical advice based on our experience in this field.

Are catecholamine assays dependable?

The first requirement for the use of plasma NA as a marker for sympathetic nerve activity is, of course, that the assay result is correct. This is far from always the case, as clearly illustrated by a comparison of analytical results obtained in a number of laboratories considered to be experienced in the field (Figures 1 and 2) (Hjemdahl, 1984b). Plasma ADR (Figures 1 and 2) and dopamine data (not shown) also varied considerably. This study demonstrates considerable inter- and intralaboratory variation, which highlights the analytical challenge at hand and makes one question the validity of pooling results from different studies or drawing too firm conclusions on the basis of 'negative' results from individual studies. The latter aspect is also influenced by physiological considerations (see below).

Most assays are validated with regard to sensitivity and reproducibility, which are essential for good results but which do not prove accuracy. An erroneous result caused by an interference can be reproduced as exactly as a correct result! Analytical results should, in my opinion, also be validated by comparative studies aimed at proving specificity. There is no 'golden standard' in this respect, but if two assays *based on sufficiently different assay principles* yield similar results, both assays may be considered to be appro-priate. Some examples of such validations have been reported (Hjemdahl et al, 1979; Allenmark et al, 1980; Goldstein et al, 1981a,b; Causon et al, 1983; Hjemdahl, 1984a; Van der Hoorn et al, 1989). Good results usually come out of such validations, even though performance in the above-mentioned interlaboratory comparison was poor (Hjemdahl, 1984b). If results differ, the assay yielding the lowest values probably comes closest to the 'truth'.

Despite this, some authors may choose to favour the method yielding the higher values (Causon et al, 1983).

The biggest analytical challenge lies in measuring the low basal levels of ADR and dopamine in plasma, as assay coefficients of variation increase when one approaches the limit of detection. However, as illustrated in Figure 2, poor sensitivity is not the only problem with plasma catecholamine determinations: lack of specificity and reproducibility are also problems.

In our experience basal supine plasma NA levels are usually approximately 0.8–2 nmol/litre (135–150 pg/ml) in arterial and antecubital venous samples from healthy volunteers; few individuals have values exceeding

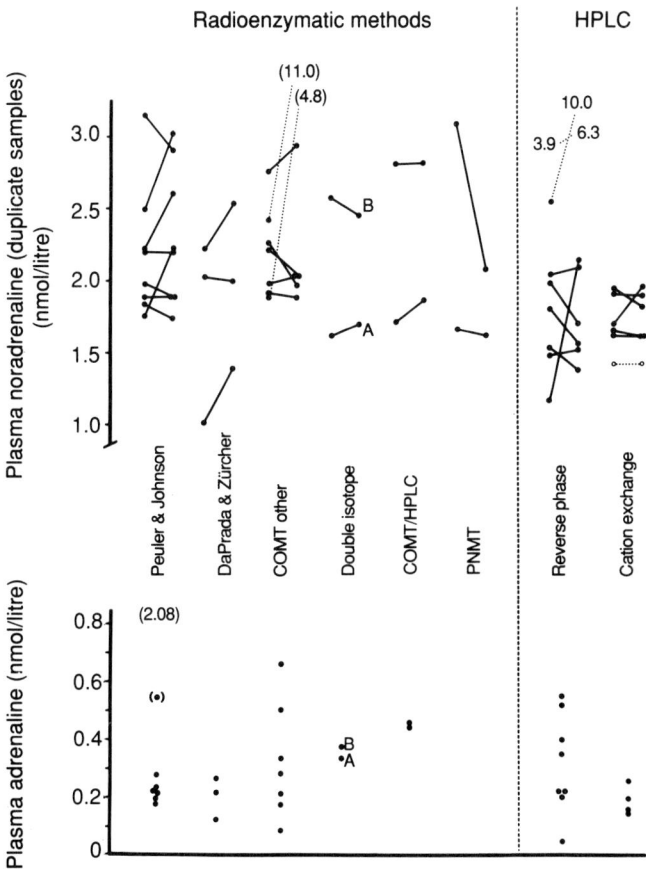

Figure 1. Plasma NA and ADR concentrations measured by various techniques in 34 different laboratories. Results were grouped together according to methodologies used (see centre row). NA data represent blind duplicate measurements (one sample was spiked with ADR). These values represent basal resting levels in a pool of plasma from healthy volunteers. It may be seen that duplicate determinations of NA showed occasional large variation and that the levels of NA and ADR varied considerably between laboratories. HPLC = high pressure liquid chromatography. For further details, see Hjemdahl (1984b).

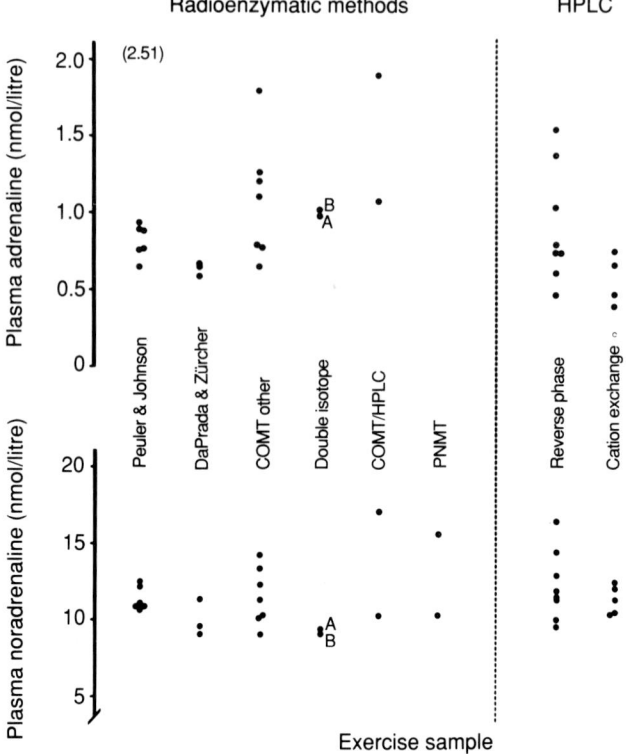

Figure 2. Data from the same interlaboratory comparison of catecholamine assays as illustrated in Figure 1. This figure shows results obtained on pooled plasma obtained from healthy volunteers after dynamic exercise. It can be seen that the variability evident in Figure 1 is not much reduced at the higher levels of NA and ADR seen in plasma after exercise. Abbreviations as for Figure 1. For further details, see Hjemdahl (1984b).

2.5 nmol/litre (see Figure 3). ADR levels are approximately 0.2–0.4 nmol/ litre (35–70 pg/ml) in arterial plasma and half this value in venous plasma; free dopamine levels in plasma are below 0.1–0.2 nmol/litre (20–30 pg/ml), on average. Examples of basal catecholamine levels in arterial plasma are given in Table 1. If basal catecholamine levels are high, either poor assay precision or unsatisfactory conditions of the experiment (especially lack of basal, unstressed conditions) may have influenced the results.

Every publication of catecholamine data should be accompanied by relevant references to the method used *and* any modifications introduced, as well as data on detection limits and coefficients of variation in the relevant concentration range (i.e. nanomolar to subnanomolar concentrations) in the laboratory performing the assay. This is not always adhered to since plasma catecholamine data are so common and the problems are not always appreciated. It is also valuable to know if and how the assay has been

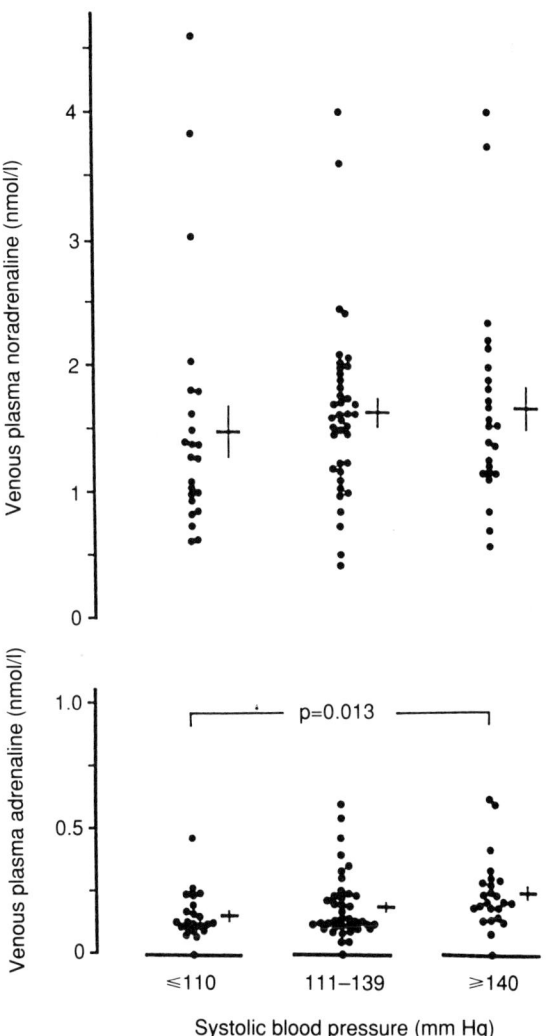

Figure 3. Forearm venous NA and ADR levels in healthy subjects in relation to blood pressure levels. Sampling was performed via an indwelling catheter after resting for 1 h. Individual data and means ± SEM are indicated. Data from Theorell et al (1985).

validated to show its accuracy (i.e. specificity). The latter is, in my opinion, seldom checked in an adequate manner.

Assay principles

Catecholamine assays may be based on several different principles, the two main ones being radioenzymatic and high performance liquid chromatography. Many modifications of each principle exist. More details on

Table 1. Renal vascular resistance (peripheral resistance units; PRU), arterial and renal venous plasma concentrations of catecholamines (nM), renal noradrenaline and dopamine overflows (pmol/min) and fractional extraction (FE) of adrenaline over the kidney (%) in studies of responses to isometric handgrip exercise (Tidgren and Hjemdahl, 1988), mental stress (Tidgren and Hjemdahl, 1989) and dynamic exercise (Tidgren et al. 1991) in healthy volunteers. Renal blood flows were measured by a renal venous thermodilution technique after visualization of renal venous anatomy in each individual (Tidgren and Hjemdahl, 1988). Renal vascular resistance was calculated on the basis of these flows and intra-arterially determined blood pressures. Plasma catecholamines were measured by cation exchange high performance liquid chromatography with amperometric detection (see Hjemdahl, 1987a). Mean values ± SEM for resting and peak values are shown ($n = 8$–12 in the various studies). For details concerning statistics, study designs and other variables, please see individual references.

Condition	Renal vascular resistance	Noradrenaline			Dopamine			Adrenaline	
		Arterial	Renal venous	Overflow	Arterial	Renal venous	Overflow	Arterial	FE
Rest	0.163 ± 0.016	0.98 ± 0.13	1.24 ± 0.14	228 ± 34	0.09 ± 0.01	0.14 ± 0.02	29 ± 3	0.24 ± 0.03	40 ± 4
Isometric exercise	0.196 ± 0.027	1.49 ± 0.16	2.36 ± 0.29	508 ± 73	0.09 ± 0.01	0.14 ± 0.02	30 ± 5	0.38 ± 0.04	42 ± 4
$P<$	0.05	0.001	0.001	0.001	NS	NS	NS	0.001	NS
Rest	0.147 ± 0.007	0.78 ± 0.06	1.09 ± 0.10	252 ± 29	0.05 ± 0.01	0.09 ± 0.01	24 ± 2	0.26 ± 0.04	46 ± 4
Mental stress	0.216 ± 0.021	1.34 ± 0.11	2.93 ± 0.54	708 ± 79	0.06 ± 0.02	0.14 ± 0.01	34 ± 4	0.68 ± 0.11	60 ± 3
$P<$	0.001	0.001	0.001	0.001	NS	0.001	0.05	0.001	0.05
Rest	0.141 ± 0.022	0.87 ± 0.08	1.05 ± 0.11	201 ± 33	0.08 ± 0.01	0.12 ± 0.01	26 ± 3	0.32 ± 0.07	42 ± 4
Dynamic exercise (max intensity; 188W)	0.334 ± 0.031	11.4 ± 2.45	19.8 ± 5.69	3039 ± 806	0.33 ± 0.06	0.84 ± 0.33	135 ± 52	2.12 ± 0.54	61 ± 7
$P<$	0.001	0.001	0.001	0.01	0.001	0.01	0.05	0.001	0.001

NS = not significant.

methodologies and references to published methods than those given here can be found in Johnson et al (1980) for radioenzymatic assays and Hjemdahl (1984a, 1987a), Krstulovic (1982) and Mefford (1981) for HPLC assays.

Radioenzymatic assays

Radioenzymatic assays (REAs) are based on methylation of the catecholamines with a radiolabelled methyl donor (usually *S*-adenosyl-methionine with a tritiated methyl group) under the influence of a methyltransferase prepared from an animal tissue. The most common approach is to use catechol-O-methyltransferase (COMT), the enzyme responsible for the extraneuronal metabolism of catecholamines to metanephrines. COMT methylates all three catecholamines. If phenylethanolamine-*N*-methyltransferase (PNMT), the enzyme which synthesizes ADR from NA, is used, only NA is measured (Henry et al, 1975). After methylation (under well-defined conditions), the methylated compounds are usually subjected to organic extraction and back-extraction into an aqueous phase, followed by thin-layer chromatography (TLC) to separate the methylated catecholamines and various contaminants. The relevant spots on the TLC plate are then removed and counted in a liquid scintillation counter. The most commonly used COMT assay is that of Peuler and Johnson (1977), which is available commercially.

We started our work in the field with an REA, but have no recent experience of this approach. REAs work well in many laboratories, although problems evidently exist (see Figures 1 and 2). In our experience the quality of the radiolabelled methyl donor was a major problem—different batches from the same manufacturer gave variable blank values and results. The commercial kit should be standardized from this point of view, which implies an advantage with regard to the dependability of assay results. Another problem is that so many steps are involved in a REA and that derivatization, extractions, etc. are seldom quantitative. Thus variability, which is not seen unless an internal standard is used, may well emerge. There are REA methods which include internal standards (i.e. double isotope techniques), but most laboratories use single isotope methods which rely on minute attention to each and every one of all the steps involved for good results.

High performance liquid chromatography

These assays are based on extraction of the catecholamines from the sample in order to purify and concentrate them, followed by separation on a high performance liquid chromatography (HPLC) column and, finally, quantitation in a sensitive detector, which also contributes to the specificity of the assay.

The method of *extraction* is governed by the requirements on purification set by the following steps; no general guidelines can be given. With our method, a simple alumina extraction (Anton and Sayre, 1962) may be used, as the HPLC columns used have a relatively high selectivity for catechol-amines. With reverse phase separation that may not be the case. For example, uric acid has been reported to interfere with NA when an inadequate extraction step is combined with inadequate separation by reverse phase HPLC (Davis et al, 1981). Many other endogenous and exogenous substances may also create problems (e.g. Bouloux et al, 1985). In any event, the extraction and separation steps should be based on different physicochemical principles to achieve good selectivity for the analytes. Many different extraction methods (and modifications of them) have been described. Before adopting one particular method it should be optimized with regard to recovery of the analytes and the degree of 'clean-up' afforded by it. The choice of extraction procedure must be integrated with choices regarding other aspects of the assay.

An internal standard should be included in the assay (before the extraction step or, if tissue levels are measured, before the tissue homogenization step) to correct for individual losses in the work-up of each sample. It is important to handle internal and external standards appropriately for good results (Candito et al, 1990). The latter authors suggested that this may be one of the reasons for poor performance in the interlaboratory comparison (Hjemdahl, 1984b), but this cannot be the sole explanation.

The specificity of the *separation* step (i.e. the HPLC column and the conditions under which it is used) is the next important aspect to consider. Reverse phase columns are the type most commonly used, due to their versatility and their general dominance in biochemical assays based on HPLC. Reverse phase chromatography separates mainly on the basis of lipophilicity, but adsorption to the silica particles which are coated with carbon chains (usually 18 carbon atoms in length, i.e. C_{18} columns) may also be of importance. In fact, C_{18} columns from different manufacturers (sometimes even different batches from the same manufacturer) yield different chromatographic separation. The separation is easily influenced by the conditions under which the reverse phase chromatography is run (mainly the mobile phase composition), which for many is an attractive feature. When separation is poor one can alter the mobile phase in order to get 'cleaner' chromatograms. This is usually done by altering the concentration of the organic modifier or the ion-pairing counter-ion in the buffer, both of which determine the partition coefficient for the analyte between the hydrophilic mobile phase and the lipophilic stationary phase of the column (i.e. the capacity factors). However, modifications aimed at solving problems may alter the chromatographic behaviour of other interfering substances and thus create new problems. For further information on reverse phase chromatography, see, for example, Bartlett (1989), Hjemdahl (1984a) and Krstulovic (1982).

Cation exchange chromatography is an old and well-established principle for the separation of catecholamines (Häggendal, 1962). With the availability of HPLC column material with reactive groups resulting in a strong cation exchanger, it seemed logical to use this principle. Hallman and coworkers (1978) described a plasma catecholamine assay based on a long cation exchange column with rather large particles and thus limited efficiency. We and others subsequently used microparticulate columns (Hjemdahl et al, 1979; Allenmark et al, 1980; Hjemdahl, 1987a), which enhanced the efficiency of separation. Later, a modification was suggested by Eriksson and Persson (1982), whereby 10% methanol was added to the mobile phase of this system. We have tested this, but have not adopted it as it seems to reduce retention times without providing improved specificity of separation. Retention times can also be altered by changing the column length or the flow rate of the mobile phase through the column. Individual batches of column material should be tested before use, as there is batch-to-batch variability (although it has been reduced over the years). Cation exchange columns do not provide as narrow peaks as reverse phase columns. In our experience the cation exchange principle nonetheless offers greater selectivity for catecholamines and we consider the cation exchange separation to be essential for our good assay results.

Another development which should be mentioned is microbore column technology, since this increases the sensitivity of the assay (in terms of absolute peak heights per concentration of analyte in the injectate) due to the reduction of dead space and band broadening in the column. This is useful for the analysis of trace amounts in small sample volumes (Durkin et al, 1985), and has been used successfully in, for example, microdialysis studies. However, microbore columns cannot handle large volumes of injectate. The microbore approach works well with reverse phase column material, but we have had problems with poor durability when attempting to pack microbore columns (≤ 1 mm inner diameter (i.d.)) with cation exchange material. Intermediate column widths (2–3 mm i.d.) can also be used, and provide some increase in sensitivity compared with the conventional column widths (which are ≥ 4 mm i.d.).

With regard to *detection*, either electrochemical or fluorimetric detection may be used—both have advantages and disadvantages. Fluorimetric detection is used by some laboratories; for descriptions and references, see Hjemdahl (1984a), Krstulovic (1982) and Van der Hoorn et al (1989). However, electrochemical detection (Kissinger et al, 1981; Mefford, 1981; Krstulovic, 1982) seems to be the dominating principle in this field. Electrochemical detection is based on the liberation of electrons when catechols are oxidized to orthoquinones (under the influence of an appropriate oxidating potential); the conversion can be either stoichiometric (coulometric detection) or partial (amperometric detection) (Kissinger et al, 1981; Hjemdahl, 1984a). Minute currents (picoamperes) are thus created and amplified, which implies that stability and low background noise are important when using electrochemical detectors. The mobile phase can never be completely free from other oxidizable substances, which results in a background current which should be minimized by using highly purified buffer constituents. Due to the creation of a background current from the mobile phase itself, flow through the detector must be as stable as possible to obtain a good signal-to-noise ratio; in practice the HPLC pump is critical for good results (see Hjemdahl, 1987a).

The electrochemical detector provides a certain degree of selectivity for catecholamines due to their susceptibility to electrochemical (and spontaneous) oxidation. The oxidating potential should be as low as possible, in order to enhance detector selectivity (Mefford, 1981). Factors such as the mobile phase composition influence detector responses (Hjemdahl, 1984a; Bartlett, 1989). If uncertain as to which oxidating potential should be used in a certain system, one may perform a voltamogram (Kissinger et al, 1981) in order to establish the right criteria (i.e. the highest possible selectivity with an adequate yield).

Coulometric detection provides a stronger signal, due to complete conversion of the analyte. However, this need not enhance the signal-to-noise ratio, which is the important aspect to consider. Coulometric detectors are available in designs allowing multiple steps (oxidation and reduction), which can be set so as to increase the selectivity for the analyte and improve the signal-to-noise ratio. Assays based on such multiple electrode designs have been described (e.g. Goldstein et al, 1984). Amperometric detection also offers good selectivity for catecholamines, provided that the oxidation potential is kept low enough. The designs and, consequently, the sensitivities of electrochemical detectors vary. If uncertain about a specific apparatus, demand to test it before buying—claims of excellence are not always borne out in practice, at least not in our laboratory.

Validation of catecholamine assays

As mentioned above, new assays should be validated by comparing analytical results with those of another well-documented assay. There are such comparisons in the literature (see above), but most assays lack this type of documentation. When examining comparative data it is important to look at the equation of the regression line (Do results fall on the line of identity and intercept at the origin?), and not only the r value for the regression line. If interlaboratory variability is possible (i.e. if the conditions of the assay are not reproduced exactly), it is wise to revalidate the assay in the new laboratory— even if it has been validated before! In particular, I would like to reiterate that any change in assay conditions results in a new assay with unproven specificity, even if results look good (Hjemdahl, 1984a). This is especially relevant to keep in mind when, as I have encountered several times, reverse phase HPLC is used in such a way that the chromatographic conditions are varied on a day-to-day basis in order to attain the desired results. Commercial kits containing all the reagents should maintain a certain standard, and should be reproducible if all the instructions are adhered to.

There are situations where perhaps even study samples should be assayed by more than one method. For example, one group has found basal venous ADR levels of approximately 0.08 nmol/litre and physiologically regulated ADR secretion in adrenalectomized humans (Shah et al, 1984), whereas others find unmeasurable ADR levels (<0.05 nmol/litre) in their adrenal-ectomized patients (Smits et al, 1986). Are such discrepancies due to assay problems or differences between the patients?

Practical comments based on our experience

We have retained the assay based on cation exchange HPLC and amperometric detection, using the simple alumina extraction procedure and α-methyldopamine as an internal standard (Hjemdahl et al, 1979). We abandoned the REA as it was tedious and expensive to run. Furthermore, we encountered the above-mentioned problems with variable quality radiolabelled S-adenosyl-methionine. The main advantage of REAs is their sensitivity (when working well), enabling measurements in small sample volumes (important, for example, when performing experiments in small animals). The most compelling incentive to switch entirely to HPLC was not that this technique was without its problems, but that problems were immediately apparent in the chromatograms. With an REA one ends up with radioactivity counts (and no information on how they got there through all the analytical steps), so it is quite difficult to identify and solve possible problems. With an HPLC assay one can check that all conditions (including sensitivity) are adequate before injecting the sample onto the column, and can then verify that the chromatogram is as 'clean' as it should be. In addition, an HPLC method is cheaper to run after the initial investment in equipment.

The main difference between our assay (Hjemdahl and Eliasson, 1979; Hjemdahl, 1987a) and most other HPLC assays is the cation exchange separation. We believe this offers more dependable separation than reverse phase chromatography, for reasons stated above. The interlaboratory comparison of analytical results illustrated in Figures 1 and 2 support this contention. We obtained further support for this opinion when setting up a urinary HPLC assay, which showed better dependability with cation exchange compared with reverse phase chromatography (Hjemdahl et al, 1989b). In this study most assay results agreed well between the two methods, but one sample showed an ADR value that was much too high with reverse phase chromatography. In the case of urine there is no sensitivity problem—the faulty result was due to an interference, as judged by a third assay used. Thus, the risk of encountering occasional interferences seems smaller with cation exchange separation.

We have experience with equipment and materials from different companies, and a detailed description of all procedures used by us has been updated once (Hjemdahl, 1987a). Since then, we have had additional experience with an HPLC pump (Kontron 422, Kontron Instruments, Everett, Massachusetts) which gives more stable flow than other pumps tested by us so far. This is most valuable, as the electrochemical detector is an extremely sensitive 'flow meter' and any check valve leak or other problem with the pump results in poor baseline stability. A good HPLC pump reduces baseline noise and the time spent on identifying and alleviating pump malfunctioning.

We have retained the amperometric principle for electrochemical detection, since the coulometric detector tested by us could not handle the mobile phase (slightly acidic and with a high ionic strength) needed for our cation exchange separation. This is an important contributor to the specificity of our assay. We have, however, recently obtained an amperometric detector with a wall-jet flow cell design (Antec, Leiden, The Netherlands), and a better signal-to-noise ratio than the ones previously used or tested by us. The Antec detector yields higher conversion of the analyte than conventional amperometric detectors. The oxidating potential may be set at a slightly lower value, as the greater sensitivity also entails a greater risk of interferences. When run appropriately, the Antec detector provides clean chromatograms and excellent signal-to-noise ratios. Due to its higher efficiency it is worthwhile adding ethylenediaminetetraacetic acid (EDTA) to the mobile phase to reduce baseline noise further (we found no advantage with this previously). We have compared analytical results with this detector and our previous ones (mainly the Waters M460, Waters Assoc., Milford, Massachusetts) and found excellent agreement (unpublished data). Thus, these modifications with regard to equipment can be recommended.

Stability of catecholamines in plasma

Catecholamines are easily oxidized and plasma samples should be stored under appropriate conditions to avoid decay with time. In our experience the most important factor is the temperature. We have reanalysed samples from the interlaboratory comparison of analytical results (Hjemdahl, 1984b) after storage at −80°C up to 6 years after the study without observing any decay for NA, ADR or dopamine, even though the samples were only taken with heparin as anticoagulant in order to be compatible with all assay methodologies used. This is at variance with a recent report (D'Alesandro et al, 1990), but in agreement with the opinion of others (Krstulovic, 1982). At −20°C, on the other hand, we have found almost blank values for catecholamines in plasma with EDTA after 1 year's storage. Claims in the literature also vary in this respect (Bouloux et al, 1985), but it seems as if heparinized plasma can be stored for at least 6 weeks at −20°C (Bouloux et al, 1985). We routinely store our samples at −80°C to be on the safe side.

If uncertain about stability, it is wise to take the precaution of adding an antioxidant to the blood upon sampling. We usually use EDTA, which has mild antioxidative properties (Hjemdahl, 1987a), as this is useful for our other assay purposes as well. EGTA and glutathion (Peuler and Johnson, 1977) probably provide the best protection for catecholamines.

With regard to the acute stability upon sampling, we have seen that samples may be left on ice (with EDTA) for a few hours without influencing the results, but there is a claim (based on an REA) that catecholamines in plasma can be left for hours even at room temperature (Rumley, 1988); however, when scrutinizing the latter data one cannot exclude a rather rapid decay (NA levels tended to decrease after only 2 h, and the coefficient of variation (C.V.) of the assay was 10.3% compared with 1–2% for our assay at basal NA levels).

STANDARDIZATION OF EXPERIMENTAL CONDITIONS

When performing plasma catecholamine studies it is important to standardize the conditions of sampling in order to minimize confounding influences. For this reason I am rather sceptical about clinical 'routine' measurements of catecholamines in plasma. Catecholamines are rapidly eliminated from the plasma, which means that one obtains 'snap-shot' information from such measurements, and failure to standardize the conditions of sampling may result in greater variation than that caused by the intervention studied. For example, in stress research the most important measurement of all may be the basal one—failure to attain basal conditions will diminish the amplitudes of responses measured!

In order to obtain good basal measurements, it is advisable to use indwelling catheters (arterial and/or venous) which are inserted at least 20–30 min before sampling. Acute venipunctures or arterial punctures are practised by some, but this introduces an element of uncertainty, as some subjects may have anticipatory responses or experience pain during the puncture. If variables with longer half-lives in plasma, such as renin or β-thromboglobulin, are to be assessed as well, the resting period may have to be extended even further to attain basal values. The subject should be comfortably placed in a quiet room at a pleasant ambient temperature and left undisturbed to attain basality before the basal measurements. It is also important that the subject is informed about the procedures involved and has the possibility to ask questions about them in order to reduce anxiety and uncertainty.

Spontaneous variation over time

There are several studies showing diurnal variation of plasma catecholamine levels (e.g. Levin et al, 1979; Mullen et al, 1980; Linsell et al, 1985), apparently with additional more rapid fluctuations over shorter periods of time (Levin et al, 1979). Thus, studies should be standardized with respect to time of day. Furthermore, increasing the number of baseline samples may increase the power of detecting stress-induced changes (Åkerstedt et al, 1983). The use of at least two baseline samples taken 5–10 min apart (the means of which may be used if there is no systematic decrease over time) is recommended to increase the dependability of basal measurements. Stricter criteria can be employed if possible. In fact, averaged baseline data can be obtained by continuous blood sampling with special equipment (Zadic et al, 1980).

Other sources of variability

In premenopausal women there is significant variation of plasma NA concentrations during the menstrual cycle (Goldstein et al, 1983a); contraceptive hormones might also be expected to influence such data. Various drugs, food and nutrients, and other commonly ingested substances (such as caffeine and nicotine) may also influence sympathetic activity and/or the turnover of catecholamines in plasma. Age, sex, body composition, posture and physical activity (as well as fitness) are other factors known to influence sympathetic activity. Thus, controls should be matched as well as possible to patient groups for all these factors, and measurements should be performed after standardized periods of rest in a standardized body position. Without going into detail, it is important to remember these aspects when attempting to minimize variability unrelated to the primary goal of the study.

It is also important to choose control groups, if needed, from relevant populations. For example, laboratory staff may have lower plasma NA levels than more appropriate controls due to familiarization with all the procedures involved (Jones et al, 1979). Comparative studies should preferably recruit patients and controls from as similar populations as possible. It is not optimal to use aggregated data from different studies for comparative purposes, especially if different methodologies (such as assay methodologies, for reasons evident from the above) and procedures/ personnel were involved in the different studies. Important inferences should be tested in new studies specifically designed to test hypotheses based on such aggregated data.

Time courses for catecholamine responses

When comparing plasma catecholamine responses to different stimuli and/or in different groups of individuals it is advisable to know what the time courses of the responses are. Even if, for example, NA in plasma may respond very quickly to a stimulus, if the stimulus is short-lasting one may miss the peak response due to the delay between its release into the neuro-effector junction and its appearance in plasma. Plasma NA is a much more 'sluggish' variable than sympathetic nerve activity.

We have observed more or less (not absolutely) stable stimulated conditions for catecholamines sampled 4–5 min after onset, compared with 8–10 min or later with orthostatic testing (arterial: Linde and Hjemdahl, 1982), lower body negative pressure (arterial and venous: Hjemdahl et al, 1982 and unpublished data), isometric contralateral handgrip exercise (arterial and venous: Hjemdahl et al, 1982 and unpublished data; arterial and renal venous: Tidgren and Hjemdahl, 1988), as well as during sub-maximal dynamic exercise at moderate intensities ($\sim 50\%$ of maximum Vo_2: Jansson et al, 1986). With more intense exercise there was, however, a progressive increase over time, probably related to progressively increased exertion ($\sim 65\%$ of maximum Vo_2: Jansson et al, 1982; $\sim 70\%$ of maximum Vo_2: Pernow et al, 1986). When stimuli such as these produce more or less steady state conditions the exact time of sampling is not critical. During mental stress we found peak responses after about 3 min, followed by somewhat lower but similar responses after 10 and 17 min (arterial and venous: Freyschuss et al, 1988 and Hjemdahl et al, 1984; arterial and renal venous: Tidgren and Hjemdahl, 1989).

When stimuli are short-lasting, on the other hand, the exact timing may be quite important. For example, with isometric contralateral handgrip exercise lasting 2 min we found that NA in forearm venous plasma peaked 1–2 min afterwards, even though muscle sympathetic nerve activity peaked at the end of the stimulus (Figure 4) (Wallin et al, 1987). A detailed analysis of NA overflow from the contralateral resting arm shows the same pattern and a 1–2 min delay between the progressively developing vasoconstriction and the NA overflow (L. Kaijser, B. Eklund and P. Hjemdahl, unpublished data).

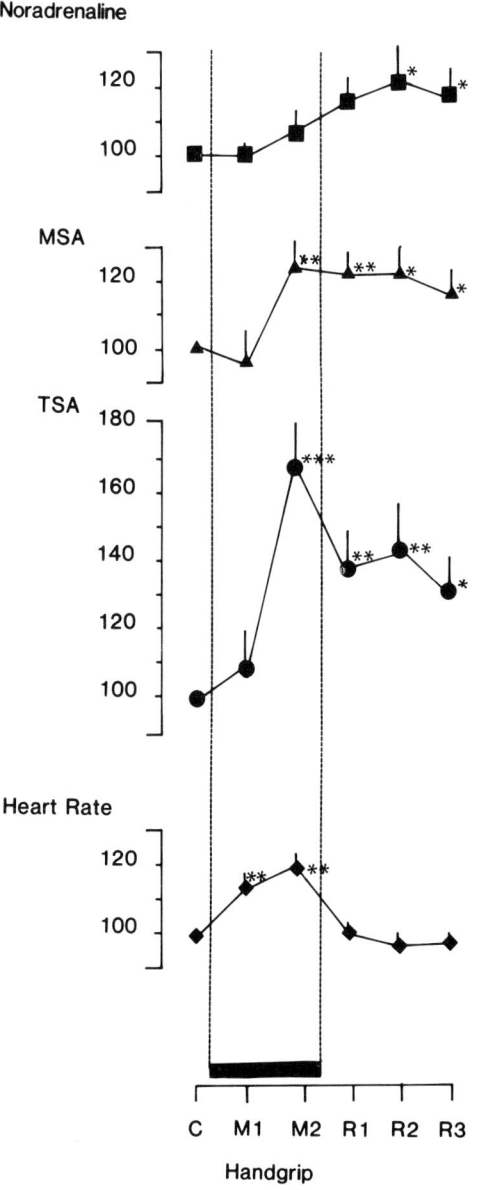

Figure 4. Time courses for relative changes of forearm venous plasma NA (noradrenaline), peroneal muscle sympathetic burst activity (MSA), 'total' muscle sympathetic activity (TSA; i.e. MSA × burst amplitudes) and heart rate during and after contralateral isometric handgrip exercise. Each time point was separated by 1 min. There may be discrepancies between arm and leg MSA, even if the two agree well at rest (Wallin and Fagius, 1988). Note the delay of the plasma NA response, which peaks 2 min after the stimulus. From Wallin et al (1987) with permission.

Other examples include graded dynamic exercise, where venous catechol-amine concentrations also peak after the exercise (Dimsdale et al, 1984); however, exact time courses were not given in that study. In agreement with this, we have seen a delayed overflow of NA from blood-perfused skeletal muscle in the dog in connection with nerve stimulation during 2 min at different frequencies (Kahan et al, 1984).

Thus, the wash-out time for NA from its site of release to the plasma may be important for the timing of sampling during short-lasting non-steady state stimuli—a 1–2 min delay should be considered. The magnitude of the delay may, of course, vary with the vascular permeability and the blood flow through the organ in question.

SHOULD CATECHOLAMINE CONCENTRATIONS, CATECHOLAMINE TURNOVER IN PLASMA OR REGIONAL NA OVERFLOW TO PLASMA BE MEASURED?

The answer to this question obviously depends on the situation under consideration. All three approaches have their virtues and drawbacks.

Kinetic aspects of catecholamines in plasma

The levels of any substance in plasma will be determined by its delivery to and elimination from this compartment, according to basic pharmacokinetic principles. In neurohormonal studies, concentration measurements domi-nate by far, due to the increased complexity and need for radiotracers in turnover studies. However, there are situations where the clearance of catecholamines (both NA and ADR) from plasma may be altered in such a way that simple concentration measurements do not give correct assess-ments of their appearance in plasma following release from sympathetic nerves and/or the adrenal medulla. Perhaps the most striking example is orthostatic testing, where reduced NA clearance from plasma and a reduced volume of distribution for the NA appearing in plasma make an important contribution to the elevation of plasma NA (Linares et al, 1987; Esler et al, 1988; Baily et al, 1990). These problems are addressed in detail in Chapter 6. A few comments are, however, pertinent here.

Radiotracer techniques can be used to study the appearance of endogenous NA in plasma and the elimination of NA in the whole body or in an individual organ (Figure 5). Esler and coworkers (1979) provided a breakthrough when they described the technique based on tritiated NA (^{3}H-NA) infusions to steady state in plasma with subsequent calculations of NA 'spillover' to plasma and NA clearance from plasma, based on measurements of radiolabelled and endogenous NA and knowledge of the infused amount of tracer. ADR release can also be more precisely assessed with radiotracer techniques (Kjaer et al, 1985); this has shown, for example, that exercise reduces ADR clearance from plasma.

Initially, measurements of NA spillover were made in venous plasma, which has the drawbacks discussed below, but measurements were later also

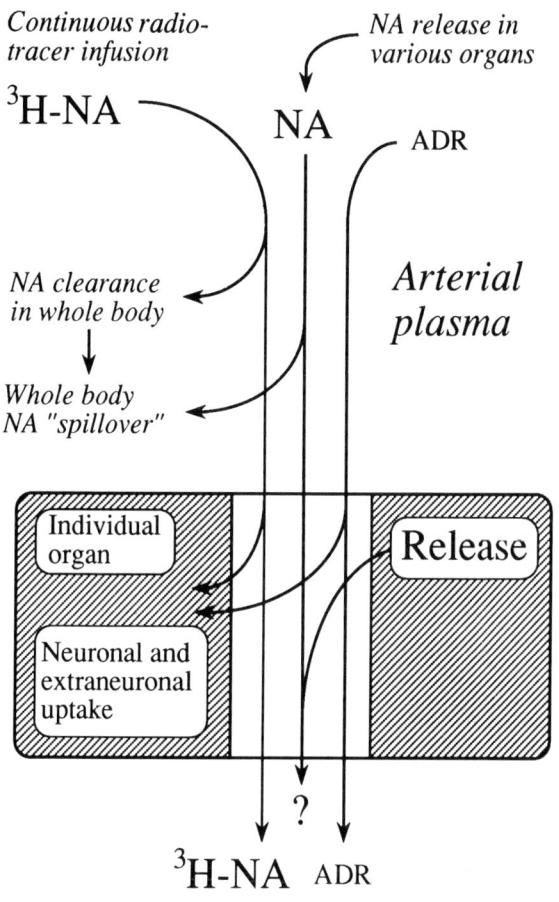

Continuous radio-
tracer infusion

NA release in
various organs

^{3}H-NA   NA

ADR

NA clearance
in whole body

Arterial
plasma

Whole body
NA "spillover"

Individual
organ

Release

Neuronal and
extraneuronal
uptake

?

^{3}H-NA ADR

Regional venous plasma

Figure 5. A schematic representation of NA turnover in the body. Whole body NA clearance and 'spillover' can be calculated on the basis of known amounts of infused ^{3}H-NA, and the levels of endogenous and radiolabelled NA determined in plasma. Overflow from an individual organ can be calculated on the basis of ^{3}H-NA or ADR extraction in the organ, arterial and venous NA concentrations and plasma flow through the organ, using the formula given in the text.

performed in arterial plasma and regional venous plasma from various organs (Esler et al, 1988). There was initially a problem with the measurement of pulmonary NA extraction caused by sampling from the right atrium instead of the pulmonary artery (in which the mixed venous plasma is truly mixed), which resulted in very high pulmonary 'spillovers' of NA. The figures obtained with atrial sampling yielded calculations showing that some 30% of the NA in arterial plasma was derived from the lungs (Esler et al, 1984), whereas data based on pulmonary arterial sampling showed much lower extraction rates for ^{3}H-NA over the lungs (Henriksen et al, 1986a; Hjemdahl et al, 1989a) and consequently much lower pulmonary NA spill-over. Thus, both analytical techniques and sampling must be handled correctly.

A limitation which has been pointed out is that the radiotracer technique assumes that there is negligible back-diffusion into the plasma of tracer taken up into the tissues. Such back-diffusion or re-release of NA may, however, influence the calculated data when infusion periods are prolonged (Henriksen and Christensen, 1989; Henriksen et al, 1989) and in organs with large tissue volumes relative to blood flow (Henriksen et al, 1989). This methodological objection has been refu.ed by Eisenhofer and coworkers (1991), as discussed further below.

Drawbacks with the radiotracer technique are ethical (exposure of subjects to radioactivity, even if Isotope Committees approve the doses given), economical (the costs of the tracer and the extra analytical work are considerable) and practical (extra access to the bloodstream is needed and, usually, extended periods of rest). These drawbacks are easily counter-balanced by crucial scientific problems, but radiotracer infusions cannot replace conventional measurements of catecholamines in plasma. There is, in my mind, no doubt that turnover studies provide valuable information on NA spillover to arterial plasma. However, one can frequently rely on the simpler concentration measurements, as variable clearance is not usually a major confounder. For crucial questions, and when no information on clearance is at hand, it is advisable to perform turnover studies as well. Regional studies of NA overflow are very important, but they can also be performed without radiotracer infusions (see below).

How generalizable are plasma catecholamine data?

When measuring catecholamines in plasma it is most important to under-stand the physiological determinants of the catecholamine concentrations at the location from which the sample was derived (Figure 6). One may aim at elucidating overall (generalized) or regional sympathetic nerve activity by NA measurements in various ways. A basic requirement when using plasma NA as a marker for sympathetic nerve activity is, of course, that the NA measured is derived from the organ(s) of interest in the investigation.

Arterial or mixed venous (i.e. pulmonary arterial) plasma NA levels or spillover are useful for studies of *overall sympathetic activity*. These indices of NA release reflect NA overflow from all organs, the relative importance of which will be determined by organ size, blood flow, vascular permeability and local sympathetic activity, all of which may vary considerably. Esler et al (1984, 1988) have calculated that of the NA in arterial plasma *at rest*, some 2–3% is derived from the heart, 20–30% from the kidneys, 9% from the hepatomesenteric region, 2% from the adrenals, 25% from skeletal muscle and 5% from skin. The initial estimate of 30% from the lungs is grossly exaggerated (see above). Approximately 20% of the human adrenal catecholamine content is NA, and there is no evidence for selective release of NA from the adrenals in humans (Ungar and Phillips, 1983). Thus, ADR

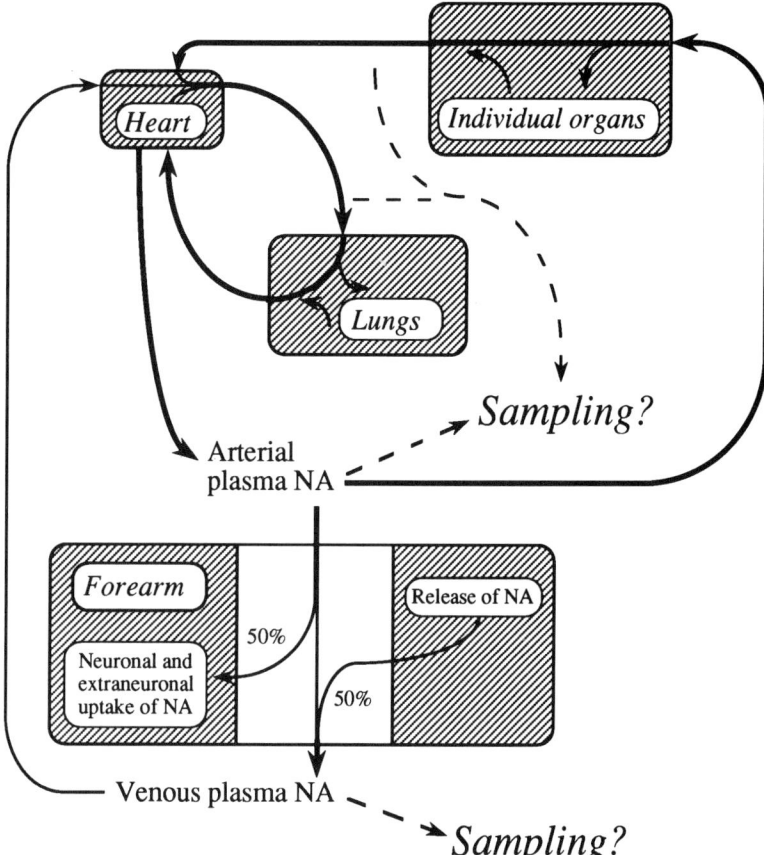

Figure 6. A schematic representation of NA overflow and removal in the body. Arterial or mixed venous (pulmonary arterial) NA measurements yield information on whole body contributions to levels in or spillover to plasma, whereas approximately one-half of the forearm venous plasma NA is derived from the forearm tissues. Venous sampling from any organ will overemphasize NA derived from the organ in question.

levels in plasma may be used to estimate the adrenal contribution to NA in arterial plasma; at rest this should be minimal. For other organs, regional NA overflow data will have to be collected to establish their importance for arterial NA levels at rest.

Arterial (or mixed venous) plasma NA levels or spillover, as measures of overall NA release, have limitations when one tries to interpret sympathetic contributions to a physiological or pathophysiological phenomenon being studied, due to the differentiated pattern in which sympathetic activity may occur (Folkow et al, 1983). The organs contributing most to NA in arterial plasma may not be those primarily engaged in the condition studied. In fact, it is my opinion that the term 'sympathetic tone' should be abandoned!

Individual organ contributions to elevations of arterial NA in response to stimuli have not been worked out in detail, but may vary considerably from the contributions at rest. When adrenaline secretion is considerable, such as during hypoglycaemia (Cryer, 1980), the adrenal contribution to NA in arterial plasma may be important. Otherwise, the kidney, splanchnic region and skeletal muscle may be more important, depending on the stimulus.

Arterial versus venous catecholamine measurements

The concentration of NA in a venous sample from any organ will be determined by the arterial contribution (NA in arterial plasma that passed through the organ without being removed) and the local overflow of NA (Figure 6). The proportions will vary with local nerve activity, removal mechanisms and flow.

Arterial and forearm venous concentrations of NA usually differ little at rest (e.g. Hjemdahl et al, 1984; Chang et al, 1986; Kjeldsen et al, 1986b; Freyschuss et al, 1988; Grossman et al, 1991), but extraction of NA during one passage through the arm is about 40–50% (see below). Thus, approximately half of the NA in venous plasma is derived from the forearm and only half from the rest of the body (Hjemdahl et al, 1984; Hjemdahl, 1987b). All would be well if the arm behaved like the rest of the body, but that is not always the case (see below).

It must be realized that conventionally sampled venous 'plasma NA' is disproportionately influenced by forearm sympathetic nerve activity and is not a generalizable marker for sympathetic activity in humans. For example, cardiologists or nephrologists should be aware of this when discussing the importance of 'sympathetic tone' for cardiac or renal function on the basis of venous plasma NA levels—in these cases quite marked differences between the organ of interest and the forearm may occur! Nonetheless, cardiac pathology or blood pressure regulation may be discussed in terms of sympathetic influences measured in terms of forearm venous plasma NA. Conversely, when relationships are found to be poor, it is often stated that 'plasma NA' is a poor marker for sympathetic activity. Indeed it may be when used in this way. However, when used (or at least interpreted) in a physiologically sensible way, NA measurements can provide relevant and valuable information.

Arterial sampling thus has definite advantages over conventional forearm venous sampling when assessing overall activity, even if venous plasma catecholamine data have increased our knowledge about sympathoadrenal activity (Cryer, 1980). Apart from circumventing the distorting influences of the forearm, arterial sampling has the advantage of providing correct estimates of the circulating catecholamine concentrations that the organs are actually exposed to. It is also more precise when assessing ADR responses to stressors. The advantages with arterial sampling have been pointed out repeatedly (e.g. Brown et al, 1981; Best and Halter, 1982; Åkerstedt et al, 1983; Hjemdahl et al, 1984; Henriksen et al, 1986b; Kjeldsen et al, 1986; Goldstein et al, 1987; Hjemdahl, 1987b), but venous sampling remains the technique most commonly used.

The drawbacks with arterial sampling are mainly practical and ethical. The risk involved is, however, minimal when catheterization is performed by an experienced physician. Ethics Committees, at least in Sweden, are rather tolerant in this respect due to the minimal risk involved. In my opinion, the advantages outweigh the risks (if the catheters are handled properly) and it is important to seek the best information possible. Venous sampling is a compromise which has to be accepted many times, but one should then interpret the data obtained accordingly.

Assessment of catecholamine removal from arterial plasma in individual organs

Catecholamines have a rapid turnover (half-life in plasma of approximately 1–2 min) due to neuronal uptake and extraneuronal uptake and metabolism, which implies that extraction from arterial plasma should be quite pronounced in most tissues and that simple veno-arterial concentration differences for NA do not reflect the contribution of the organ studied (Figure 6). Instead, one must assess the removal of NA from arterial plasma to calculate the overflow of NA from the organ in question.

The fractional extraction of catecholamines varies between individuals, between organs, and to some extent also within organs under different circumstances; there seems to be a dependence on flow (or, rather, the complex interactions of vascular tone, blood flow distribution in the organ, vascular permeability and transit time) in this respect. The confounding influence of variations in local catecholamine handling in an organ should be minimized by individual estimates in connection with each sampling. Figures for catecholamine extraction given below indicate mean values—the ranges can be considerable.

NA extraction

Forearm extraction of unlabelled NA during intra-arterial infusions was found to be 57–84%, depending on the dose of NA administered (Chang et al, 1986); a reduction of 40% was seen during nitroprusside-induced vaso-dilatation. This group found an extraction of $65 \pm 5\%$ when infusing ^{3}H-NA intra-arterially (Chang et al, 1991). Using intravenous infusions ^{3}H-NA extraction values of 48–54% were found by Goldstein et al (Goldstein et al, 1985; Grossman et al, 1991), and we recently found extractions of approximately 41% at rest (M. Lindqvist et al, unpublished data). A dependence of ^{3}H-NA extraction on flow (decreasing with increased flow and vice versa) has been found in several studies (Chang et al, 1986; Goldstein et al, 1987; Grossman et al, 1991).

The forearm extraction of locally infused ^{3}H-NA is higher than that of intravenously infused ^{3}H-NA (61 versus 48%), a difference attributed to rapid binding to non-plasma constituents in blood (Grossman et al, 1991). Thus, local infusions of tracer overestimate the removal of ^{3}H-NA from plasma in the tissue. Intravenous infusions of tracer, enabling the tracer to equilibrate between plasma and other constituents of blood before passing through the tissue, are thus preferable to local infusions.

[3]H-NA extraction over the leg has been found to be approximately the same as in the forearm, i.e. 33–40% (Savard et al, 1987; Henriksen et al, 1989) or around 55% (Hjemdahl et al, 1989a). In another study we found ^{3}H-NA extractions over the leg of 35–40%, which decreased to 25–30% during ADR infusion (Persson et al, 1989). Also in the leg there is variation of ^{3}H-NA extraction, with moderate decreases during mental stress (54 to 41%) (Hjemdahl et al, 1989) or ADR infusion (Persson et al, 1989) and pronounced, probably flow-dependent, decreases (down to 3%) during exercise (Savard et al, 1987).

Forearm or leg data do not represent skeletal muscle only, as adipose tissue, skin and other tissues are present; skeletal muscle dominates, however. Esler et al (1984) quote a figure of 46% for NA extraction over skeletal muscle based on iliac vein sampling. Extraction over skin is slightly lower (25–30%) (Esler et al, 1984). This will vary with blood flow, which is thermoregulated and easily influenced by emotions, etc. In fact, arterialization of dorsal hand vein blood by local heating is sometimes used as a substitute for arterial sampling. Figures for NA extraction in other limb tissues are lacking.

With regard to other important organs, the kidney extracts approximately 35–40% of ^{3}H-NA in arterial plasma (Esler et al, 1984; Henriksen et al, 1989; Friberg et al, 1990), whereas the hepatomesenteric region extracts some 60–65% (Esler et al, 1984; Henriksen et al, 1989). In the heart ^{3}H-NA extraction was 45% in the first report by Esler et al (1984), and later 56% (Friberg et al, 1990). Higher figures have been reported in patients with cardiac diseases (65–79%) (Goldstein et al, 1988). We found cardiac ^{3}H-NA extractions of 55–60% in a study of older patients with pacemakers (Hedman et al, 1990). In that study extraction decreased to around 50% during mental stress and 42% during dynamic exercise of moderate intensity.

ADR extraction

It is interesting to compare the extractions of ADR to those of ^{3}H-NA over various organs, due to the possibility of using endogenous ADR as a marker for NA removal from arterial plasma in the organ.

With regard to the limbs, we have found similar extractions of ^{3}H-NA and ADR (~50%) over the leg (Hjemdahl et al, 1989a) and forearm (41%) (M. Lindqvist et al, unpublished data). Savard et al (1987) found slightly higher ADR extraction compared with ^{3}H-NA extraction over the leg, but concluded that ADR extraction was probably more reliable due to recirculation of ^{3}H-NA (Savard et al, 1989). ADR extraction over the forearm increased from 46 to 55% during orthostasis (Kjeldsen et al, 1986) and from 42 to 61% during isometric exercise (Jörgensen et al, 1985). Best and Halter (1982) found ADR extractions of only 26% over the forearm at rest, which increased to 51% during ADR infusion and then dropped to 35% when propranolol was added. These data are at variance with our ADR (and ^{3}H-NA) extraction data over the leg during ADR infusion, with values decreasing from approximately 50% to 35% for ADR (Persson et al, 1989); other data also suggest inverse relationships between flow and catecholamine extraction from plasma.

Renal extractions of ADR are very similar to the values reported for ^{3}H-NA (see above) in healthy volunteers (Table 1). Interestingly, vaso-constrictor responses to mental stress and dynamic exercise were accompanied by increased renal ADR extraction (Table 1). Special care was taken in these studies to avoid admixture of adrenal blood by visualizing the catheter position and the renal venous anatomy in each experiment (Tidgren and Hjemdahl, 1988). A detailed investigation of catecholamine extraction in the dog kidney showed that ADR extraction was slightly higher (82–88%, depending on if the nerves were acutely cut or not) than that of ^{3}H-NA (73–79%) or ^{3}H-dopamine (Bradley and Hjemdahl, 1986). In our hands, cardiac ADR extraction was approximately 30% and fell to about 10% during exercise in pacemaker-treated patients (Pehrsson et al, 1988; Hedman et al, 1990), but did not change during mental stress (Hedman et al, 1990). Splanchnic ADR extraction is similar (67%) to NA extraction (Henriksen et al, 1989).

Thus, ADR extraction mimics the extraction of ^{3}H-NA quite well and can also pick up changes in extraction evoked by different physiological stimuli. The slightly higher extractions of ADR compared with ^{3}H-NA under some circumstances may be related to reappearance of the labelled NA previously removed by the tissue. An important aspect when using endogenous ADR as a marker for NA removal in tissues is assay variability, which may be greater than that of ^{3}H-NA at the low endogenous ADR concentrations prevailing. The assay used must have good precision down to about 0.05 nmol/litre (10 pg/ml) if this method is to be used with reasonable reliability.

Regional NA overflow

Regional studies of NA overflow are needed for detailed and relevant information on sympathetic activity in individual organs. This is important at rest, but even more so during stress, as both basal sympathetic activity and the degree of sympathetic activation during a stimulus may vary consider-ably from one organ to another and from one individual to another. Regional NA overflow studies require assessments of local NA handling by the organ studied (as discussed above) and blood flow measurements.

When equipped with data on the fractional extraction (FE) of ^{3}H-NA or ADR in the organ of interest one can calculate a 'corrected' veno-arterial concentration difference and multiply this by the plasma flow through the organ according to the formula:

NA overflow to plasma = [venous NA − arterial NA × (1 − FE)] × plasma flow

This will result in an estimate of NA overflow which has several methodo-logical errors in it (analytical variations for NA in arterial and venous plasma, analytical variations for ^{3}H-NA or ADR measurements on which the FE is based, and errors in blood flow measurements). All measurements involved should therefore be optimized. Blood flow measurements should, for example, be replicated in order to ensure that a single measurement is not unrepresentative due to methodological or physiological variation.

How representative then is NA overflow from an organ of the sympathetic nerve activity and transmitter release in that organ? There is no simple relationship between NA concentrations in the neuroeffector junction and in the plasma. Attempts have been made to evaluate these relationships, but at present it is doubtful whether we can obtain correct estimates of junctional or even interstitial NA concentrations. An estimate of 'intra-synaptic' (i.e. junctional) NA concentrations in humans arrived at a value of 3.3 nmol/litre using pharmacological tools (Goldstein et al, 1986). This estimate is surprisingly low and is probably confounded by mismatches between the receptors studied and the sites of NA release. NA appears to be non-uniformly released in a quantal manner (Stjärne, 1989), and junctional concentrations of NA in discrete areas are probably much higher than the average interstitial concentration of NA. Furthermore, Cousineau et al (1984, 1986) applied a sophisticated model with different tracers reflecting exchange between different compartments in the heart, and found complex diffusion barriers between cardiac tissue and blood for NA. Thus, I do not believe that at present we can obtain any sensible idea about the NA concentrations at the sites of release.

Nonetheless, NA overflow studies can give good *reflections* of NA release upon sympathetic activation. In animals, electrical stimulation of sympathetic nerves to, for example, the kidney (Oliver et al, 1981; Bradley and Hjemdahl, 1984), heart (Blombery and Heinzow, 1983), skeletal muscle (Kahan et al, 1984; Pernow et al, 1988) and liver (Yamaguchi and Garceau, 1980) evokes frequency-dependent overflows of NA to the plasma from the respective organs. Renal NA overflow mirrors recorded renal nerve activity (Noshiro et al, 1991). Stimulation of the entire sympathetic outflow in pithed animals produces frequency-dependent elevations of arterial plasma NA (Yamaguchi and Kopin, 1979). Thus, NA diffuses into plasma in a manner reflecting nerve activity quite well, provided that the blood sampled represents the stimulated region, even if NA release within the tissue is not exactly mirrored by NA overflow.

The above-mentioned flow-dependent variation of catecholamine extraction is probably paralleled by variations of NA diffusion from the neuro-effector junction. Indeed, vasodilatation may enhance the wash-out of neurally released NA from skeletal muscle (Folkow et al, 1967). Chang et al (1991) observed flow-dependent spillover of NA from the human forearm and suggested, on the basis of assumptions concerning different 'compartments' for NA removal, that the spillover of NA should be corrected (a second time) for NA extraction in the tissue, according to the formula:

$$\text{NA plasma 'appearance rate'} = \frac{\text{NA spillover}}{(1 - \text{FE})}$$

This mathematical correction cancelled out the NA spillover enhancing effect of sodium nitroprusside (Chang et al, 1991), but the proposed model has too little experimental support as yet to be generally adopted. In addition, the calculations are based on intra-arterial infusions of ^{3}H-NA, which may not be optimal (intra-arterial infusions would be more susceptible to the non-equilibrium problem discussed above and flow effects would thus be more pronounced).

Even if forearm venous plasma NA overemphasizes local sympathetic activity, it is not an adequate measure of such activity unless the arterial contribution to the NA measured is determined. Thus, as for all organs, veno-arterial concentration differences taking local NA extraction from arterial plasma into account are needed for local studies of forearm sympathetic nerve activity. Studies of the local handling of catecholamines are therefore important.

Antecubital (Wallin and Fagius, 1988) and femoral venous (Hjemdahl et al, 1989a; Persson et al, 1989) plasma NA concentrations, both of which to a large extent would be derived from skeletal muscle, correlate with microneurographically recorded axonal muscle sympathetic activity (MSA) in the peroneal nerve in humans. NA overflow from the leg also correlates reasonably well with MSA (Hjemdahl et al, 1989a) when considering the complexity of the different measurements; NA overflow measurements involve several methodological errors (see above) and MSA measurements do not yield exact estimates of nerve impulse traffic, as they are multi-unit recordings and exact frequency estimates would require single-unit recordings from several individual nerve fibres. In addition, nerve impulses reaching sympathetic varicosities do not regularly release the transmitter—the probability of release actually occurring is quite small (Brock and Cunnane, 1987; Stjärne, 1989). It is encouraging that neurophysiological and biochemical estimates of MSA agree so well, despite methodological complexities, confounding influences of local prejunctional mechanisms modulating transmitter release and diffusion problems for the transmitter into blood.

With regard to the use of ADR as a marker for NA removal from arterial plasma, the above-mentioned data support this approach, which was first suggested by Brown et al (1981) on the basis of results from phaeochromocytoma patients with high ADR levels. When directly compared, we have found quite similar calculated local NA overflows when based on ADR and ^{3}H-NA extractions in the human heart (Hedman et al, 1990), calf (Hjemdahl et al, 1989a) and forearm (M. Lindqvist et al, unpublished data), as well as in canine kidneys (Bradley et al, 1987). We have not performed direct comparisons in human kidneys, but our ADR extraction based basal NA overflow values (Table 1) agree well with data on NA spillover obtained by Esler et al (1984) at rest.

ADR extraction may be a bit more imprecise than ^{3}H-NA extraction, partly due to small differences in neuronal and extraneuronal uptake (Iversen, 1975) and partly due to lower analytical precision at basal (sub-nanomolar) ADR levels compared with that obtained at reasonably high radioactivity levels (for ^{3}H-NA). However, with a good ADR assay it is clearly possible to use ADR as a substitute for ^{3}H-NA. There may even be a case for ADR being preferable to ^{3}H-NA if re-release of tracer occurs in significant amounts (Henriksen et al, 1989; Savard et al, 1989). Eisenhofer et al (1991) claim that the findings of Henriksen and coworkers are confounded by co-determination of radiolabelled alumina extractable NA metabolites, and that recycling of ^{3}H-NA is less than 5% at normal levels of sympathetic activity. Preferential release of newly taken up ^{3}H-NA has, however, been demonstrated during nerve stimulation (e.g. Kahan et al, 1984). Wash-out or re-release of ^{3}H-NA may occur during high levels of nerve activity, and thus lead to underestimation of NA removal from arterial plasma. Re-release of ADR is, of course, also a possibility.

Taken together, it is possible to obtain a good biochemical estimate of sympathetic nerve activity using measurements of regional NA overflow from individual organs. ADR and/or ^{3}H-NA extraction should be monitored. The main aims are to catheterize the organ accurately, to obtain good measurements of blood (plasma) flow and to have good analytical precision. This approach can also be used in areas where nerve activity recordings cannot be made and enables studies of differentiated activity patterns in the sympathetic nervous system. In particular, studies of the heart and kidneys are of considerable interest.

PLASMA CONCENTRATION-EFFECT STUDIES FOR ADRENERGIC AGONISTS

Other aspects of sympathoadrenal function which require evaluation in vivo are receptor sensitivity and the levels of catecholamines in plasma which are required to activate a certain physiological mechanism. Plasma concentration-effect studies during infusions are very useful for these purposes, since there are inter- and intraindividual variations in catecholamine concentrations in plasma when dosed according to body weight.

The example probably receiving the greatest attention with regard to intraindividual variation of catecholamine kinetics is β-adrenoceptor blockade, which has repeatedly been shown to reduce catecholamine clearance from plasma. However, this effect differs for NA and ADR and also with the β-blocker studied. In a study of NA and ADR infusions with placebo, propranolol and metoprolol, we found that the main interaction was between propranolol and ADR, probably due to inhibition of ADR's powerful vasodilating effect (Hjemdahl et al, 1983). However, the explanation may not be so simple, since we recently observed that the α-blocker phentolamine, which enhances ADR-induced vasodilatation, elevated ADR concentrations further during infusion (Larsson et al, 1992).

Marked interindividual variation of NA kinetics can also be seen without drug treatment; for example, we found that poor responsiveness to circulating NA in one individual had a kinetic explanation (Hjemdahl et al, 1983). Isoprenaline (isoproterenol *USP*), which is used for β-adrenoceptor sensitivity studies in vivo, shows up to a six-fold interindividual variation of plasma concentrations (Hjemdahl et al, 1986b). The confounding influences of inter- and intraindividual variability of isoprenaline kinetics in plasma will thus be reduced by performing plasma concentration-effect studies rather than dose-effect studies (Martinsson et al, 1985, 1989).

Biochemical studies in vitro are valuable for the evaluation of adrenoceptors and indicate if a certain mechanism might be regulated by one of the catecholamines. They allow the use of full dose-response curves, and analysis of the receptor and its function in detail. However, its physiological importance cannot be judged only by in vitro studies, especially when supraphysiological concentrations of catecholamines are required for effects in the assay system. For example, micromolar or even higher concentrations of isoprenaline are frequently used to stimulate β-receptors in vitro, whereas subnanomolar concentrations of isoprenaline in plasma are associated with marked responses in humans in vivo (Martinsson et al, 1985; Hjemdahl et al, 1986b). Thus, assay systems may be artefactually insensitive in vitro. Conversely, findings with high agonist concentrations in vitro may have little physiological relevance in vivo.

Receptor sensitivity studies in vivo are, however, complex, and reflexogenic mechanisms may come into play in the intact organism. If we take the non-selective β-agonist isoprenaline as an example, heart rate is the most frequently monitored variable. Heart rate responses to a combined vasodilator and cardiac β-agonist such as isoprenaline may be influenced by reflexogenic sympathetic activation and/or vagal withdrawal, and vascular responses may be influenced by reflexogenic vasoconstrictor nerve activation.

Isoprenaline may be administered as bolus injections and heart rate responsiveness may be expressed in terms of the CD_{25}, i.e. the 'chronotropic dose' that increases heart rate by 25 beats/min (Cleaveland et al, 1972). Alternatively, isoprenaline may be given by intravenous infusion, which allows steady-state measurements and measurements of variables other than heart rate. Vagal withdrawal seems to contribute to the non-steady state responses to bolus injections of isoprenaline (Arnold and McDevitt, 1983), whereas vagal activation may attenuate the tachycardia elicited by infusions (Arnold and McDevitt, 1984), as judged by the effects of atropine. However, we found that isoprenaline concentrations in plasma were higher after blockade of the autonomic reflexes by clonidine and atropine (Jennings et al, 1981), and that the enhanced heart rate response after autonomic blockade had a mainly pharmacokinetic explanation (Martinsson et al, 1989). Blood pressure responses to isoprenaline were buffered by sympathetic vasoconstrictor nerve activation (Martinsson et al, 1989). Plasma cyclic adenosine monophosphate (AMP), which is elevated by β_2-adrenoceptor stimulation and is a sensitive indicator of ADR actions (Hjemdahl et al, 1983), may provide a useful index of β_2-adrenoceptor sensitivity in humans (Martinsson et al, 1985, 1989).

Agonist infusion studies may provide data on receptor sensitivity in vivo, provided that confounding reflexogenic mechanisms are not prominent. One can, of course, circumvent reflexogenic effects by local intra-arterial infusions, for example when studying vascular responsiveness.

Plasma concentration-effect studies are also needed to document whether ADR or NA function as circulating hormones. For example, the importance of ADR as a 'stress hormone' cannot be evaluated merely by observing elevated concentrations during stress and correlations between increases in plasma ADR and a physiological response, such as heart rate. As will be discussed below, ADR may be a good marker for stress reactions (arousal) without actually being an important mediator of responses.

CAN PREJUNCTIONAL MODULATION OF NEUROTRANSMITTER RELEASE BE ASSESSED BY PLASMA NA MEASUREMENTS?

During recent years several studies have attempted to evaluate the prejunctional modulation of NA release from sympathetic nerves in humans, as animal studies have shown that such modulation may be important for sympathetic neuroeffector function (e.g. Langer, 1981; Stjärne, 1989). One of the hypotheses attracting most interest is the possibility that ADR acts as a cotransmitter with NA (after having been taken up into the nerves), thereby facilitating NA release through prejunctional β_2-adrenoceptor stimulation (see Floras, 1992). Such a reinforcing effect of cotransmitter ADR on sympathetic neurotransmission is thought by some to contribute to the development of hypertension. Studies in humans have mainly concerned one of the following: (a) plasma NA responses to ADR infusions, (b) after-effects on heart rate following termination of ADR infusion, or (c) enhancement of neurogenic vasoconstrictor responses in the forearm after local infusion of ADR (the non-infused arm serving as control).

Plasma NA responses to ADR infusions

Plasma NA levels increase during infusions of ADR (e.g. Musgrave et al, 1984; Freyschuss et al, 1986). The pure β-agonist isoprenaline, which is not taken up into the nerves, similarly elevates plasma NA concentrations (e.g. Vincent et al, 1984; Martinsson et al, 1989). Slight differences between studies may be related to the doses given, the duration of infusions, etc. These plasma NA responses to ADR or isoprenaline infusion are sometimes claimed to be caused by prejunctional β_2-mediated facilitation of NA release, even though the experimental model lacks the first requirement for an analysis of the regulation of neurotransmitter release, namely that the nerve impulse activity is known.

  It is well known that vasodilators elicit reflexogenic increases in vasoconstrictor nerve activity when central venous pressure and/or arterial pressure is reduced. ADR is an efficient vasodilator in humans (Freyschuss et al, 1986) and might be expected to have these effects. Indeed, ADR infusion increases muscle sympathetic nerve activity (Persson et al, 1989), and findings with autonomic blockade indicate that isoprenaline activates vasoconstrictor nerves reflexogenically (Martinsson et al, 1991). Increases in nerve activity do not seem to be generalized, as the overflows of NA from the kidney (Tidgren and Hjemdahl, 1989) or the heart (Roca et al, 1993) were unchanged during ADR infusion. The venous sampling usually employed overemphasizes muscle sympathetic nerve activity, which is easily influenced by reflexogenic mechanisms (Beiser et al, 1970; Zoller et al, 1972; Wallin and Fagius, 1988). This may amplify the reflexogenic NA responses to vasodilatation. Thus, increases in axonal impulse activity (especially to skeletal muscle) may be quite important for the elevations of NA in plasma seen during infusions of β_2-adrenoceptor agonists.

NA overflow from the leg increased somewhat more than muscle sympathetic nerve activity (Persson et al, 1989), which might be taken as evidence that NA release was also facilitated. However, the diffusion of NA from the perivascular nerves to plasma may well have been altered by the vasodilatation produced by ADR. Increased wash-out of NA from skeletal muscle has been shown to occur during exercise-induced vasodilatation (Folkow et al, 1967). In canine skeletal muscle, with blood perfused at a constant flow rate, circulating ADR (6–10 nmol/litre in arterial plasma) does not influence NA overflow elicited by electrical nerve stimulation whether neuronal uptake is inhibited (Kahan et al, 1987) or not (Schwieler et al, 1992), or even in the presence of irreversible α-adrenoceptor blockade (Schwieler et al, 1992); the latter means that β-mediated facilitatory effects of ADR were not counteracted by α-mediated inhibitory effects. Prejunctional β-adrenoceptors are present in the model (Kahan and Hjemdahl, 1987; Kahan et al, 1987), but β-mediated facilitation of NA release seems to be much less important than α-mediated inhibition.

The evidence that circulating ADR, in the relevant concentration range, enhances NA release by prejunctional β_2-stimulation is thus not very firm. Whether true or not, it is quite clear that intravenous infusions of ADR or isoprenaline cannot be used to document prejunctional mechanisms in the intact organism, as nerve impulse activity is not controlled.

After-effects of ADR

The elevation in heart rate may persist much longer than the increased ADR concentrations in plasma after an infusion; this has been taken as evidence for uptake into sympathetic nerves and a subsequent facilitatory action of ADR as a cotransmitter after the infusion (see Floras, 1992). Again, other phenomena may explain the findings. For example, there is a sudden and persisting drop in central venous pressure after an ADR infusion (Persson et al, 1989), which may well trigger the elevation of heart rate. There are also long-lasting after-effects on electrolyte metabolism, which may be of importance; the hypokalaemia subsides rapidly, but reductions in magnesium and calcium in plasma are quite long-lasting (Joborn et al, 1990b). Thus, postjunctional events may be involved, and the ADR cotransmitter theory would seem to require documentation that physiological alterations influencing postjunctional sensitivity or nerve activity are not responsible for the after-effects of ADR.

Enhancement of vasoconstrictor responses

It is intriguing that vasoconstrictor responses in the forearm are enhanced after a local ADR infusion, and that neuronal uptake inhibition by desipramine reduces this effect (Floras, 1992). However, in this case postjunctional alterations may also contribute; desipramine will enhance the tissue concentrations and postjunctional effects of ADR.

The best human model for studies of prejunctional effects is probably to measure the local overflow of NA from one arm (intervention arm), with the other arm serving as control. When studying the effects of drugs that alter blood flow, it is advisable to include infusions of other vasodilators or vasoconstrictors, so that the actual effects on the sympathetic nerves can be distinguished from non-specific effects. Using tyramine-induced NA release as a model, it has been shown that α_2-mediated inhibition may occur in the human forearm (Jie et al, 1987).

In animals, NA overflow (endogenous or radiolabelled) evoked by nerve stimulation may be studied in isolated blood-perfused organs. Variable catecholamine handling in the tissue and the diffusion problems already mentioned still need to be addressed. Overflow of NA to arterial plasma levels in pithed animals is another common model; however, the exact sources of this NA are unknown and tissue contributions may differ due to blood flow redistribution, etc., following drug treatment. Nevertheless, studies of prejunctional mechanisms may be performed using plasma NA measurements in the in vivo setting, provided that the model is well characterized.

DIFFERENTIATION OF SYMPATHETIC NERVE ACTIVITY IN HUMANS

Interest in this problem emanates from observations that mental stress influences venous plasma NA concentrations little, despite marked cardio-vascular responses and feelings of stress and increases in plasma and urinary ADR (Hjemdahl and Eliasson, 1979; Åkerstedt et al, 1983; Eliasson et al, 1983). Early studies had shown that venous plasma NA responds to various stimuli in a manner that indicated that this variable would reflect sympa-thetic nerve activity (Robertson et al, 1979; Cryer, 1980). Some authors defended the opinion that venous plasma NA was a good indicator of sympathetic nerve activity (e.g. Goldstein, 1983a; Goldstein et al, 1983b), whereas others were critical of the value of 'plasma NA' (Bravo and Tarazi, 1982; Mancia et al, 1983; Floras et al, 1986). At least one early report discussed the possibility that the origin of the plasma was of importance for the NA response (Henry et al, 1979), but the dominating view was that 'plasma NA' should reflect 'sympathetic tone'.

It has long been known that various organs respond differently to various physiological and pathophysiological alterations (for example, Folkow, 1982; Folkow et al, 1983; Rowell, 1984; Shepherd and Mancia, 1986). Direct comparisons of the vascular responses of the upper and lower limb to a series of stressors even revealed important differences between these otherwise so similar regions in the body (Rusch et al, 1981). Thus, it would be reasonable to assume that the sympathetic nerve activity and the overflow of NA to plasma would also vary and that the site of measurement (in view of the above) would be important for NA responses in plasma. Mental stress and essential hypertension clearly illustrate the differentiated manner in which the sympathetic nervous system operates, and will therefore be used as examples when discussing this problem.

Responses to mental stress in humans

Elegant studies by Brod and coworkers demonstrated that mental stress (forced arithmetics) elicits a pattern of responses resembling that of the 'defence reaction', with cardiac activation, vasoconstriction in the kidneys, splanchnic area and skin, and vasodilatation in skeletal muscle (Brod et al, 1959; Brod, 1963). There is also venoconstriction, which may increase venous return to the heart (Brod et al, 1976). For more recent overviews on cardiovascular responses to stress, see Herd (1991) and Hjemdahl (1991).

We have performed a series of studies using a modified Stroop colour-word conflict test (CWT) (Frankenhaeuser et al, 1968), which has proved to be powerful and reproducible. This test produces the same response pattern as that described by Brod. We find quite marked elevations of heart rate and blood pressure (Eliasson et al, 1983; Freyschuss et al, 1988), along with increases in stroke volume and decreases in systemic vascular resistance (Freyschuss et al, 1988), and vasodilatation in the leg (Hjemdahl et al, 1989a; Linde et al, 1989), forearm (M. Lindqvist et al, unpublished data) and in adipose tissue in different locations (Linde et al, 1989). The kidney responds with pronounced vasoconstriction (Table 1) (Tidgren and Hjemdahl, 1989). There is also splanchnic vasoconstriction (Juhlin-Dannfelt et al, 1986). Thus, vascular responses are quite variable and agree with the defence reaction-like pattern described by Brod and coworkers. Plasma minerals change little (Joborn et al, 1990b); plasma potassium actually increased, contrary to expectations based on ADR infusion data. In addition, platelets are activated (see Hjemdahl et al, 1991).

Thus, mental stress elicits a blood pressure elevation which is the composite effect of cardiac stimulation and systemic vasodilatation. The latter is caused by vasodilatation in large tissue masses such as skeletal muscle and adipose tissue, which is not balanced by vasoconstriction in the kidneys and splanchnic area (Figure 7). The cardiac response to stress is complicated and involves vagal withdrawal, sympathetic stimulation and, probably, an increase in venous return which supports the cardiac output elevating effect of stress. What consequence does this reaction pattern have for plasma catecholamine responses and what are the autonomic mechanisms regulating the cardiovascular responses?

Plasma NA responses to mental stress

Forearm venous plasma NA increases little, if at all (average changes have been 0–20% increases), during a CWT (Hjemdahl and Eliasson, 1979; Åkerstedt et al, 1983; Eliasson et al, 1983; Hjemdahl et al, 1984; Freyschuss et al, 1988). We have found a similar lack of forearm venous plasma NA responses during forced arithmetic (Lindvall et al, 1991) and a more complex arithmetic task (Bohlin et al, 1986) (Figure 8). Thus, it is a consistent finding of ours that forearm venous plasma NA changes little during mental stress. After stress, however, there may be an elevation of NA in this region (Åkerstedt et al, 1983; Eliasson et al, 1983; Bohlin et al, 1986; Freyschuss et al, 1988); this may reflect baroreflex-induced sympathetic activation when the blood pressure falls immediately after the stress period.

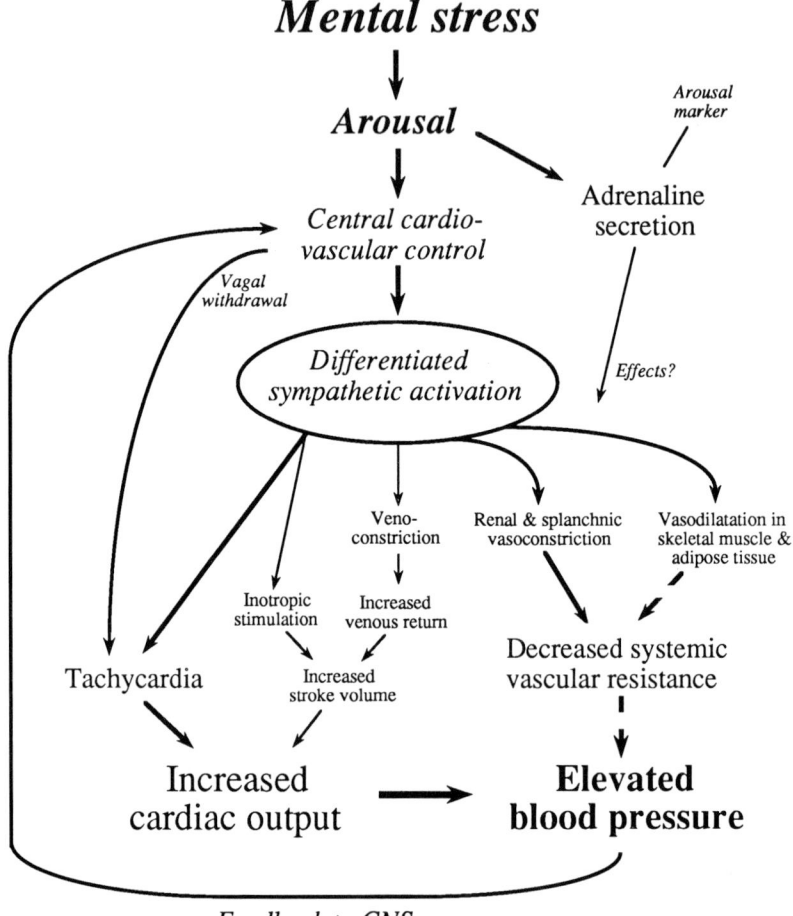

Figure 7. A schematic representation of cardiovascular responses to mental stress. The arousal reaction may be monitored by plasma ADR measurements (preferably in arterial plasma, but also in venous plasma or in urine) and leads to differentiated changes in efferent sympathetic nerve activity to various organs. The blood pressure elevation is cardiac output dependent in the absence of blocking drugs, but remains similar after β-blockade, despite marked attenuation of the cardiac output response. Thus there seems to be feedback to the central nervous system (CNS) which serves to achieve a certain blood pressure response to stress (Freyschuss et al, 1988; Julius, 1988). Individual organs respond quite differently to stress. The role of ADR as a mediator of stress responses can be questioned (see text).

With these data it would be tempting to say that stress does not activate sympathetic nerves in humans, but the situation changes when samples are obtained elsewhere during mental stress.

Femoral venous plasma NA concentrations and NA overflow from the leg increase by about 25% during a CWT (Hjemdahl et al, 1989a), in agreement

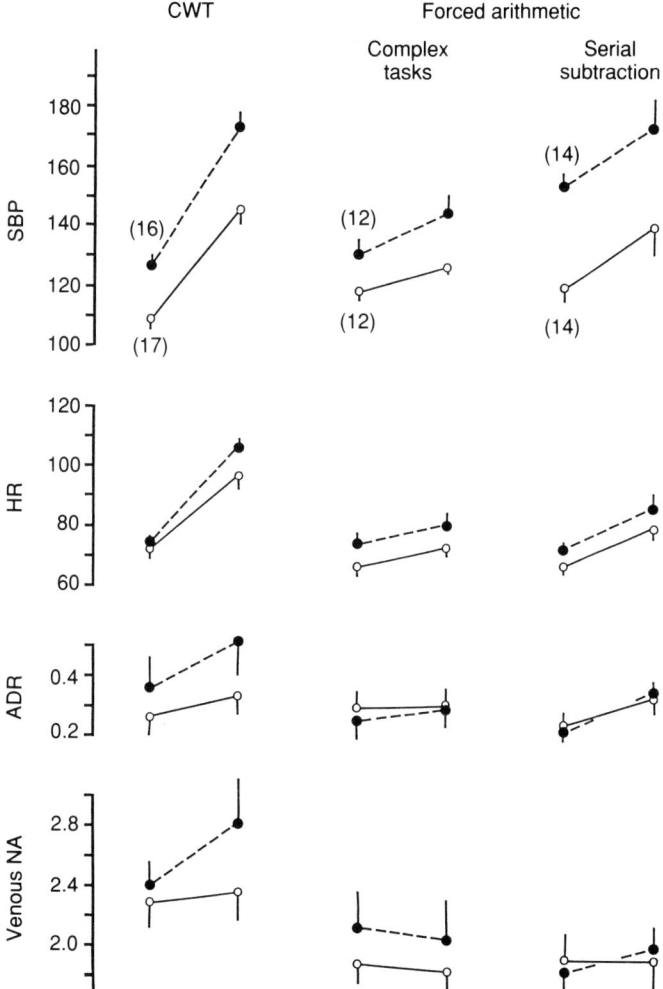

Figure 8. A compilation of data from our laboratory on venous plasma NA and ADR concentrations (nmol/litre), heart rate (HR; beats/min) and systolic blood pressure (SBP; mmHg) in normotensives (solid lines) and mild hypertensives (broken lines) with three different mental stress tests. The numbers of individuals in each group is shown. The tests were the CWT (modified colour word conflict test; Eliasson et al, 1983) and forced arithmetic by simple serial subtraction (Lindvall et al, 1991) or more complex tasks (Bohlin et al, 1986). It may be seen that the CWT, in our hands, is the most powerful stressor (as judged by heart rate and blood pressure responses) and that neither of the tests elicit marked venous plasma NA or ADR responses.

with a similar increase in peroneal MSA. Arterial plasma NA concentrations increase by 40–50% (Freyschuss et al, 1988; Tidgren and Hjemdahl, 1989) (Table 1) and the spillover of NA to arterial plasma increases as well (Goldstein et al, 1987; Hjemdahl et al, 1989a; M. Lindqvist et al, unpublished data). The elevation of arterial NA during stress was in these studies not greatly influenced by alterations in NA clearance from plasma. Renal venous NA concentrations increase more markedly than arterial ones and the renal overflow of NA is enhanced almost three-fold during a CWT (Table 1).

In studies by others, Goldstein et al (1987) found arterial but not forearm venous NA elevations in response to a video game. Jörgensen et al (1985) found no elevation of either arterial or forearm venous NA, but their stress test produced very mild pressor responses. NA spillover from the heart increases (Esler et al, 1989). Thus, sympathetic activation during mental stress can certainly be detected by NA measurements if the test is powerful enough and measurements are performed in plasma representing an activated organ.

Plasma ADR responses to stress

As seen in Figure 8, the venous plasma ADR responses to mental stress are modest. In 30 healthy volunteers undergoing invasive haemodynamic monitoring, we found elevations of arterial ADR from 0.40 to 0.88 nmol/litre (peak values after 3 min of a CWT; steady state values at 10–17 min were 0.73 nmol/litre); venous ADR levels increased from 0.26 to 0.43 nmol/litre during steady state (Freyschuss et al, 1988). Responses were similar in the renal study, but the levels were lower on the whole (Table 1) (Tidgren and Hjemdahl, 1989). In our experience, which encompasses several hundred experiments, it is extremely rare to find an ADR level in venous plasma exceeding 1 nmol/litre during mental stress. Even arterial levels rarely exceed 1 nmol/litre.

Plasma ADR responses to other stressors are usually also modest. Table 1 shows responses to isometric exercise, with less than a doubling of arterial ADR (Tidgren and Hjemdahl, 1988). Not shown are data during lower body negative pressure, which elicited only minor elevations of ADR (Tidgren et al, 1990), and data at lower exercise levels, which also showed modest elevations of ADR (Tidgren et al, 1991). As summarized by Cryer (1980), venous ADR levels increase quite differently during different stimuli, hypoglycaemia being one of the most potent. However, large increases are only seen with intense stimulation, such as exhaustive exercise, pronounced hypoglycaemia (i.e. neuroglycopenia), fainting reactions or the like. Even in acute myocardial infarction most patients do not have particularly high ADR levels (Karlsberg et al, 1981; Bertel et al, 1982); only two out of 34 patients had venous ADR levels above 1 nmol/litre in venous plasma in our study (Joborn et al, 1990a).

Thus, the physiologically interesting plasma concentration range for ADR seems to be up to approximately 1(–2) nmol/litre in arterial plasma, as higher levels are seen only under more extreme conditions. These levels are produced by intravenous infusions of approximately $0.03–0.1$ nmol $\cdot$ kg^{-1} $\cdot$ min^{-1} (about $5–15$ ng $\cdot$ kg^{-1} $\cdot$ min^{-1}) of ADR (Freyschuss et al, 1986; Tidgren and Hjemdahl, 1989), which is noteworthy when examining the literature on responses to ADR infusion.

Is ADR an important 'stress hormone'?

ADR is certainly capable of eliciting marked responses of many kinds. With regard to cardiovascular actions, there is a marked and dose-dependent vasodilatation in the systemic circulation, skeletal muscle and adipose tissue (Freyschuss et al, 1986), as well as a mainly stroke volume dependent increase in cardiac output (Stratton et al, 1985; Freyschuss et al, 1986). The skin responds with vasoconstriction during both stress and ADR infusion (Östergren et al, 1992). Mean blood pressure changes little during ADR infusion, as the vasodilatation is balanced by the increase in cardiac output (which probably is related, in part, to the reduction of afterload), but pulse pressure is widened.

When examining various responses to infused ADR at the plasma concentrations attained during mental stress, it becomes clear that only minor contributions can be made by ADR to the responses elicited by stress (Hjemdahl et al, 1986a; Hjemdahl, 1991). ADR increases heart rate little at 'stress' levels in plasma (Hjemdahl et al, 1983; Stratton et al, 1985; Freyschuss et al, 1986). Furthermore, the response patterns during mental stress and ADR infusion differ markedly. For example, the cardiac output response to stress is two-thirds heart rate dependent, but the response to ADR is two-thirds stroke volume dependent. Thus, one might expect that stress responses are mainly neurogenic. Data from adrenalectomized women also suggest a limited role for ADR as a mediator of responses to mental stress (Lenders et al, 1988). For more extensive comments on neurogenic versus hormonal mechanisms in cardiovascular regulation during stress, see Hjemdahl (1991) and Hjemdahl and Kahan (1993).

ADR is β_2-selective as a circulating hormone (Ariëns and Simonis, 1983; Hjemdahl et al, 1991), whereas (neurogenic) β-responses to NA are β_1-mediated (Lands et al, 1967). Thus, the differential effects of β_1-selective and non-selective β-blockade on responses to stress might reveal the ADR component of the response. With this approach we found that ADR contributes to, but does not fully explain, the cardiac or vasodilator responses to mental stress (Freyschuss et al, 1988; Linde et al, 1989). Vagal withdrawal and sympathetic neural activation explain most of the tachycardia (Freyschuss et al, 1988). A complicating factor is that it seems as if the primarily regulated variable during mental stress is blood pressure (Freyschuss et al, 1988; Julius, 1988). Thus, inhibition of the cardiac response to stress by β-blockade produces feedback to the central nervous system and reflexogenic alterations in the periphery which are unrelated to ADR.

Similar studies of other responses, such as platelet activation (Hjemdahl et al, 1991) or plasma mineral responses (Joborn et al, 1990b), again show that circulating ADR is of minor importance in the physiological responses to stress. Nonetheless, correlations between plasma ADR and, for example, heart rate responses to stress have been shown repeatedly (and have often been overinterpreted). Such correlations may simply reflect the value of ADR as a marker for arousal and the 'defence reaction'-like neurogenic response pattern elicited by stress, as suggested by us some time ago (Åkerstedt et al, 1983; Eliasson et al, 1983). In fact, we have recently found a close correlation ($r = 0.92$) between increases in arterial ADR and cardiac NA overflow during mental stress, but not during dynamic exercise (Hedman et al, 1990). Thus, ADR may reflect arousal and cardiac neurogenic activation without actually being all that important as a mediator of stress responses.

Mediation of limb blood flow responses to mental stress

There may also be non-adrenergic neurogenic vasodilatation during mental stress. Sympathetic cholinergic fibres seem to be activated, as atropine attenuates forearm blood flow responses to stress (Blair et al, 1959; Barcroft et al, 1960). There may also be non-cholinergic, possibly peptidergic, neurogenic vasodilatation in skeletal muscle (Hilton et al, 1979; Öhlén et al, 1990), but this cannot, in the absence of specific antagonists, be studied in humans.

Thus, vasodilatation in the limbs (i.e. mainly skeletal muscle) may be caused by the combined effects of ADR and neurogenic vasodilator influences which are partly balanced by an increase in sympathetic nerve activity, at least in the leg (Anderson et al, 1987; Hjemdahl et al, 1989a). Sympathetic nerve activity in the arm may respond differently from the leg during mental stress, as shown by increased activity in MSA recordings in the leg only (Anderson et al, 1987), and more pronounced vasodilator responses in the forearm (Rusch et al, 1981).

Essential hypertension

Essential hypertension displays a circulatory pattern resembling a mild 'defence reaction', especially in its earlier stages (Brod et al, 1959; Brod, 1963; Folkow, 1982; Folkow et al, 1983; Julius, 1991). There is an elevation of cardiac output in the early (hyperkinetic) stages of hypertension, and an elevation of heart rate is a fairly constant finding in hypertensives. The kidney is of considerable interest in hypertension and it seems that even the children of those with hypertension have an exaggerated renal vasoconstrictor response to stress (Hollenberg et al, 1981). Thus, uniform activation of the sympathetic nervous system might not be expected in hypertensive subjects. Forearm venous NA levels, which are markedly influenced by skeletal muscle nerve activity, would then have little predictive value of · more relevant pathophysiological alterations present in the disease (Folkow et al, 1983).

A large number of studies of venous plasma NA levels in hypertension has been performed, and the earlier ones were reviewed by Goldstein (1983b). The conclusion was that only young individuals with hypertension had higher NA levels. However, positive findings (i.e. higher NA levels) were more likely to occur with older fluorimetric catecholamine assays than with REAs (73 versus 33%). Few HPLC data were then available. The selection of patients and controls, experimental conditions and catecholamine assay performance may have influenced the results in the reviewed studies. In our hands, venous NA levels have not been higher in patients with mild hypertension (Figure 8), but there was a tendency towards enhanced levels during stress in the hypertensive individuals in two of the studies (Figure 8). Arterial or regional NA levels might have given a different picture in these patients, especially during stress.

Esler et al have performed a series of investigations with arterial and regional NA spillover measurements and have found increased cardiac and renal NA spillover in patients with essential hypertension (Esler et al, 1988; Esler, 1991); these signs of cardiorenal sympathetic activation even at rest were confined to younger patients. Thus, when NA overflow from the target organs in hypertension is more specifically assessed a clear and logical picture emerges. This is not the case when forearm venous blood is sampled.

Pharmacological autonomic blockade experiments have demonstrated that the elevation of cardiac output in hyperkinetic hypertension is related to sympathetic stimulation and vagal withdrawal (Julius and Esler, 1975), or perhaps only the latter (Korner et al, 1973). Thus, as is the case during stress, one should not forget vagal control of the heart when interpreting autonomic mechanisms.

Comparisons of renal responses to various stressors

Table 1 shows some of the data from our renal projects. Renal vasoconstriction is elicited by a variety of stimuli, three of which are illustrated. In addition, lower body negative pressure elicited stimulus-dependent increases in arterial NA and renal vascular tone (Tidgren et al, 1990); however, the increased renal overflow of NA was not stimulus dependent. Angiotensin II may be more important in the renal vascular response to pronounced stimulation by lower body negative pressure (Tidgren et al, 1990). Dynamic exercise showed graded and quite marked increases in arterial NA, renal NA overflow and renal vascular tone (only maximum values at 80–90% of each individual's work capacity are shown in Table 1) (Tidgren et al, 1991). Vasodilatation induced by dihydralazine evoked reflexogenic increases in NA overflow concomitantly with renal vasodilatation (Tidgren and Hjemdahl, 1988). Graded infusions of ADR, up to high arterial ADR levels (6.4 nmol/litre), enhanced renin overflow markedly, but did not influence renal blood flow or renal NA overflow (Tidgren and Hjemdahl, 1989).

Interestingly, two subjects in these studies had fainting reactions (Tidgren and Hjemdahl, 1988; Tidgren et al, 1990); both subjects showed complete cessation of renal NA overflow and pronounced elevations of ADR and renin. In one of them a very high plasma angiotensin II level could also be documented (Tidgren et al, 1990). Thus, the subjects seemed to switch from neural to hormonal support of renal vascular resistance during these fainting reactions. Esler (1991) observed abolition of regional NA spillover in both the heart and the kidney during syncope accompanied by a shut-down of muscle sympathetic nerve activity. 'Vasovagal' reactions may thus be characterized by sympathetic withdrawal, marked ADR stimulation and an activation of the renin–angiotensin system; again the situation is more complex than often believed.

This comparison of renal responses to different stimuli shows that renal nerves are easily activated by various physiological stimuli. There seems to be a relationship between renal NA overflow and other renal responses. The complexity of this organ is, however, considerable, and angiotensin II is another important regulator in this respect. More studies need to be performed to assess regional sympathetic activity in various other organs, and the influences of physiological and pathophysiological alterations on regional sympathetic activity in relation to other possible mediators of changes observed.

CONCLUDING REMARKS

This overview has mainly dealt with methodological issues involved in studies of autonomic mechanisms in humans, with special emphasis on catecholamine measurements in plasma. A major issue has been to illustrate that the sympathetic nervous system does not operate in a synchronized fashion. Rather, I believe the term 'sympathetic tone' should be abandoned. The above described effects of mental stress illustrate that different organs may respond quite differently to the same stimulus and that even the same organ (skeletal muscle) in two different locations may respond differently. This is not unique to mental stress, as forearm and calf vascular responses to other stimuli may differ as well (Rusch et al, 1981). The concept of highly localized changes in the activity of the autonomic nervous system is not new—it has been pointed out by, for example, Brod (1963), Wolf (1970), Folkow (1982) and others without having an impact on the way modern biochemical tools such as plasma catecholamine analysis often are used.

Studies of plasma catecholamine levels are numerous, and it is still common to see misinterpretation of data. Most studies are performed with antecubital venous plasma sampling, which introduces an error with regard to circulating ADR levels (variable tissue extraction) and distorts the image of sympathetic activity provided by plasma NA (the sampling site over-emphasizes forearm nerve activity). The possible sympathetic contribution to physiological and pathophysiological alterations should often be sought in the heart, kidneys and splanchnic region, rather than in skeletal muscle. Therefore, regional NA overflow studies reflecting these organs at rest and during stress would seem most appropriate. Few such studies have, due to technical difficulties, been performed. If regional studies cannot be undertaken, overall sympathetic function should preferably be studied in terms of NA levels in and spillover to arterial or mixed venous plasma, which will reflect NA overflow from all organs, in proportion to their sizes, innervation and nerve activity, as well as their blood flows.

If conventional venous sampling is employed, the plasma NA results should at least be discussed in a manner acknowledging their physiological limitations. Poor relationships between such 'plasma NA' and function merely reflect this indirect relationship. The most marked changes occur in the target organ, as illustrated by the acute adaptation to different pacing modes during exercise (a doubled cardiac NA overflow when the ventricular rate is kept constant as compared with variable; Pehrsson et al, 1988). In that case less pronounced changes occurred in the periphery. Poor relationships may also be caused by analytical shortcomings and it is important to scrutinize catecholamine data and assay validation when interpreting results. Without giving examples, it is not very surprising if venous plasma NA does not 'reflect sympathetic activity' when venous sampling is performed and/or the levels presented are far too high. Plasma catecholamines are still difficult to measure accurately and the analytical challenge should be kept in mind.

Finally, I would like to reiterate the need for a physiological approach to catecholamine measurements in plasma by recommending caution when using them for purposes such as studies of prejunctional receptors. The intact organism is regulated in a complex fashion and reflexogenic mechanisms may impose considerable confounding influences. When correctly measured (whether in terms of turnover or regional overflow from an organ or, as is often sufficient, in terms of concentrations), plasma NA data may provide very useful clues to sympathetic function in humans. I have argued that ADR may be valuable as a marker for arousal, even if it is not always so important as a mediator of stress responses. Therefore, ADR measurements in plasma can also provide valuable information.

SUMMARY

Catecholamines in plasma may be measured to assess sympathoadrenal activity. Numerous assay methodologies have been published, illustrating the fact that there are many analytical problems. Different methodologies are discussed briefly. A plea for better validation, especially with regard to specificity (which should not be confused with sensitivity or reproducibility), is made. Plasma NA is a frequently used marker for sympathetic nerve activity in humans, but the data obtained are often misinterpreted due to lack of appreciation of the physiological determinants of the NA concentration measured. NA overflow from an organ gives a good reflection of nerve activity in that organ. However, sympathetic nerve activity is highly differentiated, particularly during stress, and conventional plasma NA levels (usually forearm venous samples) cannot be taken as an indication of 'sympathetic tone' in the whole individual. NA is rapidly removed from plasma, resulting in meaningless net veno-arterial concentration differences over organs unless its removal from arterial plasma is taken into account. In the forearm, for example, 40–50% of catecholamines are removed during one passage; about half of the NA in a venous sample is derived from the arm and half from the rest of the body. Therefore, conventional venous sampling overemphasizes local (mainly skeletal muscle) nerve activity. Whole-body sympathetic nerve activity may be monitored in arterial or mixed venous (i.e. pulmonary arterial) samples, which reflect NA overflow from all organs in the body. NA levels are determined both by overflow to plasma and clearance from plasma. NA turnover studies with ^{3}H-NA infusions may be needed to assess clearance, but the simpler concentration measurements usually yield adequate information if the sampling site is relevant. NA overflow from an organ can be assessed (using ^{3}H-NA or ADR as a marker for NA extraction in the organ) and provides valuable information on local sympathetic activity. Mental stress elicits marked circulatory responses, with mainly cardiorenal sympathetic activation and minor elevations of conventional venous plasma NA levels, thus illustrating the differentiated firing pattern of the sympathetic nerves. Circulating ADR is less important than neurogenic mechanisms in the responses to stress. Concentration-effect studies for infused catecholamines may be used for receptor sensitivity studies in vivo, but reflexogenic contributions to responses need to be determined. However, prejunctional mechanisms cannot be assessed without knowledge of the nerve activity present; for example, ADR infusion leads to increased nerve activity.

When correctly sampled, measured and interpreted, plasma catecholamines can yield very valuable information on sympathoadrenal activity.

REFERENCES

Åkerstedt T, Gillberg M, Hjemdahl P et al (1983) Comparison of urinary and plasma catecholamine responses to mental stress. *Acta Physiologica Scandinavica* 117: 19–26.

Allenmark S, Hedman L & Söderberg A (1980) Microanalysis of catecholamines in human plasma by high-performance liquid chromatography as compared to a radioenzymatic method. *Microchemical Journal* 25: 567–575.

Anderson EA, Wallin BG & Mark AL (1987) Dissociation of sympathetic nerve activity in arm and leg muscle during mental stress. *Hypertension* 9(supplement 3): 114–119.

Anton A & Sayre DF (1962) A study of the factors affecting the aluminium oxide-trihydroxy-indole procedure for the analysis of catecholamines. *Journal of Pharmacology and Experimental Therapeutics* 138: 360–374.

Ariëns EJ & Simonis AM (1983) Physiological and pharmacological aspects of adrenergic receptor classification. *Biochemical Pharmacology* 32: 1539–1545.

Arnold JMO & McDevitt DG (1983) Contribution of the vagus to the haemodynamic responses following intravenous boluses of isoprenaline. *British Journal of Clinical Pharmacology* 15: 423–429.

Arnold JMO & McDevitt DG (1984) Vagal activity is increased during intravenous isoprenaline infusion in man. *British Journal of Clinical Pharmacology* 18: 311–316.

Baily RG, Prophet SA, Shenberger JS et al (1990) Direct neurohumoral evidence for isolated sympathetic nervous system activation to skeletal muscle in response to cardiopulmonary baroreceptor unloading. *Circulation Research* 66: 1720–1728.

Barcroft H, Brod J, Hejl Z et al (1960) The mechanism of the vasodilatation in the forearm during stress (mental arithmetic). *Clinical Science* 19: 577–586.

Bartlett WA (1989) Effects of mobile phase composition on the chromatographic behaviour of catecholamines and selected metabolites. *Journal of Chromatography: Biomedical Applications* 493: 1–14.

Beiser GD, Zelis R, Epstein SE et al (1970) The role of skin and muscle resistance vessels in reflexes mediated by the baroreceptor system. *Journal of Clinical Investigation* 49: 225–231.

Bertel O, Bühler FR, Baitsch G et al (1982) Plasma adrenaline and noradrenaline in patients with acute myocardial infarction. *Chest* 82: 64–68.

Best JD & Halter JB (1982) Release and clearance rates of epinephrine in man: importance of arterial measurements. *Journal of Clinical Endocrinology and Metabolism* **55**: 263–268.

Blair DA, Glover WE, Greefield ADM & Roddie IC (1959) Excitation of cholinergic vasodilator nerves to human skeletal muscles during emotional stress. *Journal of Physiology* **148**: 633–647.

Blombery PA & Heinzow BGJ (1983) Cardiac and pulmonary norepinephrine release and removal in the dog. *Circulation Research* **53**: 688–694.

Bohlin G, Eliasson K, Hjemdahl P et al (1986) Personal control over work pace—circulatory, neuroendocrine and subjective responses in borderline hypertension. *Journal of Hypertension* **4**: 295–305.

Bouloux P, Perrett D & Besser GM (1985) Methodological considerations in the determination of plasma catecholamines by high-performance liquid chromatography with electrochemical detection. *Annals of Clinical Biochemistry* **22**: 194–203.

Bradley T & Hjemdahl P (1984) Further studies on renal nerve stimulation induced release of noradrenaline and dopamine from the canine kidney in situ. *Acta Physiologica Scandinavica* **122**: 369–379.

Bradley T & Hjemdahl P (1986) Renal extractions of endogenous and radiolabelled catecholamines in the dog. *Acta Physiologica Scandinavica* **126**: 505–510.

Bradley T, Hjemdahl P & DiBona GF (1987) Increased release of norepinephrine and dopamine from canine kidney during bilateral carotid occlusion. *American Journal of Physiology* **252**: F240–F245.

Bravo EL & Tarazi RC (1982) Plasma catecholamines in clinical investigation: a useful index or a meaningless number? *Journal of Laboratory and Clinical Medicine* **100**: 155–160.

Brock JA & Cunnane TC (1987) Relationship between the nerve action potential and transmitter release from sympathetic postganglionic nerve terminals. *Nature* **326**: 605–607.

Brod J (1963) Haemodynamic basis of acute pressor reactions and hypertension. *British Heart Journal* **25**: 227–245.

Brod J, Fencl V, Hejl Z & Jirka J (1959) Circulatory changes underlying blood pressure elevation during acute emotional stress (mental arithmetic) in normotensive and hypertensive subjects. *Clinical Science* **18**: 269–279.

Brod J, Cachovan M, Bahlman J et al (1976) Haemodynamic response to an emotional stress (mental arithmetic) with special reference to the venous side. *Australian and New Zealand Journal of Medicine* **6(supplement 2)**: 19–25.

Brown MJ, Jenner DA, Allison DJ & Dollery CT (1981) Variations in individual organ release of noradrenaline measured by an improved radioenzymatic technique; limitations of peripheral venous measurements in the assessment of sympathetic nerve activity. *Clinical Science* **61**: 585–590.

Candito M, Krstulovic AM, Sbirazzuoli V & Chambon P (1990) Proposal for the standardization of the calibration method for the assay of catecholamines. *Journal of Chromatography: Biomedical Applications* **526**: 194–202.

Causon RC, Brown MJ, Bouloux PM & Perret D (1983) Analytical differences in measurements of plasma catecholamines. *Clinical Chemistry* **29**: 735–737.

Chang PC, van der Krogt JA, Vermeij P & van Brummelen P (1986) Norepinephrine removal and release in the forearm of healthy subjects. *Hypertension* **8**: 801–809.

Chang PC, Kriek E, van der Krogt JA & van Brummelen P (1991) Does regional norepinephrine spillover represent local sympathetic activity? *Hypertension* **18**: 56–66.

Cleaveland CR, Rangno RE & Shand DG (1972) A standardized isoproterenol sensitivity test—the effects of sinus arrhythmia, atropine, and propranolol. *Archives of Internal Medicine* **130**: 47–52.

Cousineau D, Goresky CA, Bach GG & Rose CP (1984) Effect of β-adrenergic blockade on in vivo norepinephrine release in canine heart. *American Journal of Physiology* **246**: H283–H292.

Cousineau D, Rose CP & Goresky CA (1986) Plasma expansion effect on cardiac capillary and adrenergic exchange in intact dogs. *Journal of Applied Physiology* **60**: 147–153.

Cryer PE (1980) Physiology and pathophysiology of the human sympathoadrenal neuroendocrine system. *New England Journal of Medicine* **303**: 436–444.

D'Alesandro MM, Gruber DF, Reed L et al (1990) Effects of collection methods and storage on the in vitro stability of canine plasma catecholamines. *American Journal of Veterinary Research* **51**: 257–259.

Davis GC, Kissinger PT & Shoup RE (1981) Strategies for determination of serum or plasma norepinephrine by reverse-phase liquid chromatography. *Analytical Chemistry* **53:** 156–159.

Dimsdale JE, Hartley LH, Guiney T et al (1984) Postexercise peril—plasma catecholamines and exercise. *Journal of the American Medical Association* **251:** 630–632.

Durkin TA, Caliguri EJ, Mefford IN et al (1985) Determination of catecholamines in tissue and body fluids using microbore HPLC with amperometric detection. *Life Sciences* **37:** 1803–1810.

Eisenhofer G, Esler MD, Goldstein DS & Kopin IJ (1991) Neuronal uptake, metabolism, and release of tritium-labeled norepinephrine during assessment of its plasma kinetics. *American Journal of Physiology* **261:** E505–E515.

Eliasson K, Hjemdahl P & Kahan T (1983) Circulatory and sympatho-adrenal responses to stress in borderline and established hypertension. *Journal of Hypertension* **1:** 131–139.

Eriksson B-M & Persson B-A (1982) Determination of catecholamines in rat heart tissue and plasma samples by liquid chromatography with electrochemical detection. *Journal of Chromatography* **228:** 143–154.

Esler M (1991) Neural regulation of the cardiovascular system. In Byrne DG & Rosenman RH (eds) *Anxiety and the Heart*, pp 159–185. New York: Hemisphere.

Esler M, Jackman G, Bobik A et al (1979) Determination of norepinephrine apparent release rate and clearance in humans. *Life Sciences* **25:** 1461–1470.

Esler M, Jennings G, Leonard P et al (1984) Contribution of individual organs to total noradrenaline release in humans. *Acta Physiologica Scandinavica Supplement* **527:** 11–16.

Esler M, Jennings G, Korner P et al (1988) Assessment of human sympathetic nervous system activity from measurements of noradrenaline turnover. *Hypertension* **11:** 3–20.

Esler M, Jennings G & Lambert G (1989) Measurement of overall and cardiac norepinephrine release into plasma during cognitive challenge. *Psychoneuroendocrinology* **14:** 477–481.

Floras JS (1992) Epinephrine and the genesis of hypertension. *Hypertension* **19:** 1–18.

Floras J, Jones JV, Hassan O et al (1986) Failure of plasma norepinephrine to consistently reflect sympathetic activity in humans. *Hypertension* **8:** 641–649.

Folkow B (1982) Physiological aspects of primary hypertension. *Physiological Reviews* **62:** 347–504.

Folkow B, Häggendal J & Lisander B (1967) Extent of release and elimination of noradrenaline at peripheral adrenergic nerve terminals. *Acta Physiologica Scandinavica Supplement* **307:** 1–38.

Folkow B, Di Bona GF, Hjemdahl P et al (1983) Measurements of plasma norepinephrine concentrations in human primary hypertension—a word of caution on their applicability for assessing neurogenic contributions. *Hypertension* **5:** 399–403.

Frankenhaeuser M, Mellis I, Rissler A et al (1968) Catecholamine excretion as related to cognitive and emotional reaction patterns. *Psychosomatic Medicine* **30:** 109–120.

Freyschuss U, Hjemdahl P, Juhlin-Dannfelt A & Linde B (1986) Cardiovascular and metabolic responses to low dose adrenaline infusion: an invasive study in humans. *Clinical Science* **70:** 199–206.

Freyschuss U, Hjemdahl P, Juhlin-Dannfelt A & Linde B (1988) Cardiovascular and sympathoadrenal responses to mental stress: influence of β-blockade. *American Journal of Physiology* **255:** H443–H451.

Friberg P, Meredith I, Jennings G et al (1990) Evidence for increased renal norepinephrine overflow during sodium restriction in humans. *Hypertension* **16:** 121–130.

Goldstein DS (1983a) Commentary (to Folkow et al, 1983). *Hypertension* **5:** 402–403.

Goldstein DS (1983b) Plasma catecholamines and essential hypertension—an analytical review. *Hypertension* **5:** 86–99.

Goldstein DS, Feuerstein GZ, Izzo JL Jr et al (1981a) Validity of liquid chromatography with electrochemical detection for measuring plasma levels of norepinephrine and epinephrine in man. *Life Sciences* **28:** 467–475.

Goldstein DS, Feuerstein GZ, Kopin IJ & Keiser HR (1981b) Validity of liquid chromatography with electrochemical detection for measuring dopamine in human plasma. *Clinica Chimica Acta* **117:** 113–120.

Goldstein DS, Levinson P & Keiser HR (1983a) Plasma and urinary catecholamines during the human ovulatory cycle. *American Journal of Obstetrics and Gynecology* **146:** 824–829.

Goldstein DS, McCarty R, Polinsky RJ & Kopin IJ (1983b) Relationship between plasma norepinephrine and sympathetic neural activity. *Hypertension* **5:** 552–559.

Goldstein DS, Stull R, Zimlichman R et al (1984) Simultaneous measurement of DOPA, DOPAC, and catecholamines in plasma by liquid chromatography with electrochemical detection. *Clinical Chemistry* **30:** 815–816.

Goldstein DS, Zimlichman R, Stull R et al (1985) Measurement of regional neuronal removal of norepinephrine in man. *Journal of Clinical Investigation* **76:** 15–21.

Goldstein DS, Zimlichman R, Stull R et al (1986) Estimation of intrasynaptic norepinephrine concentrations in humans. *Hypertension* **8:** 471–475.

Goldstein DS, Eisenhofer G, Sax FL et al (1987) Plasma norepinephrine pharmacokinetics during mental challenge. *Psychosomatic Medicine* **49:** 591–605.

Goldstein DS, Brush JE Jr, Eisenhofer G et al (1988) In vivo measurement of neuronal uptake of norepinephrine in the human heart. *Circulation* **78:** 41–48.

Grossman E, Chang PC, Hoffman A et al (1991) Tracer norepinephrine kinetics: dependence on regional blood flow and the site of infusion. *American Journal of Physiology* **260:** R946–R952.

Häggendal J (1962) On the use of strong exchange resins for determinations of small amounts of catecholamines. *Scandinavian Journal of Clinical and Laboratory Investigation* **14:** 537–544.

Hallman H, Farnebo L-O & Hamberger B (1978) A sensitive method for the determination of plasma catecholamines using liquid chromatography with electrochemical detection. *Life Sciences* **23:** 1049–1052.

Hedman A, Hjemdahl P, Nordlander R & Åström H (1990) Effects of mental and physical stress on central haemodynamics and cardiac sympathetic nerve activity during QT interval-sensing rate-responsive and fixed rate ventricular inhibited pacing. *European Heart Journal* **11:** 903–915.

Henriksen JH & Christensen NJ (1989) Plasma norepinephrine in humans: limitations in assessment of whole body norepinephrine kinetics and plasma clearance. *American Journal of Physiology* **257:** E743–E750.

Henriksen JH, Christensen NJ & Ring-Larsen H (1986a) Pulmonary extraction of noradrenaline in man. *European Journal of Clinical Investigation* **16:** 423–427.

Henriksen JH, Ring-Larsen H & Christensen NJ (1986b) Catecholamines in plasma from artery, cubital vein, and femoral vein in patients with cirrhosis. Significance of sampling site. *Scandinavian Journal of Clinical and Laboratory Investigation* **46:** 39–44.

Henriksen JH, Christensen NJ & Ring-Larsen H (1989) Continuous infusion of tracer norepinephrine may miscalculate unidirectional nerve uptake of norepinephrine in humans. *Circulation Research* **65:** 388–395.

Henry DP, Starman BJ, Johnson DG & Williams RH (1975) A sensitive radioenzymatic assay of norepinephrine in tissues and plasma. *Life Sciences* **16:** 375–384.

Henry DP, Dentino M, Gibbs PS & Weinberger MH (1979) Vascular compartmentalization of plasma norepinephrine in normal man. *Journal of Laboratory and Clinical Medicine* **94:** 429–437.

Herd JA (1991) Cardiovascular responses to stress. *Physiological Reviews* **71:** 305–330.

Hilton SM, Spyer KM & Timms RJ (1979) The origin of the hind limb vasodilatation evoked by stimulation of the motor cortex in the cat. *Journal of Physiology* **287:** 545–557.

Hjemdahl P (1984a) Catecholamine measurements by high performance liquid chromatography. *American Journal of Physiology* **247:** E13–E20.

Hjemdahl P (1984b) Inter-laboratory comparison of plasma catecholamine determinations using several different assays. *Acta Physiologica Scandinavica Supplement* **527:** 43–54.

Hjemdahl P (1987a) Catecholamine measurements in plasma by high-performance liquid chromatography with electrochemical detection. *Methods in Enzymology* **142:** 521–534.

Hjemdahl P (1987b) Physiological aspects of catecholamine sampling. *Life Sciences* **41:** 841–844.

Hjemdahl P (1991) Physiology of the autonomic nervous system as related to cardiovascular function: implications for stress research. In Byrne DG & Rosenman RH (eds) *Anxiety and the Heart*, pp 95–158. New York: Hemisphere.

Hjemdahl P & Eliasson K (1979) Sympatho-adrenal and cardiovascular response to mental stress and orthostatic provocation in latent hypertension. *Clinical Science* **57:** 189s–191s.

Hjemdahl P & Kahan T (1993) Skeletal muscle circulation. In Bennett T & Gardiner S (vol. eds) *Nervous Control of Blood Vessels* (in press). From *The Autonomic Nervous System* series ed. by G. Burnstock. Reading: Harwood Academic.

Hjemdahl P, Daleskog M & Kahan T (1979) Determinations of plasma catecholamines by high performance liquid chromatography: comparison with a radioenzymatic method. *Life Sciences* **25**: 131–138.

Hjemdahl P, Eklund B & Kaijser L (1982) Catecholamine handling by the human forearm at rest and during isometric exercise and lower body negative pressure. *British Journal of Pharmacology* **77**: 324P.

Hjemdahl P, Åkerstedt T, Pollare T & Gillberg M (1983) Influence of beta-adrenoceptor blockade by metoprolol and propranolol on plasma concentrations and effects of nor-adrenaline and adrenaline during i.v. infusion. *Acta Physiologica Scandinavica Supplement* **515**: 45–53.

Hjemdahl P, Freyschuss U, Juhlin-Dannfelt A & Linde B (1984) Differentiated sympathetic activation during mental stress evoked by the Stroop test. *Acta Physiologica Scandinavica Supplement* **527**: 25–29.

Hjemdahl P, Freyschuss U, Juhlin-Dannfelt A & Linde B (1986a) Plasma catecholamines and mental stress. In Christensen NJ, Henriksen O & Lassen NA (eds) *The Sympathoadrenal System—Adrenergic Physiology and Pathophysiology*, pp 237–248. Copenhagen, New York & Tokyo: Munksgaard, Raven Press & Nankodo.

Hjemdahl P, Martinsson A & Larsson K (1986b) Improvement of isoprenaline infusion test by plasma concentration measurements. *Life Sciences* **39**: 629–635.

Hjemdahl P, Fagius J, Freyschuss U et al (1989a) Muscle sympathetic nerve activity and norepinephrine release during mental challenge in humans. *American Journal of Physiology* **257**: E654–E664.

Hjemdahl P, Larsson PT, Bradley T et al (1989b) Catecholamine measurements in urine by high-performance liquid chromatography with amperometric detection—comparison with an autoanalyzer fluorescence method. *Journal of Chromatography: Biomedical Applications* **494**: 53–66.

Hjemdahl P, Larsson PT & Wallén NH (1991) Effects of stress and β-blockade on platelet function. *Circulation* **84(supplement 6)**: VI-44–V-61.

Hollenberg NK, Williams GH & Adams DF (1981) Essential hypertension: abnormal renal vascular and endocrine responses to a mild psychological stimulus. *Hypertension* **2**: 11–17.

Iversen LL (1975) Uptake processes for biogenic amines. In Iversen LL, Iversen SD & Snyder SH (eds) *Handbook of Psychopharmacology*, pp 381–442. New York: Plenum Press.

Jansson E, Hjemdahl P & Kaijser L (1982) Diet induced changes in sympatho-adrenal activity in relation to substrate utilization during submaximal exercise. *Acta Physiologica Scandinavica* **114**: 171–178.

Jansson E, Hjemdahl P & Kaijser L (1986) Epinephrine-induced changes in muscle carbo-hydrate metabolism during exercise in male subjects. *Journal of Applied Physiology* **60**: 1466–1470.

Jennings G, Bobik A, Esler M & Korner P (1981) Contribution of cardiovascular reflexes to differences in β-adrenoceptor mediated responses in essential hypertension. *Clinical Science* **61**: 177s–180s.

Jie K, van Brummelen P, Vermeij P et al (1987) Modulation of noradrenaline release by periph-eral alpha₂-adrenoceptors in humans. *Journal of Cardiovascular Pharmacology* **9**: 407–413.

Joborn H, Hjemdahl P, Larsson PT et al (1990a) Platelet and plasma catecholamines in relation to plasma minerals and parathyroid hormone following acute myocardial infarction. *Chest* **97**: 1098–1105.

Joborn H, Hjemdahl P, Larsson PT et al (1990b) Effects of prolonged adrenaline infusion and mental stress on plasma minerals and parathyroid hormone. *Clinical Physiology* **10**: 37–53.

Johnson GA, Kupiecki RM & Baker CA (1980) Single isotope derivative (radioenzymatic) methods in the measurement of catecholamines. *Metabolism: Clinical and Experimental* **29(supplement 1)**: 1106–1113.

Jones DH, Hamilton CA & Reid JL (1979) Choice of control groups in the appraisal of sympathetic nervous activity in essential hypertension. *Clinical Science* **57**: 339–344.

Jörgensen LS, Bönlökke L & Christensen NJ (1985) Plasma adrenaline during mental stress and isometric exercise in man. The role of arterial sampling. *Scandinavian Journal of Clinical and Laboratory Investigation* **45**: 447–452.

Juhlin-Dannfelt A, Freyschuss U & Linde B (1986) Splanchnic circulatory and metabolic responses to mental stress—the immportance of circulatory adrenaline. *Acta Pharmacologica and Toxicologica* **59(supplement V):** 62.

Julius S (1988) The blood pressure seeking properties of the central nervous system. *Journal of Hypertension* **6:** 177–185.

Julius S (1991) Changing role of the autonomic nervous system in human hypertension. *Journal of Hypertension* **8(supplement 7):** S59–S65.

Julius S & Esler M (1975) Autonomic nervous cardiovascular regulation in borderline hypertension. *American Journal of Cardiology* **36:** 685–696.

Kahan T & Hjemdahl P (1987) Prejunctional beta₂-adrenoceptor-mediated enhancement of noradrenaline release in skeletal muscle vasculature in situ. *Journal of Cardiovascular Pharmacology* **10:** 433–438.

Kahan T, Hjemdahl P & Dahlöf C (1984) Relationship between the overflow of endogenous and radiolabelled noradrenaline from canine blood perfused gracilis muscle. *Acta Physiologica Scandinavica* **122:** 571–582.

Kahan T, Hjemdahl P & Dahlöf C (1987) Facilitation of nerve stimulation evoked noradrenaline overflow by isoprenaline but not by circulating adrenaline in the dog in vivo. *Life Sciences* **40:** 1811–1818.

Karlsberg RP, Cryer PE & Roberts R (1981) Serial plasma catecholamine responses early in the course of clinical acute myocardial infarction: relationship to infarct extent and mortality. *American Heart Journal* **102:** 24–29.

Kissinger PT, Bruntlett CS & Shoup RE (1981) Neurochemical applications of liquid chromatography with electrochemical detection. *Life Sciences* **28:** 455–465.

Kjaer M, Christensen NJ, Sonne B et al (1985) Effect of exercise on epinephrine turnover in trained and untrained male subjects. *Journal of Applied Physiology* **59:** 1061–1067.

Kjeldsen SE, Westheim A, Aakesson I et al (1986) Plasma adrenaline and noradrenaline during orthostasis in man: the importance of arterial sampling. *Scandinavian Journal of Clinical and Laboratory Investigation* **46:** 397–401.

Korner PI, Shaw J, Uther JB et al (1973) Autonomic and non-autonomic circulatory components in essential hypertension in man. *Circulation* **48:** 107–117.

Krstulovic AM (1982) Investigations of catecholamine metabolism using high-performance liquid chromatography—analytical methodology and clinical applications. *Journal of Chromatography: Biomedical Applications* **229:** 1–34.

Lands AM, Arnold A, McAuliff JP et al (1967) Differentiation of receptor systems activated by sympathomimetic amines. *Nature* **214:** 597–598.

Langer SZ (1981) Presynaptic regulation of the release of catecholamines. *Pharmacological Reviews* **32:** 337–362.

Larsson PT, Wallén NH, Egberg N & Hjemdahl P (1992) α-Adrenoceptor blockade by phentolamine inhibits adrenaline-induced platelet activation in vivo without affecting resting measurements. *Clinical Science* **82:** 369–376.

Lenders JWM, Peters JHM, Pieters GFF et al (1988) Hemodynamic reactivity to sympathoadrenal stimulation in adrenalectomized women. *Journal of Clinical Endocrinology and Metabolism* **67:** 139–143.

Levin BE, Rappaport M & Natelson BH (1979) Ultradian variations of plasma noradrenaline in humans. *Life Sciences* **25:** 621–628.

Linares OA, Jacquez JA, Zech LA et al (1987) Norepinephrine metabolism in man—kinetic analysis and model. *Journal of Clinical Investigation* **80:** 1332–1341.

Linde B & Hjemdahl P (1982) Effect of tilting on adipose tissue vascular resistance and sympathetic activity in humans. *American Journal of Physiology* **242:** H161–H167.

Linde B, Hjemdahl P, Freyschuss U & Juhlin-Dannfelt A (1989) Adipose tissue and skeletal muscle blood flow during mental stress. *American Journal of Physiology* **256:** E12–E18.

Lindvall K, Kahan T, de Faire U et al (1991) Stress-induced changes in blood pressure and left ventricular function in mild hypertension. *Clinical Cardiology* **14:** 125–132.

Linsell CR, Lightman SL, Mullen PE et al (1985) Circadian rhythms of epinephrine and norepinephrine in man. *Journal of Clinical Endocrinology and Metabolism* **60:** 1210–1215.

Mancia G, Ferrari A, Gregorini L et al (1983) Plasma catecholamines do not invariably reflect sympathetically induced changes in blood pressure in man. *Clinical Science* **65:** 227–235.

Martinsson A, Larsson K & Hjemdahl P (1985) Reduced β₂-adrenoceptor responsiveness in exercise induced asthma. *Chest* **88:** 594–600.

Martinsson A, Lindvall K, Melcher A & Hjemdahl P (1989) β-Adrenergic receptor responsiveness in humans: concentration-effect, as compared with dose-effect evaluation and influence of autonomic reflexes. *British Journal of Clinical Pharmacology* **28**: 83–94.

Martinsson A, Melcher A, Lindvall K & Hjemdahl P (1991) Comparison between isoprenaline infusions and bolus injections to assess β-adrenoceptor function in man, with special reference to cardiac contractility and the influence of autonomic reflexes. *Acta Physiologica Scandinavica* **141**: 167–180.

Mefford IN (1981) Application of high performance liquid chromatography with electrochemical detection to neurochemical analysis: measurement of catecholamines, serotonin and metabolites in rat brain. *Journal of Neuroscience Methods* **3**: 207–224.

Mullen PE, Lightman S, Linsell C et al (1980) Rhythms of plasma noradrenaline in man. *Psychoneuroendocrinology* **6**: 213–222.

Musgrave IV, Bachmann AW & Gordon RD (1984) Increased plasma noradrenaline during adrenaline infusion in man. *Journal of Hypertension* **2(supplement 3)**: 135–137.

Noshiro T, Saigusa T, Way D, Dorward PK & McGrath BP (1991) Norepinephrine spillover faithfully reflects sympathetic nerve activity in conscious rabbits. *American Journal of Physiology* **261**: F44–F50.

Öhlén A, Persson MG, Lindbom L et al (1990) Nerve-induced noradrenergic vasoconstriction and vasodilatation in skeletal muscle. *American Journal of Physiology* **258**: H1334–H1338.

Oliver JA, Pinto J, Sciacca RR & Cannon PJ (1981) Basal norepinephrine overflow into the renal vein: effect of renal nerve stimulation. *American Journal of Physiology* **239**: F371–F377.

Östergren J, Kahan T, Hjemdahl P et al (1992) Effects of sympatho-adrenal activation on the finger skin microcirculation in mild hypertension. *Journal of Human Hypertension* **6**: 169–173.

Pehrsson K, Hjemdahl P, Åström H & Nordlander R (1988) A comparison of sympatho-adrenal activity and cardiac performance at rest and during exercise in patients with ventricular demand or atrial synchronous pacing. *British Heart Journal* **60**: 212–220.

Pernow J, Lundberg J, Kaijser L et al (1986) Plasma neuropeptide Y-like immunoreactivity and catecholamines during various degrees of sympathetic activation in man. *Clinical Physiology* **6**: 561–578.

Pernow J, Kahan T, Hjemdahl P & Lundberg JM (1988) Possible involvement of neuropeptide Y in sympathetic vascular control in canine skeletal muscle. *Acta Physiologica Scandinavica* **132**: 43–50.

Persson B, Andersson OK, Hjemdahl P et al (1989) Adrenaline infusion in man increases muscle sympathetic activity and noradrenaline overflow to plasma. *Journal of Hypertension* **7**: 747–756.

Peuler JD & Johnson GA (1977) Simultaneous single isotope radioenzymatic assay of norepinephrine, epinephrine and dopamine. *Life Sciences* **21**: 625–636.

Robertson D, Johnson GA, Robertson RM et al (1979) Comparative assessment of stimuli that release neuronal and adrenomedullary catecholamines in man. *Circulation* **59**: 637–643.

Roca J, Caturla MC, Hjemdahl P et al (1993) Effect of adrenaline on ventricular function and coronary hemodynamics in relation to catecholamine handling in transplanted hearts. *European Journal of Cardiology* (in press).

Rowell LB (1984) Reflex control of regional circulations in humans. *Journal of the Autonomic Nervous System* **11**: 101–114.

Rumley AG (1988) The in vitro stability of catecholamines in whole blood. *Annals of Clinical Biochemistry* **25**: 585–586.

Rusch NJ, Shepherd JT, Webb RC & Vanhoutte PM (1981) Different behaviour of the resistance vessels of the human calf and forearm during contralateral isometric exercise, mental stress, and abnormal respiratory movements. *Circulation Research* **48**: I-118–I-130.

Savard G, Strange S, Kiens B et al (1987) Noradrenaline spillover during exercise in active versus resting skeletal muscle. *Acta Physiologica Scandinavica* **131**: 507–515.

Savard GK, Richter EA, Strange S et al (1989) Norepinephrine spillover from skeletal muscle during exercise in humans: role of muscle mass. *American Journal of Physiology* **257**: H1812–H1818.

Schwieler JH, Kahan T, Nussberger J et al (1992) Influence of angiotensin II, alpha- and beta-adrenoceptors on peripheral noradrenergic neurotransmission in vivo. *Acta Physiologica Scandinavica* **145**: 333–343.

Shah SD, Tse TF, Clutter WE & Cryer PE (1984) The human sympathochromaffin system. *American Journal of Physiology* **247:** E380–E384.

Shepherd JT & Mancia G (1986) Reflex control of the human cardiovascular system. *Reviews of Physiology, Biochemistry and Pharmacology* **105:** 3–99.

Smits P, Pieters G & Thien T (1986) The role of epinephrine in the circulatory effects of coffee. *Clinical Pharmacology and Therapeutics* **40:** 431–437.

Stjärne L (1989) Basic mechanisms and local modulation of nerve impulse-induced secretion of neurotransmitters from individual nerve varicosities. *Reviews of Physiology, Biochemistry and Pharmacology* **112:** 1–137.

Stratton JR, Pfeifer MA, Ritchie JL & Halter JB (1985) Hemodynamic effects of epinephrine: concentration-effect study in humans. *Journal of Applied Physiology* **58:** 1199–1206.

Theorell T, Hjemdahl P, Ericsson F et al (1985) Psychosocial and physiological factors in relation to blood pressure at rest—a study of Swedish men in their upper twenties. *Journal of Hypertension* **3:** 591–600.

Tidgren B & Hjemdahl P (1988) Reflex activation of renal nerves in humans—effects on noradrenaline, dopamine and renin overflow to renal venous plasma. *Acta Physiologica Scandinavica* **134:** 23–34.

Tidgren B & Hjemdahl P (1989) Renal responses to mental stress and epinephrine in man. *American Journal of Physiology* **257:** F682–F689.

Tidgren B, Hjemdahl P, Theodorsson E & Nussberger J (1990) Renal responses to lower body negative pressure in humans. *American Journal of Physiology* **259:** F573–F579.

Tidgren B, Hjemdahl P, Theodorsson E & Nussberger J (1991) Renal responses to dynamic exercise in man. *Journal of Applied Physiology* **70:** 2279–2286.

Ungar A & Phillips JH (1983) Regulation of the adrenal medulla. *Physiological Reviews* **63:** 787–843.

Van der Hoorn FAJ, Boomsma F, Man in't Veld AJ & Schalekamp MADH (1989) Determination of catecholamines in human plasma by high-performance liquid chromatography: comparison between a new method with fluorescence detection and an established method with electrochemical detection. *Journal of Chromatography: Biomedical Applications* **487:** 17–28.

Vincent HH, Boomsma F, Man in't Veld AJ et al (1984) Effects of selective and non-selective β-agonists on plasma potassium and norepinephrine. *Journal of Cardiovascular Pharmacology* **6:** 107–114.

Wallin BG & Fagius J (1988) Peripheral sympathetic neural activity in conscious humans. *Annual Review of Physiology* **50:** 565–576.

Wallin BG, Mörlin C & Hjemdahl P (1987) Muscle sympathetic activity and venous plasma noradrenaline concentrations during static exercise in normotensive and hypertensive subjects. *Acta Physiologica Scandinavica* **129:** 489–497.

Wolf S (1970) Emotions and the autonomic system. *Archives of Internal Medicine* **126:** 1024–1030.

Yamaguchi N & Garceau D (1980) Correlations between hemodynamic parameters of the liver and norepinephrine release upon hepatic nerve stimulation in the dog. *Canadian Journal of Physiology and Pharmacology* **58:** 1347–1355.

Yamaguchi I & Kopin IJ (1979) Plasma catecholamine and blood pressure responses to sympathetic stimulation in pithed rats. *American Journal of Physiology* **237:** H305–H310.

Zadic Z, Hamilton BP & Kowarski AA (1980) Integrated concentration of epinephrine and norepinephrine in normal subjects and in patients with mild essential hypertension. *Journal of Clinical Endocrinology and Metabolism* **50:** 842–845.

Zoller RP, Mark AL, Abboud FM et al (1972) The role of low pressure baroreceptors in reflex vasoconstrictor responses in man. *Journal of Clinical Investigation* **51:** 2967–2972.

4

Adrenergic control of the secretion of anterior
pituitary hormones

SAAD AL-DAMLUJI

Adrenaline and noradrenaline exert significant influences on the secretion
of the hormones of the anterior pituitary, some of which have been shown to
be physiologically important in humans or experimental animals. These
effects are exerted mostly on the hypothalamic hypophysiotrophic
hormones that regulate the anterior pituitary. This chapter summarizes the
evidence that supports a role for the adrenergic system in the control of
secretion of the anterior pituitary hormones. The focus is on more recently
acquired knowledge, especially where it is likely to be relevant to human
physiology or pathology. In several places, the reader is referred to review
articles that deal with the earlier literature, which cannot be covered in the
available space.

ADRENERGIC INNERVATION OF THE HYPOTHALAMUS
AND PITUITARY

Most anatomical descriptions of the adrenergic innervation of the hypothalamus are based on observations in the rat, but the few detailed studies on
the human hypothalamus indicate a similar pattern to that described in
rodents (Nobin and Bjorklund, 1973; Pearson et al, 1983). Both the human
and the rat hypothalamus contain high concentrations of adrenaline and
noradrenaline (Vogt, 1954; Bertler, 1961) and all the hypothalamic nuclei
that regulate neuroendocrine functions are densely innervated by
noradrenergic nerve terminals. The cell bodies of the adrenergic and
noradrenergic neurones are in the brain stem. The axons ascend in the
ventral noradrenergic bundle and the nerve terminals form synapses with
the peptidergic neurones in the hypothalamus.

The magnocellular vasopressin neurones of the supraoptic and paraventricular nuclei are predominantly innervated by the A1 collection of
noradrenergic neurones in the ventrolateral medulla. The parvocellular 41
amino acid corticotrophin-releasing hormone (CRH-41) neurones (some of
which also contain vasopressin; Whitnall et al, 1987) are predominantly
innervated by the A2 collection of noradrenergic neurones (which forms
part of the nucleus tractus solitarius of the vagal complex in the dorsomedial

ISBN 0–7020–1698–5

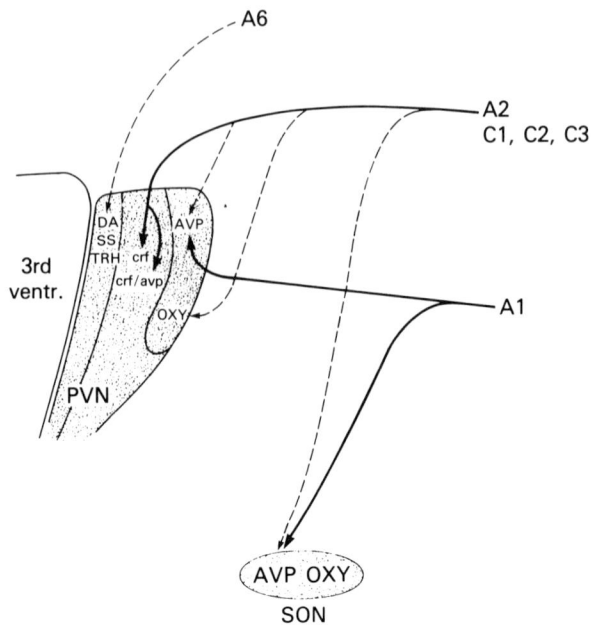

Figure 1. The adrenergic and noradrenergic innervation of the hypothalamic paraventricular and supraoptic nuclei. Major innervations are represented by heavy lines and minor innervations by broken lines. For details, see text. Based on Cunningham and Sawchenko (1988) and Cunningham et al (1990). A1, A2 and A6 = noradrenergic neurones of the ventrolateral medulla, the dorsomedial medulla and the locus coeruleus, respectively; AVP = magnocellular vasopressinergic neurones; C1, C2 and C3 = medullary groups of PNMT-immunoreactive neurones; crf = parvocellular CRH-41 neurones; crf/avp = parvocellular neurones that contain both CRH-41 and vasopressin; DA = dopaminergic neurones; OXY = oxytocinergic neurones; PVN = paraventricular nucleus; SON = supraoptic nucleus; SS = somatostatinergic neurones; TRH = thyrotrophin-releasing hormone neurones.

medulla) and by the C1, C2 and C3 collections of adrenergic, phenyl-ethanolamine-N-methyltransferase (PNMT immunoreactive) neurones (Figure 1) (Cunningham and Sawchenko, 1988; Cunningham et al, 1990). Oxytocin neurones are sparsely innervated with noradrenergic terminals. The locus coeruleus provides the paraventricular nucleus with a small supply of terminals whose distribution is predominantly in the medial part of the periventricular subdivision of the nucleus, which contains cell bodies of dopamine, somatostatin and thyrotrophin-releasing hormone (TRH) neurones (Cunningham et al, 1990). Synaptic connections are evident between these peptidergic neurones and the adrenergic and noradrenergic nerve terminals (Shioda et al, 1986; Bosler et al, 1987; Liposits et al, 1987, 1990). The cell bodies and dendrites of the growth hormone-releasing hormone (GHRH) neurones, which are in the arcuate nucleus, are also innervated by noradrenergic nerve terminals (Liposits et al, 1990), as are the gonadotrophin-releasing hormone (GnRH) cells in the medial preoptic area (Hoffman et al, 1982).

The role of adrenaline as a neurotransmitter in the brain is still unclear and there are data that suggest that the hypothalamic neurones that contain PNMT are not 'adrenergic neurones' in the conventional sense. It has been postulated that noradrenaline released from the noradrenergic neurones is taken up by 'PNMT neurones' and converted to adrenaline. This is then released back into the extracellular space, from where it is taken up and stored with noradrenaline as a cotransmitter in the noradrenergic neurones (Ross et al, 1984; Mefford, 1987). Some of the adrenaline released from the PNMT neurones may also act on α_2-adrenoceptors, which the PNMT neurones appear to innervate (Stolk et al, 1984).

The anterior pituitary is not innervated by noradrenergic neurones, but the neural and intermediate lobes of the rat contain significant quantities of dopamine and smaller amounts of noradrenaline and adrenaline. Both the neural and intermediate lobes are innervated by the brain, but the posterior pituitary receives, in addition, a noradrenergic supply from the superior cervical ganglion (Saavedra, 1985).

Dopamine is secreted into hypophysial portal plasma and its role in the tonic inhibition of prolactin secretion is established. However, there is controversy as to whether adrenaline is secreted into hypophysial portal plasma in any significant quantities (for review, see Al-Damluji, 1988). In humans undergoing pituitary surgery, catecholamine concentrations in blood from the lesioned stalk were higher than in the periphery, but mean concentrations did not exceed 1.5 nmol/litre (Paradisi et al, 1989). Higher concentrations are seen in peripheral plasma during stressful stimuli, so it appears unlikely that the anterior pituitary is exposed to much higher concentrations of adrenaline and noradrenaline than are found in the periphery. In rats too, a recent study concluded that adrenaline in the hypophysial portal circulation is derived mainly from the adrenal glands, and that the hypothalamus makes no significant contribution to portal adrenaline concentrations (Pesce et al, 1990). This observation is in accord with morphological studies showing that PNMT-immunoreactive nerve fibres are sparse in the median eminence, and are almost confined to the zona interna; only a few PNMT axons were detectable in the zona externa, where the capillary plexus is located (Bosler et al, 1987).

Both α_1 and α_2-adrenergic receptors are found in high density in most regions of the hypothalamus, including the paraventricular nucleus (Leibowitz et al, 1982; Cummings and Seybold, 1988). β-Adrenoceptors are also found in the hypothalamus, again including the paraventricular nucleus (Leibowitz et al, 1982; Petrovic et al, 1983). In the anterior pituitary, α_1-adrenoceptors are undetectable in fresh tissue obtained from pituitaries in vivo (Battaglia et al, 1983; De Souza and Kuyatt, 1987). The appearance of α_1-adrenoceptors in cultured pituitary cells (Giguere et al, 1981; Peters et al, 1983) is presumably due to upregulation of the receptors in the absence of catecholamines in the culture medium. Studies on rat and porcine pituitaries have shown α_1 binding sites only in the posterior lobe and these appear to be innervated by the superior cervical ganglion (De Souza and Kuyatt, 1987). β-Adrenergic receptors have been detected by autoradiography in the anterior and posterior lobes of humans and rats (De Souza, 1985) and in the intermediate lobe of rats (Schimchowitsch and Pelletier, 1988).

ADRENERGIC CONTROL OF THE SECRETION OF ADRENOCORTICOTROPHIN

The hypothalamus secretes a mixture of peptides that act synergistically with each other to stimulate the secretion of adrenocorticotrophin (ACTH) (Gillies et al, 1982). These peptides are referred to as the 'corticotrophin-releasing factor (CRF) complex'. Two of the main constituents of the CRF complex are CRH-41 and vasopressin. The synergistic action of these two peptides has been shown to be important in the physiological control of ACTH secretion (Linton et al, 1985). Several other hypothalamic peptides can stimulate the secretion of ACTH, but their physiological significance has not yet been established (for review, see Antoni, 1986). It is possible that the hypothalamus may release different ACTH secretagogues in response to different stimuli (Plotsky et al, 1989).

Experiments on pituitary cells in vitro have shown that CRH-41 is the most potent known ACTH secretagogue, being much more potent than vasopressin (Vale et al, 1983). However, CRH-41 and vasopressin are equipotent in stimulating ACTH secretion when injected into rats in vivo (Rivier and Vale, 1983). This difference is likely to be due to exogenous vasopressin interacting synergistically with endogenous CRH-41 when it is injected in vivo (Rivier and Vale, 1983).

The cell bodies of the CRH-41 neurones are in the parvocellular part of the paraventricular nucleus, and the axons project to the zona externa of the median eminence, where the hormone is secreted into portal plasma. Under basal conditions, approximately half the CRH-41 neurones also contain vasopressin, but following adrenalectomy, vasopressin appears in most of the CRH-41 neurones (Whitnall et al, 1987). This indicates the ability of these neurones to respond to perturbations of homeostasis by appropriately altering the identity of their neurosecretory products. Vasopressin is also present in the magnocellular neurones of the supraoptic and paraventricular nuclei, whose axons project to the posterior pituitary. The secretory products of the posterior pituitary can reach the anterior lobe via the short portal vessels that connect these two lobes (Oliver et al, 1977). CRH-41 is also present in some of the magnocellular oxytocinergic neurones (Dreyfuss et al, 1984), which may play a role in the control of ACTH secretion.

Stressful conditions stimulate the secretion of both catecholamines and glucocorticoids, so the interaction of these two hormonal systems has been of interest for some decades. The issue was the subject of a long controversy that is now coming to an end (for discussion of the historical background, see Al-Damluji, 1988; Plotsky et al, 1989).

α_1-Adrenoceptors

In the brain, α_1-adrenoceptors are located postsynaptically. The following evidence indicates that activation of α_1-adrenoceptors that are located in the brain stimulates the secretion of ACTH:

1. In humans, the secretion of ACTH can be stimulated by methoxamine, an α_1-agonist that crosses the blood–brain barrier, but not by an

equipotent dose of noradrenaline, an α_1-agonist that reaches the pituitary gland and the median eminence following an intravenous infusion but does not cross the blood–brain barrier (Al-Damluji and Grossman, 1985; Al-Damluji et al, 1985, 1986). Further studies demonstrated that the α_2- and β-agonist properties of noradrenaline did not account for the differences from methoxamine (Al-Damluji et al, 1987a). This provided the first evidence that activation of α_1-adrenoceptors, located in the brain, could stimulate the secretion of ACTH. Prior to this work, it had been known that certain drugs such as the amphetamines (Rees et al, 1970) and methoxamine (Nakai et al, 1973) could stimulate the secretion of ACTH, but the location of the responsible receptors was unknown.

2. In patients with hypothalamic disease but with responsive pituitary corticotroph cells, methoxamine had no stimulant action on ACTH secretion (Figure 2) (Al-Damluji and Rees, 1987; Al-Damluji and Francis, 1993). This confirmed that the stimulant α_1-adrenoceptors are not located in the anterior pituitary.

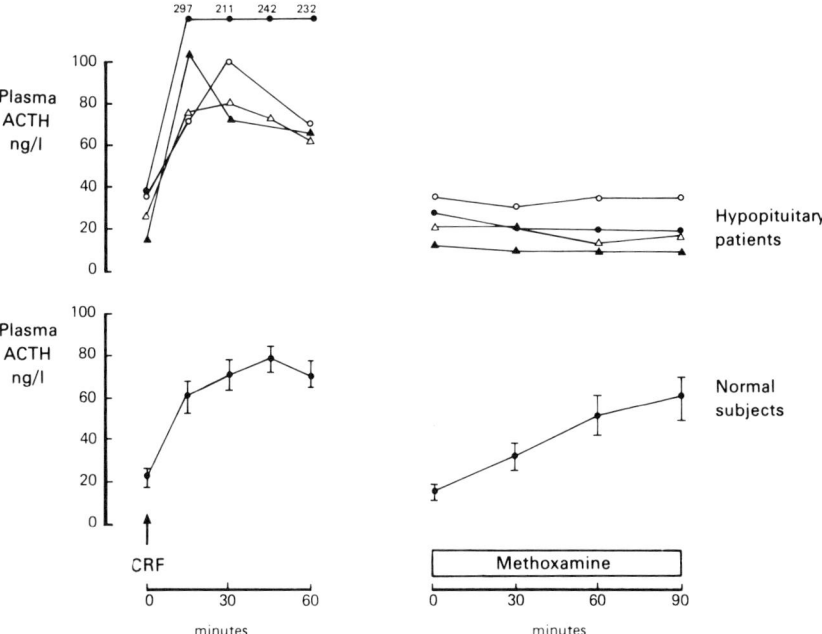

Figure 2. The effects of synthetic ovine CRH-41 (CRF; 100 µg over 1 min) and methoxamine (20 mg intravenously from 0 to 90 min) on plasma ACTH concentrations in four patients with hypopituitarism due to hypothalamic dysfunction (upper panels) and in six normal volunteers (lower panels). The data from the normal volunteers are expressed as the means ± SEM and those from the patients are plotted individually. The hypopituitary patients responded to CRH-41, indicating that they have responsive pituitary corticotroph cells; however, they did not respond to methoxamine. This supports other evidence that indicates that the α_1-adrenoceptors that stimulate ACTH secretion are not located directly on the corticotrophs, but are in the brain. From Al-Damluji and Francis (1993).

3. In rats, intracerebroventricular infusion of α_1-agonists also stimulates the secretion of ACTH (Szafarczyk et al, 1987); methoxamine was more potent in stimulating ACTH secretion when it was administered intracerebroventricularly than intravenously (Al-Damluji et al, 1990a).

The identity of the hypothalamic peptides that mediate the effects of the α_1-adrenoceptors has been the subject of investigation. As described above, the hypothalamus secretes a CRF complex, the constituents of which appear to act synergistically in stimulating ACTH secretion. Activation of α_1-adrenoceptors stimulates the secretion of several hypothalamic peptides, including CRH-41 and vasopressin (Hiwatari and Johnston, 1985; Plotsky, 1987; Szafarczyk et al, 1987; Calogero et al, 1988; Hillhouse and Milton, 1989). It appears that the effect of the α_1-adrenoceptors is exerted primarily on neurones secreting vasopressin, which in turn stimulates the secretion of ACTH, acting synergistically with CRH-41. The evidence for this was obtained in rats: the ACTH response to an intracerebroventricular infusion of an α_1-agonist could be reduced by a vasopressin antagonist but not by an equipotent dose of a CRH-41 antagonist (Al-Damluji et al, 1990a). Confirmation of the essential role of vasopressin was obtained from the finding that Brattleboro rats, which are deficient in bioactive vasopressin but not in other CRFs such as CRH-41 or oxytocin, had no ACTH response to a central infusion of an α_1-agonist (Al-Damluji et al, 1990b). Figure 3 is a representation of the hypothetical model of the complex interaction between the noradrenergic neurones and the hypothalamic peptidergic neurones that influence the secretion of ACTH.

The physiological significance of the stimulant α_1-adrenoceptors has been demonstrated in two situations in humans: the cortisol secretory pattern during waking hours and the ACTH and cortisol responses to feeding have been shown to be mediated by stimulant α_1-adrenoceptors (Al-Damluji et al, 1987b,c). However, catecholamines do not mediate all stimuli to ACTH secretion in humans, as the nocturnal cortisol surge and the response to hypoglycaemia are unaffected by α_1-adrenoceptor blockade (Al-Damluji et al, 1987b; Cuneo et al, 1987). Although physiological stimuli have not been studied in the rat, the corticosterone response to immobilization stress, the ACTH response to ether and the CRH-41 response to haemorrhage can be reduced by α_1-adrenergic antagonists (Gibson et al, 1986; Plotsky, 1987; Szafarczyk et al, 1987; Aguilera et al, 1992). These findings indicate that α_1-adrenoceptors mediate the ACTH responses to various stimuli in humans and rats.

α_2-Adrenoceptors

In the brain, as in the periphery, α_2-adrenoceptors are believed to be located both presynaptically (on the noradrenergic neurone) and postsynaptically (on the target neurone). Activation of these receptors is believed to inhibit the firing of the neurones on which they are located.

In dogs, activation of α_2-adrenoceptors that are located in the brain inhibits the secretion of ACTH in response to stress (Ganong et al, 1982). In humans, the α_2-adrenoceptors are not activated under basal conditions

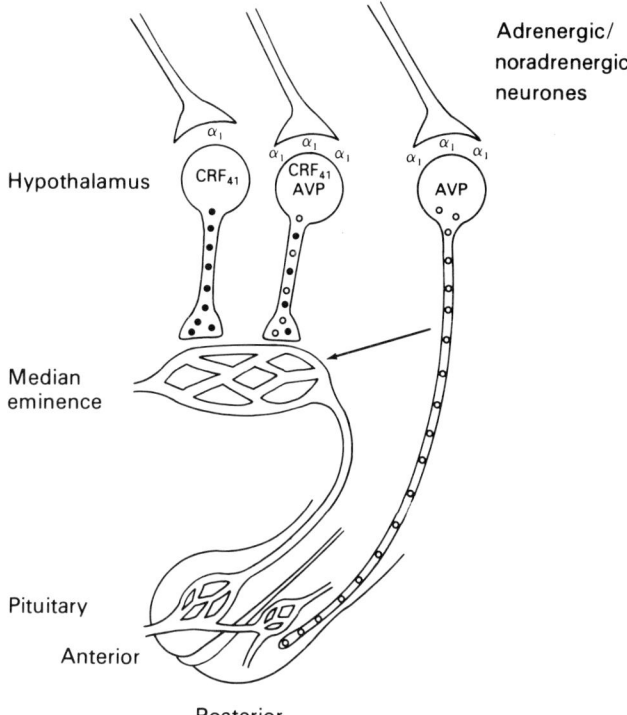

Figure 3. Proposed model of the relationship between the α_1-adrenoceptors, the vasopressin neurones (AVP) and the CRH-41 neurones (CRF$_{41}$) that stimulate ACTH secretion. When α_1-adrenoceptors are activated, at least three types of neurones may be stimulated: magnocellular vasopressin neurones that supply the neurohypophysis, whose secretions may reach the anterior pituitary via the short portal vessels or the median eminence; parvocellular neurones that contain CRH-41; and parvocellular neurones that contain both CRH-41 and vasopressin. The available data suggest that when α_1-adrenoceptors are activated, the primary response is from neurones that secrete vasopressin, but that the presence of CRH-41 is important for vasopressin to exert its full effect, presumably by the known synergy between the two peptides. It is possible that the vasopressin neurones may have a lower threshold for activation. As the intensity of the α_1-stimulus increases, CRH-41 neurones will presumably be activated, and CRH-41 will be secreted into the long portal vessels. From Al-Damluji et al (1990b).

(Al-Damluji et al, 1988, 1990c), i.e. with subjects lying supine in a darkened room, with no auditory or visual stimulation. Under such conditions, administration of an α_2-antagonist has no effect on the secretion of noradrenaline or ACTH (Al-Damluji et al, 1988, 1990c). This is presumably because noradrenaline release from the neurones is minimal under such circumstances, so the presynaptic α_2-adrenoceptors are not occupied by noradrenaline to a significant extent. In contrast, when ACTH secretion is stimulated by an agent that exerts its action on central noradrenergic neurones, administration of an α_2-antagonist enhances the ACTH response to that stimulus (Al-Damluji et al, 1988, 1990c).

It seems likely that the α_2-adrenoceptors provide a central negative feed-back mechanism that prevents excessive glucocorticoid responses to stress. This effect presumably complements the inhibitory effects of corticosteroids on the secretion of ACTH and the 'CRF complex'. In addition to this presynaptic α_2 inhibition of ACTH secretion, there is evidence in rats that, under some circumstances, activation of postsynaptic α_2-adrenoceptors may stimulate the secretion of CRH-41 (Calogero et al, 1988; Assenmacher et al, 1992).

β-Adrenoceptors

In humans, activation of β-adrenoceptors with intravenous infusions of selective agonists does not stimulate ACTH secretion (Al-Damluji et al, 1987a). It has not been possible to study the effects of activation of central β-adrenoceptors in humans due to the lack of agonists with adequate penetration of the blood–brain barrier. Most investigators have found that β-blockade has no effect on the adrenocortical response to hypoglycaemia in humans (for review, see Al-Damluji, 1988) and no evidence has been presented as yet of a physiological role for these receptors in the control of ACTH secretion in humans. The situation in the rat is less clear. Some investigators found that activation of central β-adrenoceptors stimulates the secretion of CRH-41 or ACTH, whereas others found an inhibitory effect (Plotsky, 1987; Szafarczyk et al, 1987; Takao et al, 1988; Tsagarakis et al, 1988; Widmaier et al, 1989). The role (if any) of β-adrenoceptors in the control of ACTH secretion in the rat remains ambiguous.

Circulating catecholamines

In 1947, Long proposed that circulating adrenaline, derived from the adrenal medulla, stimulated the secretion of ACTH by a direct action on the pituitary corticotrophs. Some investigators subsequently reported that adrenaline enhanced the action of CRH-41 on cultured rat adenohypo-physial cells in vitro (for review, see Al-Damluji, 1988). However, in normal human volunteers, intravenous infusions of adrenaline and noradrenaline that increase plasma catecholamine concentrations to the upper limit of the physiological range do not stimulate ACTH secretion, nor do they enhance the stimulant effects of CRH-41 or vasopressin on ACTH secretion (Milsom et al, 1986; Al-Damluji et al, 1987d; Jackson et al, 1987). It is therefore clear that, in humans, peripheral circulating catecholamines have no stimulant effect on ACTH secretion, and the ACTH response to stress in humans is unlikely to be mediated by the concomitant sympathoadrenal response. In contrast, a stimulant action of circulating catecholamines acting on β_2-adrenoceptors in the rat intermediate lobe may be physiologically relevant in the responses of that lobe to some stressful stimuli (Berkenbosch et al, 1983). The intermediate lobe is vestigial in adult humans.

The role of dietary tyrosine

Tyrosine is a dietary amino acid that is also the precursor in the catecholamine

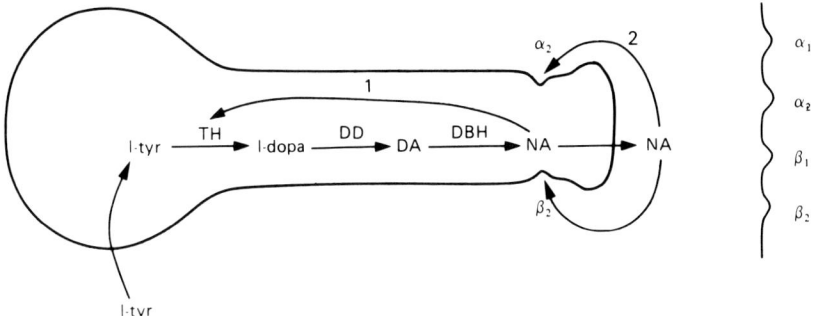

Figure 4. Schematic representation of the negative feedback mechanisms that are involved in the regulation of noradrenaline synthesis and release. 1 = inhibition of tyrosine hydroxylase by the products of the catecholamine synthesis pathway; 2 = inhibition of noradrenaline release by presynaptic α_2-adrenoceptors. l-tyr: L-tyrosine; TH = tyrosine hydroxylase; L-dopa = L-dihydroxyphenylalanine; DD = 'dopa decarboxylase' (L-neutral amino acid decarboxylase); DA = dopamine; DBH = dopamine-β-hydroxylase; NA = noradrenaline; α_1 = postsynaptic α_1-adrenoceptor; α_2 = pre- and postsynaptic α_2-adrenoceptors; β_1 = postsynaptic β_1-adrenoceptor; β_2 = pre- and postsynaptic β_2-adrenoceptors. From Al-Damluji (1991).

synthesis pathway (Figure 4). The large neutral amino acids, including tyrosine, share a common, competitive mechanism for transport across the blood–brain barrier and into the neurones (Pardridge and Oldendorf, 1977; Morre and Wurtman, 1981). The possible effects of dietary intake of tyrosine on the central noradrenergic system have been the subject of considerable interest and some controversy.

In the early studies following the discovery of tyrosine hydroxylase, it was reported that the products of the catecholamine synthesis pathway (e.g. noradrenaline) exerted an inhibitory effect on the activity of this enzyme (Nagatsu et al, 1964; Udenfriend et al, 1965). This was thought to act as a negative feedback process, whereby noradrenaline limits its own rate of synthesis. Administration of tyrosine was therefore not expected to increase the rate of turnover of noradrenaline unless the animals were stressed, as stress increases the neuronal discharge rate, resulting in increased activity of tyrosine hydroxylase (Gordon et al, 1966). However, more recently it was proposed that the synthesis of catecholamines may be dependent on the availability of tyrosine (Wurtman et al, 1974; Carlsson and Lindqvist, 1978). This proposal was based upon experiments in which tyrosine was administered to animals that had been pretreated with a dihydroxyphenylalanine (dopa) decarboxylase inhibitor to inhibit the conversion of dopa to dopamine and noradrenaline. In view of the confusion regarding the role of tyrosine, we examined the effect of tyrosine in humans, using the secretion of ACTH as an index of the release of noradrenaline in the hypothalamus (see below).

Tyrosine was administered in doses that were similar to the estimated tyrosine content of an average meal and also in supraphysiological doses. The secretion of ACTH and the release of noradrenaline into plasma were unaffected by administration of any of the doses of tyrosine (Al-Damluji et al, 1988). The reasons for the lack of effect of tyrosine were then investigated. We postulated that this may have been due to activation of one of the negative feedback processes that control the rate of synthesis and release of the catecholamines (Figure 4). Whereas tyrosine on its own had no effect on the release of noradrenaline or the secretion of ACTH, following pretreatment with an α_2-antagonist, idazoxan, administration of tyrosine caused a significant increase in the release of noradrenaline and the secretion of ACTH (Al-Damluji et al, 1988). It therefore seems that the lack of effect of tyrosine under basal conditions is due in part to activation of presynaptic α_2-adrenoceptors that inhibit the release of noradrenaline.

In conclusion, administration of tyrosine under basal conditions has no effect on the release of noradrenaline. The lack of effect of tyrosine is due to two main factors: inhibition of tyrosine hydroxylase by intracellular noradrenaline (Nagatsu et al, 1964; Udenfriend et al, 1965) and activation of presynaptic α_2-adrenoceptors, which inhibit noradrenaline release (Al-Damluji et al, 1988). The likely explanation for the stimulant effect of tyrosine following blockade of the dopa decarboxylase enzyme (Wurtman et al, 1974; Carlsson and Lindqvist, 1978) is that blockade of the enzyme prevented the increase in intracellular noradrenaline concentrations that would inhibit tyrosine hydroxylase under physiological conditions.

The ACTH response to adrenergic drugs as an index of activation of the hypothalamic noradrenergic system

An important problem in pharmacology is the absence of a method for assessing the activation of adrenergic receptors in the human brain. For example, it is not possible currently to assess whether a drug in development as a potential antidepressant is capable of increasing the release of noradrenaline in the human brain. It is therefore difficult to screen a series of drugs or to determine suitable doses in humans without carrying out long-term placebo-controlled therapeutic trials, which consume much time and resources. Based on the findings described above, it was proposed that the ACTH response to adrenergic drugs might serve as an in vivo marker of the release of endogenous catecholamines and of activation of α_1-adrenoceptors in the hypothalamus (Al-Damluji, 1989, 1991).

The ACTH response to the release of endogenous catecholamines may also serve as a marker of damage to the hypothalamic noradrenergic system in various diseases in humans, which is currently inaccessible to clinical investigation. However, it is not known whether a hypothalamic noradrenergic lesion might result in denervation hypersensitivity of the postsynaptic α_1-adrenoceptors, which might restore the ACTH response to the release of endogenous catecholamines. Rats with disruption of noradrenergic nerve terminals induced by 6-hydroxydopamine were examined for their responsiveness to stimuli that evoke ACTH release, either via release of endogenous catecholamines or with the selective exogenous α_1 agonist methoxamine, which is not subject to uptake by noradrenergic neurones (Al-Damluji and White, 1992). The postsynaptic α_1-adrenoceptors that modulate ACTH secretion did not undergo denervation hypersensitivity, and were therefore unable to compensate for the loss of noradrenergic nerve terminals. The ACTH response to the combination of catecholamine precursor and α_2-agonist was reduced, enabling detection of the hypothalamic noradrenergic lesion in the rats in vivo (Al-Damluji and White, 1992).

This work is at an early stage, but the ACTH response to the release of endogenous catecholamines promises to be useful for screening drugs, such as antidepressants, that are intended to increase the release of noradrenaline in the human brain. As the ACTH response to the combination of a catecholamine precursor and an α_2-antagonist requires an intact hypothalamic noradrenergic system (Al-Damluji and White, 1992), this method should also be useful for the detection of hypothalamic noradrenergic lesions in humans.

ADRENERGIC CONTROL OF THE SECRETION OF PROLACTIN

The predominant hypothalamic neurotransmitter in the control of prolactin secretion is dopamine. The cell bodies of the dopaminergic neurones are in the arcuate nucleus and the periventricular part of the paraventricular nucleus. These 'tuberoinfundibular' neurones project to the zona externa of the median eminence, where dopamine is secreted into the long portal vessels. Dopamine exerts a tonic inhibitory effect on the secretion of prolactin that is readily demonstrable in both humans and rats (for review, see Ben-Jonathan, 1985). Increased concentrations of prolactin stimulate the activity of the tuberoinfundibular neurones, which in turn inhibit the secretion of prolactin, acting as a negative feedback mechanism (Hokfelt and Fuxe, 1972). Several hypothalamic peptides are capable of stimulating the secretion of prolactin, including TRH and vasoactive intestinal peptide (VIP), and oestrogens also stimulate the synthesis of prolactin in the lactotrophs.

In humans, the adrenergic control of prolactin secretion seems to operate on similar principles to those described for ACTH. The role of adrenergic mechanisms in the control of prolactin secretion in experimental animals has been controversial, but it is possible to interpret some of the data from experimental animals to support the conclusions reached in the human studies.

α_1-Adrenoceptors

In humans, the secretion of prolactin is stimulated by intravenous infusion of methoxamine, the α_1-adrenergic agonist that can cross the blood–brain barrier (Al-Damluji et al, 1989). The effect is not reproduced by equipotent doses of noradrenaline, which reaches the pituitary gland and the median eminence but does not cross the blood–brain barrier (Figure 5) (Al-Damluji

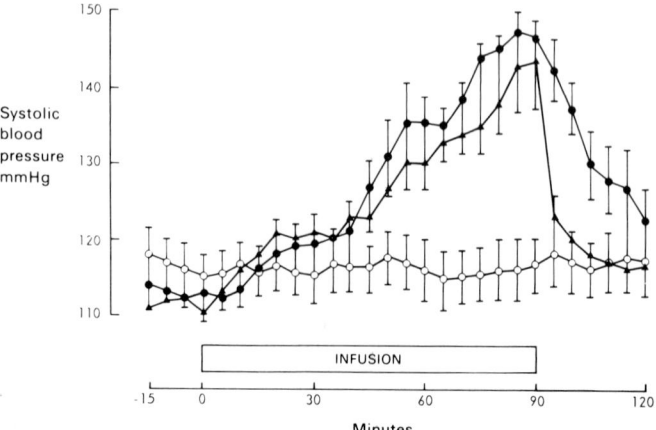

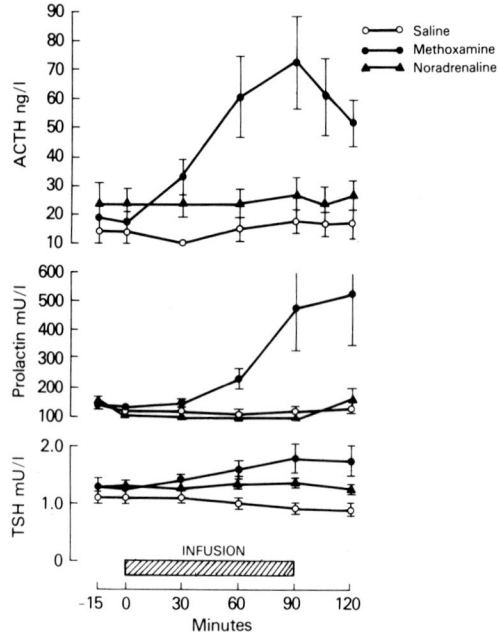

Figure 5. The effects of methoxamine, noradrenaline and saline on systolic blood pressure (upper panel) and plasma ACTH, prolactin and TSH concentrations (lower panel) in six volunteers. Methoxamine was given as a continuous intravenous infusion of 20 mg over 90 min. Noradrenaline was infused at an initial rate of 4.8 μg/min ($0.08\ μg\cdot kg^{-1}\cdot min^{-1}$) and the rate of the infusion was adjusted to mimic the changes in systolic blood pressure that had been observed during the methoxamine infusion given on a previous day. Final noradrenaline infusion rates ranged from 7.2 to 19.8 μg/min (mean ± SEM of $12.2 ± 1.8\ μg/min = 0.2 ± 0.03\ μg\cdot kg^{-1}\cdot min^{-1}$). From Al-Damluji and Francis (1993).

and Francis, 1993). This indicates that the α_1-adrenoceptors that stimulate prolactin secretion are located in the brain rather than in the periphery or directly in the pituitary. The α_2- and β-adrenergic agonist properties of noradrenaline did not account for the differences from methoxamine (Al-Damluji and Francis, 1993). As methoxamine also stimulated the secretion of thyroid-stimulating hormone (TSH), it is possible that the α_1-adrenoceptors act on hypothalamic TRH neurones; in humans, TRH is equipotent in stimulating the secretion of TSH and prolactin, and the smallest doses of TRH that stimulate TSH secretion will also stimulate the secretion of prolactin (Noel et al, 1974; Figure 6).

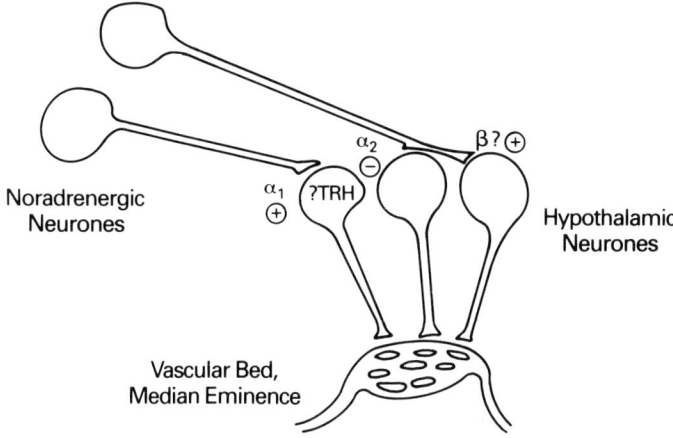

Figure 6. Schematic representation of a hypothetical model of the effects of central noradrenergic neurones on the secretion of prolactin. Activation of central α_1-adrenoceptors stimulates the secretion of prolactin. There is a concomitant increase in the secretion of TSH, suggesting that the effect may be exerted via an increase of the secretion of TRH into portal plasma. During certain stimuli to prolactin secretion, such as hypoglycaemia, noradrenaline also activates postsynaptic α_2-adrenoceptors that are inhibitory. These α_2-adrenoceptors appear to dampen the prolactin response to certain stimuli. There is evidence in the rat that activation of β-adrenoceptors stimulates the secretion of prolactin, but this effect has not been demonstrable in humans.

There is evidence for a stimulant effect of α_1-adrenoceptors on the secretion of prolactin in rats. In the early studies, peripheral administration of the noradrenaline precursor DL-dihydroxyphenylserine (DOPS) stimulated the secretion of prolactin in rats (Donoso et al, 1971), while central infusion of 6-hydroxydopamine reduced serum prolactin concentrations (Kizer et al, 1975). This suggested that a central noradrenergic pathway stimulates prolactin secretion in the rat. Although there is no direct evidence that activation of brain α_1-adrenoceptors stimulates the secretion of prolactin in the rat, there are several studies that would be compatible with this suggestion. The most convincing was the finding that intraperitoneal injection of prazosin prevented the elevation of serum prolactin concentrations on the afternoon of pro-oestrus (Clemens and Shaar, 1980). This suggested that this physiological effect was mediated by α_1-adrenoceptors, although the location of these receptors was not investigated. Infusion of adrenaline into the preoptic hypothalamic area or into the lateral cerebral ventricle stimulated the secretion of prolactin in rats and the effect was blocked by phentolamine (Willoughby et al, 1986; Koshiyama et al, 1989); the authors assumed that the effects of adrenaline were mediated by α_2-adrenoceptors, but it was not possible to reach a definitive interpretation in view of the non-selective nature of the drugs used. The prolactin response to cerebroventricular infusion of nicotine appears to be blocked by antagonists of α_1-, α_2- and β-adrenoceptors (Matta and Sharp, 1992). Thus, while there are no reports on the effects on prolactin secretion of cerebroventricular infusions of selective α_1-adrenergic agonists in the rat, the above studies make it likely that in rats, as in humans, activation of α_1-adrenoceptors located in the brain stimulates the secretion of prolactin.

The physiological significance of the stimulant α_1-adrenoceptors in the control of prolactin secretion in humans is as yet unknown. The prolactin response to hypoglycaemia was unaffected by the selective α_1-antagonist prazosin, even though it was given in doses that caused drowsiness, indicating blockade of central adrenergic receptors (Tatar and Vigas, 1984). Further studies in humans should be directed at more physiological stimuli of the secretion of prolactin. The findings that phenoxybenzamine and prazosin prevented the elevation of serum prolactin concentrations on the afternoon of pro-oestrus (Subramanian and Gala, 1976a,b; Clemens and Shaar, 1980) suggest that α_1-adrenoceptors may play a role in the physiological control of prolactin secretion in the rat.

α_2-Adrenoceptors

The available evidence in humans suggests that, as in the case of ACTH, α_2-adrenoceptors are not involved in the control of prolactin secretion under basal conditions, but they exert an inhibitory influence under some situations when prolactin secretion is stimulated.

In humans under basal conditions, the secretion of prolactin is unaffected by the α_2-antagonists yohimbine, idazoxan and atipamezole (Bouloux et al, 1986; Al-Damluji et al, 1988; Karhuvaara et al, 1990), or by the α_2-agonists clonidine and guanfacine (Lal et al, 1975; Lancranjan and Marbach, 1977). This suggests that there is no tonic inhibition of prolactin secretion by α_2-adrenoceptors in humans. However, it seems that such an inhibitory effect may operate when secretion of the hormone is increased by certain stimuli. Thus, the prolactin response to hypoglycaemia in humans was inhibited by the α_2-agonist guanfacine (Lancranjan et al, 1978) and enhanced by the α_2-antagonist yohimbine (Tatar and Vigas, 1984). Enhancement of the prolactin response to hypoglycaemia by yohimbine (Tatar and Vigas, 1984) suggests that, during this stimulus, brain adrenaline or noradrenaline exert an inhibitory effect on the secretion of prolactin.

The site of this α_2-inhibition is likely to be in the brain, rather than directly in the pituitary; guanfacine does not inhibit prolactin secretion in humans who have been given the dopaminergic antagonist metoclopramide, which increases serum prolactin concentrations by a direct action on the pituitary (Lancranjan et al, 1978). Although a recently developed lactotroph cell line from a rat pituitary tumour has been found to possess α_2-adrenoceptors whose activation inhibits prolactin secretion (Judd and MacLeod, 1991), the available evidence suggests that this effect does not operate in humans (see below). In humans the prolactin response to hypoglycaemia is not mediated by adrenergic mechanisms (Lauridsen et al, 1983; Tatar and Vigas, 1984); it therefore seems likely that the inhibitory α_2-adrenoceptors (Lancranjan et al, 1978) are located postsynaptically.

Clonidine was also reported to inhibit prolactin secretion in suckling rats (Lien et al, 1986). However, the role of α_2-adrenoceptors in the control of prolactin secretion in experimental animals has been the subject of considerable controversy. Particularly puzzling has been the finding in some experiments that peripheral administration of both α_2-agonists and α_2-antagonists stimulates prolactin secretion in rats; this has been described as the 'α_2 paradox' (Jurcovicova et al, 1989a,b; Krulich et al, 1989). Furthermore, idazoxan, which is one of the most selective and potent α_2-antagonists (Ruffolo et al, 1988), inhibits secretion of prolactin (Jurcovicova et al, 1989b; Preziosi et al, 1989). α_2-Adrenoceptors are a heterogeneous group (Bylund, 1988) whose activation may lead either to inhibition of adenylate cyclase or stimulation of polyphosphoinositide hydrolysis (Cotecchia et al, 1990). It is possible that the apparently paradoxical effects of the α_2-adrenergic drugs may be explicable on the basis of actions on different receptor subtypes. The reason that these 'paradoxical effects' are not seen in humans could be that larger relative doses were used in the rats, leading to activation of multiple receptors.

β-Adrenoceptors

No clear evidence exists for a role for β-adrenoceptors in the control of prolactin secretion in humans. In two placebo-controlled studies, propranolol had no effect on serum prolactin concentrations under basal conditions (Saxton et al, 1981; Dart et al, 1982) and the prolactin response to hypoglycaemia is uninfluenced by propranolol or atenolol (Lauridsen et al, 1983). However, in anaesthetized rats, the prolactin response to cerebroventricular administration of the noradrenaline precursor L-DOPS could be blocked by propranolol (Koshiyama et al, 1987). The prolactin response to cerebroventricular infusion of nicotine in awake rats appears to be blocked by antagonists of α_1-, α_2- and β-adrenoceptors (Matta and Sharp, 1992). Peripheral administration of propranolol reduced the oestrogen surge in ovariectomized, oestrogen-treated rats (Subramanian and Gala, 1976a,b), and cerebroventricular infusion of a β_2-antagonist reduced the prolactin response to immobilization stress (Haanwinckel et al, 1991). It is therefore likely that central β-adrenoceptor activation exerts a stimulant effect on prolactin secretion in the rat. Further studies on the effects of β-blockers on the prolactin responses to physiological stimuli in both humans and rats would be of interest.

Circulating catecholamines

High concentrations of adrenaline and noradrenaline inhibit the secretion of prolactin from pituitary cells in vitro (MacLeod, 1969; Birge et al, 1970; Koch et al, 1970), but these effects can be blocked by sulpiride and domperidone, indicating that they are mediated by dopaminergic receptors (Denef and Baes, 1982; Ishibashi and Yamaji, 1984). The minimum concentrations at which adrenaline and noradrenaline inhibit prolactin secretion in vitro were 24 to 100 nmol/litre (Shaar and Clemens, 1974; Hoefer et al, 1984; Ishibashi and Yamaji, 1984). These concentrations are not seen under physiological conditions in the peripheral plasma of humans or rats (Kvetnansky et al, 1978; Robertson et al, 1979), or even in plasma from the lesioned pituitary stalk of anaesthetized humans or rats (Paradisi et al, 1989; Thomas et al, 1989a). In hyperprolactinaemic states caused by prolonged interruption of the delivery of catecholamines to the pituitary, intravenous infusions of adrenaline and noradrenaline inhibit prolactin secretion in humans and sheep (Nicoletti et al, 1984; Thomas et al, 1989b). Interruption of the delivery of catecholamines to the pituitary causes upregulation of pituitary receptors (Cheung and Weiner, 1976; Heiman and Ben-Jonathan, 1983), which would have increased the sensitivity of the lactotrophs to the actions of infused catecholamines. Intravenous infusion of noradrenaline has no effect on the secretion of prolactin in humans (Al-Damluji et al, 1989; Al-Damluji and Francis, 1993), but this does not exclude the possibility that circulating catecholamines may inhibit the prolactin response to some physiological stimuli. The demonstration that intravenous infusion of an α_1-adrenergic agonist that crosses the blood–brain barrier stimulates prolactin secretion in humans (Al-Damluji and Francis, 1993) indicates that any inhibition of prolactin secretion at the pituitary is likely to be of minor importance compared with the stimulant action of central α_1-adrenoceptors.

While peripheral administration of adrenaline and noradrenaline had no stimulant effect on prolactin secretion in rats or humans (Mougey et al, 1986; Al-Damluji and Francis, 1993), activation of β-adrenoceptors on cultured rat pituitary cells was found to stimulate prolactin secretion (Denef and Baes, 1982). The effect was transient, presumably due to rapid desensitization of the response (Denef and Baes, 1982). It is likely that this effect represents supersensitivity of the adrenoceptors on the pituitary cells, which were grown in the absence of catecholamines. Thus, β-adrenergic agonists did not stimulate the secretion of prolactin from freshly dispersed pituitary cells in vitro (Perkins et al, 1985).

ADRENERGIC CONTROL OF THE SECRETION OF TSH

The secretion of TSH from the pituitary thyrotrophs is under the control of the hypothalamic TRH. TRH neurones with cell bodies in the periventricular region of the paraventricular nucleus (adjacent to the third ventricle) project to the zona externa of the median eminence and secrete their products into the long portal vessels of the hypothalamo–hypophysial portal system (Lechan and Jackson, 1982; Jackson and Lechan, 1985). These TRH neurones are innervated by adrenergic (PNMT) and noradrenergic neurones, with which they make synaptic connections (Shioda et al, 1986; Liposits et al, 1987). In addition, neurones that synthesize TRH are widely distributed in the central nervous system, including the hypothalamus, where they appear to serve a variety of other functions. Thyroid hormones exert a negative feedback effect both on the secretion of TRH from the hypothalamus (Belchetz et al, 1978) and on TSH from the pituitary (Vale et al, 1974). Somatostatin also inhibits the secretion of both TRH (Hirooka et al, 1978) and TSH (Vale et al, 1974). Dopamine exerts a modest inhibitory effect on the secretion of TSH in rats and humans, but the more powerful feedback effects of thyroid hormones tend to minimize the inhibitory action of dopamine (Scanlon et al, 1979; Tuomisto and Mannisto, 1985).

α_1-Adrenoceptors

In humans methoxamine stimulated the secretion of TSH but the effect was not reproduced by an equipotent dose of noradrenaline (Figure 5) (Al-Damluji et al, 1989; Al-Damluji and Francis, 1993). This indicated that, as in the case of ACTH and prolactin, activation of α_1-adrenoceptors that are located in the brain could stimulate the secretion of TSH. These stimulant α_1-adrenoceptors may play a role in the control of TSH secretion under some circumstances in humans; in hypothyroid patients the α_1-antagonist thymoxamine reduced the exaggerated nocturnal surge of TSH secretion, indicating that the increase in TSH secretion in hypothyroidism is mediated in part by α_1-adrenoceptors (Valcavi et al, 1987). Thymoxamine had no effect on the nocturnal pattern of TSH secretion in euthyroid subjects, indicating that the nocturnal surge of TSH secretion in humans is not mediated by α_1-adrenoceptors (Valcavi et al, 1987). This is similar to the lack of effect of α_1-antagonists on the nocturnal pattern of cortisol secretion in humans (Al-Damluji et al, 1987b).

The stimulant effect of methoxamine on the secretion of TSH was relatively weak, so the differences between the effects of methoxamine and noradrenaline were not as clear as in the case of ACTH and prolactin (Figure 5). Noradrenaline seemed to reduce the circadian fall of TSH secretion, although the effect was not statistically significant. It is possible that, in the case of TSH, the stimulant α_1-adrenoceptors are located both in the brain and in the median eminence, which is accessible to infused noradrenaline (Samorajski and Marks, 1962). Arancibia et al (1989) have obtained evidence in rats suggesting that α_1-adrenoceptors located in the median eminence may exert a stimulant effect on the secretion of TSH (see below).

The role of adrenergic mechanisms in the control of secretion of TSH in the rat has been controversial (for review, see Tuomisto and Mannisto, 1985). Adrenaline, noradrenaline and phenylephrine stimulate the secretion of TRH from hypothalamic fragments in vitro and the effects are blocked by prazosin (Grimm and Reichlin, 1973; Hirooka et al, 1978;

Tapia-Arancibia et al, 1985). Infusion of phenylephrine into the median eminence of conscious rats causes an increase in the release of TRH (Tapia-Arancibia et al, 1985). In conscious rats with cannulae in the median eminence, local infusion of prazosin inhibited the secretion of TRH in response to cold exposure (Arancibia et al, 1989), suggesting that α_1-adrenoceptors located in the median eminence may be important in the physiological control of TSH secretion in these animals. In spite of the apparently clear evidence that activation of α_1-adrenoceptors stimulates the secretion of TSH in rats, Krulich et al (1982) reported that methoxamine inhibited the secretion of TSH in rats in vivo and the effect was antagonized by prazosin. Although the data on the adrenergic control of TSH secretion in rats are controversial, there is a considerable amount of evidence that is compatible with the finding in humans that activation of α_1-adrenoceptors located in the brain stimulates the secretion of TSH.

Experiments that utilized inhibitors of PNMT in rats suggested that the α_1-adrenoceptors may be activated by endogenous adrenaline as well as noradrenaline; however, interpretation of the data was somewhat clouded by the fact that the PNMT inhibitors possess antagonist activity at α-adrenoceptors (Terry, 1986).

α_2- and β-adrenoceptors

There is no clear evidence for the involvement of α_2- or β-adrenoceptors in the control of TSH secretion in humans; under basal conditions, the secretion of TSH was unaffected by clonidine, yohimbine, idazoxan or propranolol (Lal et al, 1975; Goldberg et al, 1986; Al-Damluji et al, 1988; Birk Lauridsen et al, 1976). The evidence in the rat is less clear. The secretion of TRH from rat hypothalamic fragments was unaffected by clonidine, and yohimbine and propranolol had no effect on the TRH response to noradrenaline (Tapia-Arancibia et al, 1985). These findings are compatible with those in humans. However, peripheral administration of the α_2-agonist clonidine stimulated the secretion of TSH, and the effect was antagonized by yohimbine but not by prazosin; administration of yohimbine alone reduced plasma TSH concentrations (Krulich et al, 1982; Jaffer et al, 1991). This would imply a stimulant effect of α_2-adrenoceptors on the secretion of TSH. Some investigators found that peripheral administration of β-agonists inhibited the secretion of TSH in rats (Jaffer et al, 1991), implying that activation of β-adrenoceptors exerts an inhibitory effect on the secretion of TSH.

Thus, there is an apparent inconsistency between the lack of effect of α_2- and β-adrenoceptors on the secretion of TRH by hypothalamic fragments in vitro (Tapia-Arancibia et al, 1985), and the reported stimulant effects of α_2-adrenoceptors and the inhibitory effects of β-adrenoceptors on the secretion of TSH in vivo (Krulich et al, 1982; Jaffer et al, 1991). This may be due to the effects of the adrenergic manipulations on the secretion of somatostatin, which inhibits the secretion of TSH; activation of α_2-adrenoceptors inhibits the secretion of somatostatin (which would result in an increase in the secretion of TSH), whereas activation of β-adrenoceptors stimulates the secretion of somatostatin (which would inhibit TSH secretion). The effects of adrenergic manipulations on the secretion of somatostatin are discussed below.

Circulating catecholamines

Activation of α_1-adrenoceptors on cultured adenohypophysial cells stimulates the secretion of TSH (Klibanski et al, 1983; Peters et al, 1983). Caution is required in interpreting these data, as α_1-adrenoceptors are not demonstrable in the anterior pituitary in vivo (Battaglia et al, 1983; De Souza and Kuyatt, 1987). This suggests that pituitary cells may undergo changes in the expression of adrenergic receptors during incubation in vitro. As indicated above, intravenous infusion of noradrenaline had no stimulant effect on the secretion of TSH in humans. The TSH response to TRH was unaffected by α- or β-adrenergic agonists or antagonists in humans (Birk Lauridsen et al, 1976), suggesting that catecholamines do not modulate the secretion of TSH directly in the pituitary.

ADRENERGIC CONTROL OF THE SECRETION OF GROWTH HORMONE

The secretory activity of the pituitary somatotrophs is controlled by two important hypothalamic peptides, GHRH and somatostatin. The cell bodies of the GHRH neurones are in the arcuate nucleus and those of the somatostatin neurones are in the periventricular region of the paraventricular nucleus. The axons project to the zona externa of the median eminence, where the peptides are released into the portal circulation. Adrenergic and noradrenergic nerve terminals innervate both the arcuate nucleus and the periventricular region of the paraventricular nucleus (Bosler et al, 1987; Liposits et al, 1990).

The secretion of growth hormone is stimulated by GHRH and inhibited by somatostatin. In addition, both growth hormone itself and somatomedin, produced in the liver in response to growth hormone, exert negative feedback effects on the hypothalamo–somatotroph unit. In addition to the interaction of GHRH and somatostatin at the level of the pituitary, the GHRH neurones in the arcuate nucleus are innervated by somatostatinergic fibres (Liposits et al, 1988) and somatostatin appears to exert a tonic inhibitory effect on the secretion of GHRH (Plotsky and Vale, 1985). Generation of a growth hormone pulse appears to involve a reduction in the tonic inhibitory somatostatinergic influence, which results in a pulse of GHRH being secreted into the portal circulation (Plotsky and Vale, 1985). While somatostatin concentrations are low, this pulse of GHRH results in a pulse of growth hormone. Thus, the secretion of the two antagonistic peptides, somatostatin and GHRH, is integrated in a reciprocal manner, allowing the physiological secretion of growth hormone to take place in a characteristic pulsatile pattern, which is most evident during sleep. Emerging evidence suggests that the central adrenergic system modulates the secretion of growth hormone by dual actions on both somatostatin and GHRH.

α₂-Adrenoceptors

There is a considerable amount of evidence indicating that central adrenergic pathways acting on α₂-adrenoceptors stimulate the secretion of growth hormone in both humans and experimental animals. Muller et al (1968) reported that intracerebroventricular injection of noradrenaline depleted the growth hormone content of the pituitary, implying release of growth hormone into the bloodstream. The secretion of growth hormone was reduced by depletion of hypothalamic catecholamines with reserpine or 6-hydroxydopamine, and by inhibitors of catecholamine synthesis; under these conditions, administration of the α₂-agonist clonidine stimulated the secretion of growth hormone. These findings indicated that the central adrenergic neural pathways exerted a stimulant effect on the secretion of growth hormone by acting on postsynaptic α₂-adrenoceptors. For an expert account of these early studies, the reader is referred to the review by Muller (1987).

Adrenaline is likely to be the main endogenous catecholamine acting on the α₂-adrenoceptors; inhibition of the synthesis of adrenaline reduced the secretion of growth hormone, and the effect was reversed by clonidine (Terry et al, 1982). Activation of α₂-adrenoceptors stimulated the secretion of GHRH from rat hypothalamic slices in vitro (Kabayama et al, 1986; Tsagarakis et al, 1989), and pretreatment with antiserum to GHRH abolished the growth hormone response to clonidine in rats (Miki et al, 1984). It is likely that activation of postsynaptic α₂-adrenoceptors may, in addition, inhibit the secretion of somatostatin (Ishikawa et al, 1983). Clonidine does not stimulate the secretion of growth hormone directly from the rat pituitary (Alba-Roth et al, 1989).

Clonidine stimulates the secretion of growth hormone in humans (Lal et al, 1975). There is indirect evidence from human studies that the action of clonidine is exerted via both stimulation of GHRH (Alba-Roth et al, 1989) and inhibition of somatostatin (Valcavi et al, 1988; Devesa et al, 1990). This would be analogous to the data obtained in rats described above. Under basal conditions, administration of the selective α₂-antagonist idazoxan had no effect on the secretion of growth hormone in humans (Al-Damluji et al, 1988). However, phentolamine and yohimbine reduced the growth hormone response to hypoglycaemia (Blackard and Heidingsfelder, 1968; Tatar and Vigas, 1984). These studies indicate that activation of α₂-adrenoceptors is partly responsible for the increase in secretion of growth hormone under some circumstances in humans.

Clonidine as a treatment for short stature

While administration of growth hormone is the standard method of treating short stature, it suffers from disadvantages such as the expense of the treatment and the necessity of giving injections several times a week (Anonymous, 1989). These problems have prompted a search for pharmacological methods of stimulating the secretion of endogenous growth hormone, particularly as abnormalities of growth hormone secretion frequently appear to be due to alterations in the secretion of hypothalamic hormones and neurotransmitters rather than abnormalities of the pituitary somatotrophs (Grossman et al, 1983).

Oral administration of clonidine was proposed as a clinical test to identify children with growth hormone deficiency (Gil-Ad et al, 1979) and subsequent clinical studies investigated the possibility of using clonidine as a treatment of short stature. In preliminary, uncontrolled studies, administration of clonidine seemed to improve the growth of short children with partial growth hormone deficiency (Pintor et al, 1985, 1987; Castro-Magana et al, 1986). However, in a subsequent placebo-controlled study, clonidine had no effect on the growth of short children with normal growth hormone responses to provocative stimuli (Pescovitz and Tan, 1988). In a more recent controlled study, clonidine was reported to accelerate the growth of short children with normal growth hormone secretion, although in the dose used clonidine was not as effective as treatment with growth hormone (Volta et al, 1991).

Whether clonidine really accelerates the growth of short children is therefore still unclear, but it is possible that the drug may have a small effect in the doses that have been used. In any case, there is no information on whether the effect of clonidine observed in these short-term studies results in improved final height. Administration of drugs to normal children raises interesting ethical, clinical and social issues (Lantos et al, 1989), but the data obtained so far should encourage further studies that aim to develop improved pharmacological manipulations for stimulating the secretion of endogenous growth hormone which may be of use to patients who would genuinely benefit from such treatment (Hindmarsh and Brook, 1987; Anonymous, 1990).

α_1-Adrenoceptors

In rats, intracerebroventricular administration of methoxamine and phenylephrine inhibited the secretion of growth hormone, and the effects were antagonized by prazosin (Krulich et al, 1982). This indicated that activation of central α_1-adrenoceptors exerted an inhibitory effect on the secretion of growth hormone in rats. A similar conclusion was reached in the dog (Cella et al, 1984). The inhibitory effect of these α_1-adrenoceptors appears to be exerted via stimulation of the secretion of somatostatin, which in turn inhibits the secretion of growth hormone (Epelbaum et al, 1981). Activation of α_1-adrenoceptors stimulated the secretion of GHRH from rat hypothalamic slices in vitro (Tsagarakis et al, 1989), but it is likely that this effect is counteracted by a more prominent action of α_1-adrenoceptors on the secretion of somatostatin; the overall effect of activation of α_1-adrenoceptors in vivo is inhibition of the secretion of growth hormone in rats, dogs and humans (see below).

Imura et al (1971) reported that intravenous infusion of α_1-adrenergic agonists in humans was associated with a small increase in the secretion of growth hormone, but the changes may well have been due to the spontaneous pulsatile secretory pattern of this hormone. In our studies,

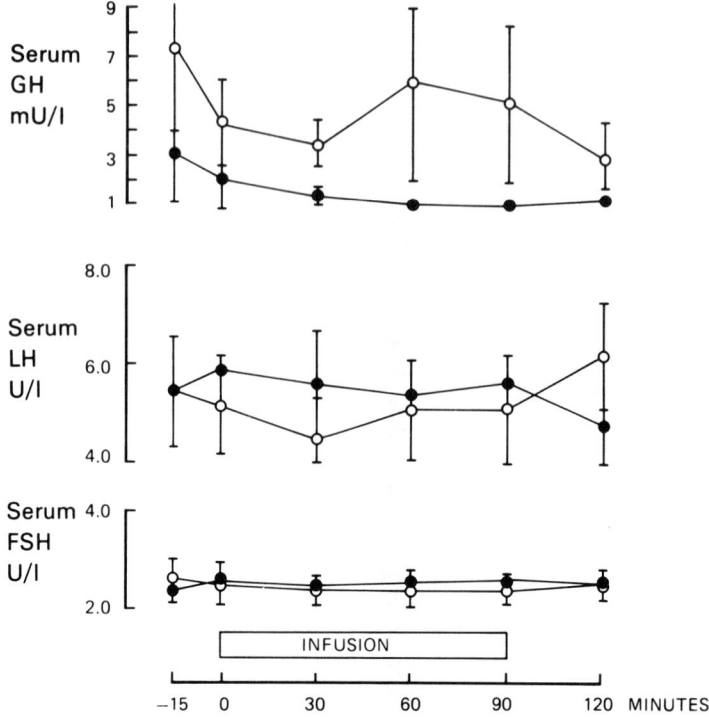

Figure 7. The effect of methoxamine and saline on the plasma concentrations of growth hormone (GH) luteinizing hormone (LH) and follicle-stimulating hormone (FSH) in six men. Methoxamine was infused as described in the legend to Figure 5. ○ = saline; ● = methoxamine.

methoxamine had no stimulant effect on the secretion of growth hormone in normal volunteers. In fact, plasma growth hormone concentrations were lower during infusion of the α_1-agonist than during placebo. The differences were not statistically significant, presumably due to the spontaneous pulsatile secretion of growth hormone during the placebo infusion (Figure 7). An inhibitory effect would be compatible with the data in rats and dogs described above. It may be possible to demonstrate an inhibitory α_1-adrenergic effect in humans if methoxamine or phenylephrine are infused during a manoeuvre that stimulates the secretion of growth hormone. Although catecholamines are clearly involved in mediating the growth hormone response to hypoglycaemia (Blackard and Heidingsfelder, 1968; Tatar and Vigas, 1984), prazosin had no effect on the growth hormone response to this stimulus in humans (Tatar and Vigas, 1984). There is no information on the effects of selective α_1-antagonists on the growth hormone responses to more physiological stimuli. However, the available data suggest that endogenous catecholamines acting on α_1-adrenoceptors are unlikely to play an important inhibitory role in the secretion of growth hormone; the inhibitory action of catecholamines appears to be exerted predominantly via β-adrenoceptors.

β-Adrenoceptors

Activation of central β-adrenoceptors inhibits the secretion of growth hormone. Administration of propranolol has no effect on the secretion of growth hormone under basal conditions in humans (Blackard and Heidingsfelder, 1968), but it does augment the growth hormone response to drugs that increase the release of endogenous catecholamines, such as amphetamines and desipramine (Rees et al, 1970; Laakmann et al, 1986). It therefore seems that release of endogenous catecholamines from the nerve terminals in the hypothalamus results in activation of both α_2-adrenoceptors which stimulate the secretion of growth hormone and β-adrenoceptors which inhibit secretion of the hormone (Figure 8). The α_2-adrenoceptors predominate, such that the overall effect of amphetamines and desipramine is to increase the secretion of growth hormone. Intravenous infusion of adrenaline has no effect on growth hormone secretion in humans, but the combination of adrenaline and propranolol stimulates the secretion of growth hormone (Massara and Strumia, 1970). It therefore seems that intravenous infusion of adrenaline

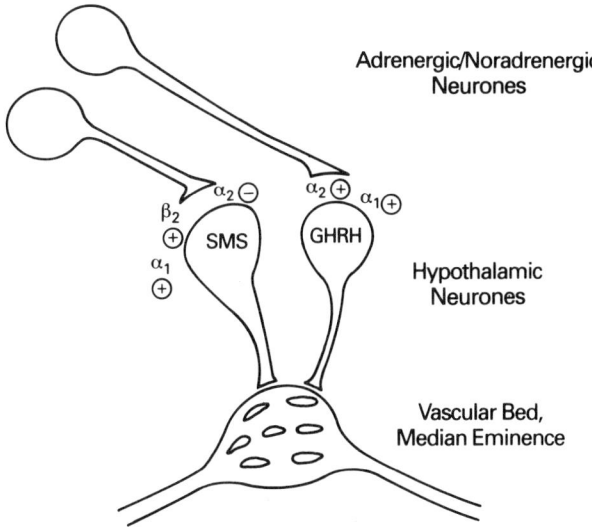

Figure 8. Schematic representation of a hypothetical model of the effects of central noradrenergic neurones on the secretion of growth hormone. When adrenaline or noradrenaline are released from the nerve terminals, both α_2- and β-adrenoceptors are activated. The α_2-adrenoceptors stimulate the secretion of GHRH and inhibit the secretion of somatostatin (SMS), resulting in an increase in the secretion of growth hormone. The β-adrenoceptors stimulate the secretion of somatostatin, which attenuates the growth hormone response. The effect of the α_2-adrenoceptors predominates, such that drugs like amphetamines and tricyclic antidepressants cause an overall increase in the secretion of growth hormone. The inhibitory action of the β-adrenoceptors is readily demonstrable, as propranolol enhances the growth hormone response to most stimuli. Activation of postsynaptic α_1-adrenoceptors also stimulates the secretion of somatostatin, resulting in inhibition of the secretion of growth hormone. However, this is a minor effect compared with the inhibitory β-adrenergic mechanism.

activates both α_2- and β-adrenoceptors; propranolol unmasks the opposing actions of these two receptors, which are presumably located in the median eminence (which is accessible to infused catecholamines; Samorajski and Marks, 1962).

The β_2-adrenergic agonist salbutamol inhibits the growth hormone response to GHRH in humans (Camanni et al, 1989). On the basis of studies on rat hypothalamic slices in vitro, it seems likely that the effect of the inhibitory β_2-adrenoceptors is exerted via stimulation of the secretion of somatostatin, which in turn inhibits the secretion of growth hormone (Epelbaum et al, 1981).

Activation of β-adrenoceptors stimulates the secretion of growth hormone from rat pituitary cells in vitro (Perkins et al, 1985). This mechanism is not evident in vivo, presumably because it is a minor effect compared with the stimulant action of β-adrenoceptors on the secretion of somatostatin, which results in an overall inhibition of growth hormone secretion (see above).

Propranolol has no significant effect on the secretion of growth hormone during waking hours in humans (Blackard and Heidingsfelder, 1968; Mauras et al, 1987), but the inhibitory β-adrenoceptors appear to attenuate the growth hormone response to various stimuli, such as exercise and hypoglycaemia (Blackard and Heidingsfelder, 1968; Hansen, 1971; Kelijman and Frohman, 1989). β-Adrenergic blockade with propranolol or atenolol also enhanced the growth hormone responses to GHRH in children of short and normal stature and in adult men (Chihara et al, 1985; Mauras et al, 1987; Kelijman and Frohman, 1989). These findings may indicate involvement of β-adrenoceptors in the negative feedback effect of growth hormone on the hypothalamo–pituitary unit; following administration of GHRH, the increase in secretion of growth hormone may increase the turnover of catecholamines in the hypothalamus, resulting in activation of β-adrenoceptors which then stimulate secretion of somatostatin. Administration of β-blockers would remove this negative feedback effect and enhance the effect of GHRH. This possible mechanism was investigated in humans (Kelijman and Frohman, 1989), but the authors were unable to reach a definitive conclusion.

Propranolol and atenolol had no effect on the spontaneous nocturnal pulsatile secretion of growth hormone in short children or in adult men (Martha et al, 1988, 1990; Kelijman and Frohman, 1989). This was a surprising finding as the same dose of β-blockers enhanced the growth hormone response to hypoglycaemia and GHRH during waking hours. The implication from these data is that the nocturnal secretion of growth hormone in humans is not regulated by the inhibitory β-adrenoceptors, but that these receptors do modulate the growth hormone response to various stimuli during waking hours. This seems analogous to the finding that central α_1-adrenoceptors are involved in controlling the secretory activity of the hypothalamo–pituitary adrenal axis during waking hours but not at night (Al-Damluji et al, 1987b). It is possible that, as in the case of ACTH, the secretion of growth hormone during sleep is regulated by different neurotransmitters from those involved during waking hours.

ADRENERGIC CONTROL OF THE SECRETION OF GONADOTROPHINS

Secretion of the gonadotrophins is stimulated by the hypothalamic GnRH. During embryonic development, the GnRH neurones arise in the olfactory placode and migrate posteriorly to the preoptic area in the medial basal hypothalamus (Schwanzel-Fukuda and Pfaff, 1989; Wray et al, 1989). The axons terminate in the zona externa of the median eminence, where GnRH is secreted into the portal vascular plexus. GnRH is secreted in a characteristic pulsatile manner, resulting in pulsatile secretion of the gonadotrophins.

Gonadal steroids influence the hypothalamo–pituitary unit in a complex manner. In addition to the classical negative feedback effects, oestrogens are capable of exerting a positive feedback action that is believed to be responsible in part for the mid-cycle surge in the secretion of luteinizing hormone (LH). Gonadal steroids may also influence the turnover of brain catecholamines by direct interactions with receptors for steroid hormones in the brain. In addition, brain enzymes may transform gonadal steroids in several ways, including aromatization of androgens to oestrogens, 5α-reduction of testosterone and catecholoestrogens production. Catecholoestrogens may in turn influence hypothalamic function by binding as competitive antagonists to oestrogen receptors, or by inhibiting the activity of some of the enzymes that degrade catecholamines in the brain.

The GnRH neurones of the rat are innervated by noradrenergic nerve terminals (Hoffman et al, 1982; Chen et al, 1989). In rats, there is a large amount of evidence indicating that brain catecholamines acting on α_1-adrenoceptors stimulate secretion of the gonadotrophins. This mechanism is important in the physiological control of the secretion of gonadotrophins in a number of circumstances in rats, including the pulsatile secretory pattern of LH, the increase in LH secretion in pro-oestrus, and the LH response to the administration of progesterone in oestrogen-primed, ovariectomized rats. Most investigators found that β-adrenergic antagonists had no effect on the secretion of gonadotrophins in rats. For a discussion of the early literature on this subject, the reader is referred to the reviews by Barraclough and Wise (1982) and Kalra and Kalra (1983); for more recent data, see Leposavic et al (1990), Jarry et al (1990) and Gearing and Terasawa (1991) and the references therein.

There is a close similarity in the menstrual cycles of women and rhesus monkeys (Knobil, 1974). In early studies, infusion of large doses of noradrenaline into the third ventricle had no stimulant effect on the secretion of LH or follicle-stimulating hormone (FSH) (Knobil, 1974), but more recent work has indicated that infusion of noradrenaline and methoxamine into the median eminence stimulates the secretion of GnRH in ovariectomized rhesus monkeys (Terasawa et al, 1988). In ovariectomized monkeys, the pulsatile secretion of LH and GnRH was interrupted by intravenous administration of phentolamine, phenoxybenzamine and prazosin, whereas yohimbine and propranolol had no effect (Bhattacharya et al, 1972; Kaufman et al, 1985; Gearing and Terasawa, 1991). These data indicated involvement of the central α_1-adrenoceptors in the pulsatile activity of GnRH neurones in ovariectomized rhesus monkeys.

Experiments on rat hypothalamic fragments in vitro suggest that the effects of the α_1-adrenoceptors may be exerted directly on the GnRH neurones (Negro-Vilar et al, 1979; Leposavic et al, 1990). However, emerging evidence suggests that noradrenaline is not directly responsible for the pulsatile secretion of LH. Thus, prazosin reduces the amplitude but not the frequency of GnRH pulses in the median eminence (Gearing and Terasawa, 1991), and the pulsatile release of noradrenaline into the preoptic hypothalamic area does not always correlate with the LH secretory pattern (Jarry et al, 1990). Further, recent evidence indicates that a GnRH neuronal cell line releases GnRH in a spontaneous pulsatile secretory pattern, independent of the presence of neurotransmitters (Escalera et al, 1992; Krsmanovic et al, 1992; Westel et al, 1992). It therefore seems likely that GnRH neurones possess an intrinsic pacemaker activity that may be modulated by catecholamines acting on α_1-adrenoceptors.

In spite of the clear evidence that central α_1-adrenoceptors stimulate the secretion of LH in rats and monkeys, it has not been possible to demonstrate such an effect in humans. α-Adrenergic receptor blockade with effective doses of phentolamine, phenoxybenzamine and thymoxamine did not diminish the pulsatile secretory pattern of LH in normal men or women (Santen and Bardin, 1973; Veldhuis et al, 1983; Paradisi et al, 1987), and thymoxamine did not reduce the elevated plasma LH concentrations observed in the polycystic ovary syndrome (Paradisi et al, 1987). Methoxamine and prazosin had no effect on the secretion of LH in normal men (Figure 7) (Al-Damluji and Francis, 1993). The doses of methoxamine and prazosin were effective at central α_1-adrenoceptors: methoxamine stimulated the secretion of ACTH, prolactin and TSH, while prazosin blocked the effects of methoxamine on the secretion of these hormones and caused the subjects to be drowsy. Noradrenaline infusions had no effect on plasma concentrations of LH or FSH (Barnes et al, 1986; Al-Damluji and Francis, 1993).

Previous investigators had speculated that the lack of effects of α_1-antagonists on the secretion of LH in humans could be due to inadequate doses of the antagonists (Veldhuis et al, 1983; Casper and Yen, 1985). However, we feel that this is an unlikely explanation as we can readily demonstrate the effects of these adrenergic manipulations on the secretion of ACTH, prolactin and TSH; these effects have been shown to be exerted at central locations.

Clonidine, in doses that caused drowsiness and stimulated the secretion of growth hormone, had no effect on the secretion of LH in men (Lal et al, 1975; Kaufman and Vermeulen, 1989) or in postmenopausal women (Tulandi et al, 1983). Women who are amenorrhoeic due to weight loss have low LH pulse frequency; clonidine had no effect on the secretion of LH in these patients (Khoury et al, 1987). However, clonidine is predominantly an α_2-agonist, with only weak activity at α_1-adrenoceptors; it would have been more appropriate to examine the effect of a more potent α_1-agonist such as methoxamine on the secretion of LH in these patients.

While most investigators used adrenergic agonists and antagonists, others examined the effects of blockade of catecholamine synthesis on the secretion of gonadotrophins in humans. The use of α-methyl-p-tyrosine (AMPT) is less selective than adrenergic receptor blockers, as inhibition of tyrosine hydroxylase interrupts the synthesis of dopamine as well as noradrenaline and adrenaline. Nicoletti et al (1981a, 1984) found that AMPT had no effect on the secretion of LH in normal women of reproductive age or in postmenopausal women. However, in a larger dose, this drug appears to stimulate the secretion of LH (Plosker et al, 1991). This may be due to the depletion of dopamine, which inhibits the secretion of LH in humans (Leblanc et al, 1976; Barnes et al, 1986), rather than by an action on the adrenergic system.

The only evidence that I am aware of suggesting involvement of catecholamines in LH secretion in humans was the finding that α-methyldopa inhibited the LH response to progesterone in oestrogen-primed, postmenopausal women (Nicoletti et al, 1981b). The authors found that clonidine did not stimulate LH secretion in these women, so they were unclear how this data should be interpreted (Nicoletti et al, 1981b). α-Methyldopa is converted to α-methylnoradrenaline, which then acts as an agonist at α_2-adrenoceptors. The correct interpretation of these interesting data seems to be that α-methylnoradrenaline, acting on presynaptic α_2-adrenoceptors, may have inhibited the release of noradrenaline from noradrenergic nerve terminals that mediate the LH response to progesterone. This interpretation would be consistent with the data that have implicated the postsynaptic α_1-adrenoceptors in mediating the LH response to progesterone in oestrogen-primed, ovariectomized rats (see above). It is possible that the hypogonadal state may increase the responsiveness of the hypothalamo–pituitary unit to the pharmacological manipulations. Alternatively, the physiological regulation by neurotransmitters may have been altered by the chronic absence of some gonadal steroids; the importance of the steroid milieu in regulating the GnRH responses to activation of α_1-adrenoceptors has been demonstrated in rat hypothalamic fragments in vitro (Leposavic et al, 1990).

In conclusion, despite intensive study, no role can be attributed to noradrenaline in the regulation of gonadotrophin secretion in normal human subjects of reproductive age. However, the suggestion that noradrenaline may be involved in mediating the LH response to progesterone in oestrogen-primed postmenopausal women (Nicoletti et al, 1981b) is consistent with much data in ovariectomized rats and monkeys.

SUMMARY

The hypothalamic hypophysiotrophic neurones are densely innervated by adrenergic and noradrenergic nerve terminals. Activation of α_1-adrenoceptors located in the brain stimulates the secretion of ACTH, prolactin and TSH. The effects of the α_1-adrenoceptors seem to be exerted on hypothalamic neurones that secrete vasopressin, CRH-41 and TRH. These mechanisms are important in the physiological control of the secretion of ACTH and TSH in humans. α_2-Adrenoceptors are not involved in the control of secretion of these hormones under basal conditions in humans. However, α_2-adrenoceptors exert an inhibitory effect that acts as a negative feedback mechanism, limiting excessive secretion of these hormones. There is no convincing evidence for the involvement of β-adrenoceptors in the control of the secretion of these three hormones in humans. Studies on cultured anterior pituitary cells suggested that adrenaline and noradrenaline may influence the secretion of ACTH, prolactin and TSH directly at the level of the pituitary. However, these effects are not demonstrable in humans, and are likely to be due to alterations in the pituitary adrenoceptors during culture.

In the case of growth hormone, activation of α_2-adrenoceptors located in the brain stimulates secretion of this hormone both by increasing the secretion of GHRH and by inhibiting the secretion of somatostatin. Activation of β-adrenoceptors inhibits the secretion of growth hormone via an increase in the secretion of somatostatin. The effects of the central α_2- and β-adrenoceptors are important in the physiological control of growth hormone secretion in humans.

A considerable amount of evidence implicates brain α_1-adrenoceptors in the control of secretion of the gonadotrophins in experimental animals, but, despite intensive study, no convincing evidence has been found in humans of reproductive age.

Acknowledgement

I thank Dr Paul Sawchenko for comments on Figure 1.

REFERENCES

Aguilera G, Kiss A, Hauger R & Tizabi Y (1992) Regulation of the hypothalamic–pituitary–adrenal axis during stress: role of neuropeptides and neurotransmitters. In Kvetnansky R, McCarty R & Axelrod J (eds) *Stress: Neuroendocrine and Molecular Approaches*, pp 363–381. New York: Gordon and Breach Science.

Alba-Roth J, Losa M, Spiess Y, Schopohl J, Muller OA & von Werder K (1989) Interaction of clonidine and GHRH on GH secretion in vivo and in vitro. *Clinical Endocrinology* **30:** 485–491.

Al-Damluji S (1988) Review: adrenergic mechanisms in the control of corticotrophin secretion. *Journal of Endocrinology* **119:** 5–14.

Al-Damluji S (1989) Measuring the activity of brain adrenergic receptors with a neuro-endocrine marker. *Journal of Endocrinology* **123(supplement):** abstract 44.

Al-Damluji S (1991) Measuring the activity of brain adrenergic receptors in man. *Journal of Endocrinological Investigation* **14:** 245–254.

Al-Damluji S & Francis D (1993) Activation of central alpha-1 adrenoceptors in humans stimulates secretion of prolactin and TSH, as well as ACTH. *American Journal of Physiology* (in press).

Al-Damluji S & Grossman A (1985) Adrenergic and opioid control of ACTH secretion in man. *Neuroscience Letters* **22:** S406.

Al-Damluji S & Rees LH (1987) Effects of catecholamines on the secretion of adrenocortico-trophin (ACTH) in man. *Journal of Clinical Pathology* **40:** 1098–1107.

Al-Damluji S & White A (1992) Central noradrenergic lesion impairs the ACTH response to release of endogenous catecholamines. *Journal of Neuroendocrinology* **4:** 319–323.

Al-Damluji S, Tomlin S, Perry L et al (1985) Alpha adrenergic stimulation of ACTH secretion by a specific central mechanism in man. *Journal of Endocrinology* **104(supplement):** abstract 48.

Al-Damluji S, Grossman A & Besser GM (1986) Central alpha-1 adrenoceptors stimulate ACTH secretion in man. *Journal of Physiology* **374:** 45P.

Al-Damluji S, Perry L, Tomlin S et al (1987a) Alpha adrenergic stimulation of corticotropin secretion by a specific central mechanism in man. *Neuroendocrinology* **45:** 68–76.

Al-Damluji S, Cunnah D, Perry L, Grossman A & Besser GM (1987b) The effect of alpha adrenergic manipulation on the 24 hour pattern of cortisol secretion in man. *Clinical Endocrinology* **26:** 61–66.

Al-Damluji S, Iveson T, Pendlebury D, Thomas J, Rees LH & Besser GM (1987c) Food induced cortisol secretion is mediated by central alpha-1 adrenoceptor modulation of pituitary ACTH secretion. *Clinical Endocrinology* **26:** 629–636.

Al-Damluji S, Cunnah D, Grossman A et al (1987d) Effect of adrenaline on basal and ovine corticotrophin-releasing factor-stimulated ACTH secretion in man. *Journal of Endocrinology* **112:** 145–150.

Al-Damluji S, Ross G, Touzell R, Perrett D, White A & Besser GM (1988) Modulation of the actions of tyrosine by alpha-2 adrenoceptor blockade. *British Journal of Pharmacology* **95:** 405–412.

Al-Damluji S, Francis D & Besser GM (1989) Activation of alpha-1 adrenoceptors stimulates prolactin and TSH secretion in man. *Journal of Endocrinological Investigation* **12(supplement 2):** 140.

Al-Damluji S, Thomas R, White A & Besser GM (1990a) Vasopressin mediates alpha-1 adrenergic stimulation of ACTH secretion. *Endocrinology* **126:** 1989.

Al-Damluji S, White A & Besser GM (1990b) Brattleboro rats have deficient adrenocorticotropin responses to activation of central alpha-1 adrenoceptors. *Endocrinology* **127:** 2849–2853.

Al-Damluji S, Bouloux P, White A & Besser GM (1990c) The role of alpha-2 adrenoceptors in the control of ACTH secretion; interaction with the opioid system. *Neuroendocrinology* **51:** 76–81.

Anonymous (1989) Alternatives to growth hormone. *Lancet* **i:** 820–822.

Anonymous (1990) How far should indications for growth hormone treatment expand? *Lancet* **335:** 764.

Antoni FA (1986) Hypothalamic control of adrenocorticotropin secretion: advances since the discovery of 41-residue corticotropin-releasing factor. *Endocrine Reviews* **7:** 351–378.

Arancibia S, Tapia-Arancibia L, Astier H & Assenmacher I (1989) Physiological evidence for alpha-1 adrenergic facilitatory control of the cold-induced TRH release in the rat, obtained by push–pull cannulation of the median eminence. *Neuroscience Letters* **100:** 169–174.

Assenmacher I, Szafarczyk A, Barbanel G et al (1992) Role of catecholaminergic and selected peptidergic systems in the control of hypothalamic–pituitary–adrenocortical responses to stress. In Kvetnansky R, McCarty R & Axelrod J (eds) *Stress: Neuroendocrine and Molecular Approaches*, pp 383–394. New York: Gordon and Breach Science.

Barnes RB, Cha KY, Lee DG & Lobo RA (1986) Modulation of luteinizing hormone immunoreactivity and bioactivity but not norepinephrine in women. *American Journal of Obstetrics and Gynecology* **154:** 445–450.

Barraclough CA & Wise PM (1982) The role of catecholamines in the regulation of pituitary luteinizing hormone and follicle-stimulating hormone secretion. *Endocrine Reviews* **3:** 91–119.

Battaglia G, Shannon M & Titeler M (1983) Initial detection of [^{3}H]prazosin-labelled alpha-1 receptors in the porcine pituitary neurointermediate lobe. *Molecular Pharmacology* **24:** 409–412.

Belchetz PE, Gredley G, Bird D & Himsworth RL (1978) Regulation of thyrotrophin secretion by negative feedback of tri-iodothyronine on the hypothalamus. *Journal of Endocrinology* **76:** 439–448.

Ben-Jonathan N (1985) Dopamine: a prolactin-inhibiting hormone. *Endocrine Reviews* **6:** 564–589.

Berkenbosch F, Tilders FJH & Vermes I (1983) Beta adrenoceptor activation mediates stress-induced secretion of beta-endorphin-related peptides from intermediate but not anterior pituitary. *Nature* **305:** 237–239.

Bertler A (1961) Occurrence and localization of catecholamines in the human brain. *Acta Physiologica Scandinavica* **51:** 97–107.

Bhattacharya AN, Dierschke DJ, Yamaji T & Knobil E (1972) The pharmacologic blockade of the circhoral mode of LH secretion in the ovariectomized rhesus monkey. *Endocrinology* **90:** 778–786.

Birge CA, Jacobs LS, Hammer CT & Daughaday WH (1970) Catecholamine inhibition of prolactin secretion by isolated rat adenohypophyses. *Endocrinology* **86:** 120–130.

Birk Lauridsen U, Faber J, Friis T, Kirkegaard C & Nerup J (1976) Thyrotropin (TSH) release during altered adrenergic alpha and beta receptor influence. *Hormone and Metabolic Research* **8:** 406–407.

Blackard WG & Heidingsfelder SA (1968) Adrenergic receptor control mechanism for growth hormone secretion. *Journal of Clinical Investigation* **47:** 1407–1414.

Bosler O, Beaudet A & Denoroy L (1987) Electron-microscopic characterization of adrenergic axon terminals in the diencephalon of the rat. *Cell and Tissue Research* **248:** 393–398.

Bouloux PMG, Grossman A, Allolio B, Delitala G & Besser GM (1986) Effects of adrenergic antagonism on the growth hormone, prolactin and cortisol response to a synthetic opioid agonist in man. *Hormone Research* **23:** 83–90.

Bylund DB (1988) Subtypes of alpha-2 adrenoceptors: pharmacological and molecular biological evidence converge. *Trends in Pharmacological Sciences* **9:** 356–361.

Calogero AE, Gallucci WT, Chrousos GP & Gold PW (1988) Catecholamine effects upon rat hypothalamic corticotropin-releasing hormone secretion in vitro. *Journal of Clinical Investigation* **82:** 839–846.

Camanni F, Ghigo E, Mazza E et al (1989) Aspects of neurotransmitter control of GH secretion: basic and clinical studies. In Muller EE, Cocchi D & Locatelli V (eds) *Advances in Growth and Growth Factor Research*, pp 263–281. Rome: Pythagora Press.

Carlsson A & Lindqvist M (1978) Dependence of 5-HT and catecholamine synthesis on concentrations of precursor amino acids in rat brain. *Archives of Pharmacology* **303:** 157–164.

Casper RF & Yen SSC (1985) Review: Neuroendocrinology of menopausal flushes: a hypothesis of flush mechanism. *Clinical Endocrinology* **22:** 293–312.

Castro-Magana M, Angulo M, Fuentes B, Castelar ME, Canas A & Espinoza B (1986) Effect of prolonged clonidine administration on growth hormone concentrations and rate of linear growth in children with constitutional growth delay. *Journal of Pediatrics* **109:** 784–787.

Cella SG, Morgese M, Mantegazza P & Muller EE (1984) Inhibitory action of the alpha-1 adrenergic receptor on growth hormone secretion in the dog. *Endocrinology* **114:** 2406–2408.

Chen WP, Witkin JW & Silverman AJ (1989) Gonadotropin releasing hormone (GnRH) neurons are directly innervated by catecholamine terminals. *Synapse* **3:** 288–290.

Cheung CY & Weiner RI (1976) Supersensitivity of anterior pituitary dopamine receptors involved in the inhibition of prolactin secretion following destruction of the medial basal hypothalamus. *Endocrinology* **99:** 914–917.

Chihara K, Kodama H, Kaji H et al (1985) Augmentation by propranolol of growth hormone-releasing hormone-(1-44)-NH$_2$-induced growth hormone release in normal short and normal children. *Journal of Clinical Endocrinology and Metabolism* **61:** 229–233.

Clemens JA & Shaar CJ (1980) Control of prolactin secretion in mammals. *Federation Proceedings* **39:** 2588–2592.

Cotecchia S, Kobilka BK, Daniel KW et al (1990) Multiple second messenger pathways of alpha-adrenergic receptor subtypes expressed in eukaryotic cells. *Journal of Biological Chemistry* **265:** 63–69.

Cummings S & Seybold V (1988) Relationship of alpha-1 and alpha-2 adrenergic binding sites to regions of the paraventricular nucleus of the hypothalamus containing corticotropin-releasing factor and vasopressin neurons. *Neuroendocrinology* **47:** 523–532.

Cuneo RC, Livesey JH, Nicholls MG, Espiner EA & Donald RA (1987) Effect of alpha-1 adrenergic blockade on the hormonal response to hypoglycaemic stress in normal man. *Clinical Endocrinology* **26:** 1–8.

Cunningham ET & Sawchenko PE (1988) Anatomical specificity of noradrenergic inputs to the paraventricular and supraoptic nuclei of the rat hypothalamus. *Journal of Comparative Neurology* **274:** 60–76.

Cunningham ET, Bohn MC & Sawchenko PE (1990) Organization of adrenergic inputs to the paraventricular and supraoptic nuclei of the hypothalamus in the rat. *Journal of Comparative Neurology* **292**: 651–667.

Dart AM, McHardy K & Barber HE (1982) The effect of propranolol on luteinising hormone and prolactin plasma concentrations in hypertensive women. *British Journal of Clinical Pharmacology* **14**: 839–841.

Denef C & Baes M (1982) Beta-adrenergic stimulation of prolactin release from superfused pituitary cell aggregates. *Endocrinology* **111**: 356–358.

De Souza EB (1985) Beta-2 adrenergic receptors in pituitary. *Neuroendocrinology* **41**: 289–296.

De Souza EB & Kuyatt BL (1987) Alpha-1 adrenergic receptors in the neural lobe of the rat pituitary: autoradiographic identification and localization. *Endocrinology* **120**: 2227–2233.

Devesa J, Arce V, Lois N, Tresguerres AF & Lima L (1990) Alpha-2-adrenergic agonism enhances the growth hormone (GH) response to GH-releasing hormone through an inhibition of hypothalamic somatostatin release in normal men. *Journal of Clinical Endocrinology and Metabolism* **71**: 1581–1588.

Donoso AO, Bishop W, Fawcett CP, Krulich L & McCann SM (1971) Effects of drugs that modify brain monoamine concentrations on plasma gonadotropin and prolactin levels in the rat. *Endocrinology* **89**: 774–784.

Dreyfuss F, Burlet A, Tonon MC & Vaudry H (1984) Comparative immunoelectron microscopic localization of corticotropin-releasing factor (CRF-41) and oxytocin in the rat median eminence. *Neuroendocrinology* **39**: 284–287.

Epelbaum J, Tapia-Arancibia L & Kordon C (1981) Noradrenaline stimulates somatostatin release from incubated slices of the amygdala and the hypothalamic preoptic area. *Brain Research* **215**: 393–397.

Escalera GM, Choi ALH & Weiner RI (1992) Generation and synchronization of gonadotropin-releasing hormone (GnRH) pulses: intrinsic properties of the GT1-1 GnRH neuronal cell line. *Proceedings of the National Academy of Sciences of the USA* **89**: 1852–1855.

Ganong WF, Chalett J, Jones H et al (1982) Further characterization of alpha-adrenergic receptors in brain that affect blood pressure and the secretion of ACTH, GH and renin in dogs. *Endocrinologia Experimentalis* **16**: 191–205.

Gearing M & Terasawa E (1991) The alpha-1 adrenergic neuronal system is involved in the pulsatile release of luteinizing hormone-releasing hormone in the ovariectomized female rhesus monkey. *Neuroendocrinology* **53**: 373–381.

Gibson A, Hart SL & Patel S (1986) Effects of 6-hydroxydopamine-induced lesions of the paraventricular nucleus, and of prazosin, on the corticosterone response to restraint in rats. *Neuropharmacology* **25**: 257–260.

Giguere V, Cote J & Labrie F (1981) Characteristics of the alpha-adrenergic stimulation of adrenocorticotropin secretion in rat anterior pituitary cells. *Endocrinology* **109**: 757–762.

Gil-Ad I, Topper E & Laron Z (1979) Oral clonidine as a growth hormone stimulation test. *Lancet* **ii**: 278–280.

Gillies GE, Linton EA & Lowry PJ (1982) Corticotropin releasing activity of the new CRF is potentiated several times by vasopressin. *Nature* **299**: 355–357.

Goldberg MR, Jackson RV, Krakau J, Island DP & Robertson D (1986) Influence of yohimbine on release of anterior pituitary hormones. *Life Sciences* **39**: 395–398.

Gordon R, Spector S, Sjoerdsma A & Udenfriend S (1966) Increased synthesis of norepinephrine and epinephrine in the intact rat during exercise and exposure to cold. *Journal of Pharmacology and Experimental Therapeutics* **153**: 440–447.

Grimm Y & Reichlin S (1973) Thyrotropin-releasing hormone (TRH): neurotransmitter regulation of secretion by mouse hypothalamic tissue in vitro. *Endocrinology* **93**: 626–631.

Grossman A, Savage MO, Wass JAH et al (1983) Growth-hormone-releasing factor in growth hormone deficiency: demonstration of a hypothalamic defect in growth hormone release. *Lancet* **ii**: 137–138.

Haanwinckel MA, Antunes-Rodrigues J & Silva EDC (1991) Role of central beta-adrenoceptors on stress-induced prolactin release in rats. *Hormone and Metabolic Research* **23**: 318–320.

Hansen AP (1971) The effect of adrenergic receptor blockade on the exercise-induced serum growth hormone rise in normals and juvenile diabetics. *Journal of Clinical Endocrinology* **33**: 807–812.

Heiman ML & Ben-Jonathan N (1983) Increase in pituitary dopaminergic receptors after monosodium glutamate treatment. *American Journal of Physiology* **245**: E261–E265.

Hillhouse EW & Milton NGN (1989) Effect of noradrenaline and gamma aminobutyric acid on the secretion of corticotrophin-releasing factor-41 and arginine vasopressin from the rat hypothalamus in vitro. *Journal of Endocrinology* **122:** 719–723.

Hindmarsh PC & Brook CGD (1987) Effect of growth hormone on short normal children. *British Medical Journal* **295:** 573–577.

Hirooka Y, Hollander CS, Suzuki S, Ferdinand P & Juan SI (1978) Somatostatin inhibits release of thyrotropin releasing factor from organ cultures of rat hypothalamus. *Proceedings of the National Academy of Sciences of the USA* **75:** 4509–4513.

Hiwatari M & Johnston CI (1985) Involvement of vasopressin in the cardiovascular effects of intracerebroventricularly administered alpha-1 adrenoceptor agonists in the conscious rat. *Journal of Hypertension* **3:** 613–620.

Hoefer MT, Heiman ML & Ben-Jonathan N (1984) Prolactin secretion by cultured anterior pituitary cells: influence of culture conditions and endocrine status of the pituitary donor. *Molecular and Cellular Endocrinology* **35:** 229–235.

Hoffman GE, Wray S & Goldstein M (1982) Relationship of catecholamines and LHRH: light microscopic study. *Brain Research Bulletin* **9:** 417–430.

Hokfelt T & Fuxe K (1972) Effects of prolactin and ergot alkaloids on the tubero-infundibular dopamine (DA) neurons. *Neuroendocrinology* **9:** 100–122.

Imura H, Kato Y, Ikeda M, Morimoto M & Yawata M (1971) Effect of adrenergic-blocking or -stimulating agents on plasma growth hormone, immunoreactive insulin, and blood free fatty acid levels in man. *Journal of Clinical Investigation* **50:** 1069–1079.

Ishibashi M & Yamaji T (1984) Direct effects of catecholamines, thyrotropin-releasing hormone, and somatostatin on growth hormone and prolactin secretion from adenomatous and nonadenomatous human pituitary cells in culture. *Journal of Clinical Investigation* **73:** 66–78.

Ishikawa K, Suzuki M & Kakegawa T (1983) Localization of alpha-2-adrenergic agonist sensitive area in the hypothalamus for growth hormone release in the rat. *Endocrinologia Japonica* **30:** 397–403.

Jackson IMD & Lechan RM (1985) Immunohistochemical localization in the rat brain of the precursor for thyrotropin-releasing hormone. *Science* **229:** 1097–1099.

Jackson RV, Jackson AJ, Grice JE, Penfold PJ, Armour MB & Bachmann AW (1987) Adrenaline infusion and adrenocorticotrophin (ACTH) and cortisol release in normotensive and hypertensive man. *Clinical and Experimental Pharmacology and Physiology* **14:** 203–208.

Jaffer A, Daniels WMU, Russell VA & Taljaard JJF (1991) The effect of medial forebrain bundle lesion on thyrotropin secretion in the rat. *Neurochemical Research* **16:** 577–581.

Jarry H, Leonhardt S & Wuttke W (1990) A norepinephrine-dependent mechanism in the preoptic/anterior hypothalamic area but not in the mediobasal hypothalamus is involved in the regulation of the gonadotropin-releasing hormone pulse generator in ovariectomized rats. *Neuroendocrinology* **51:** 337–344.

Judd AM & MacLeod RM (1991) Dopamine receptor and adrenoceptor agonists inhibit prolactin release from MMQ cells. *European Journal of Pharmacology* **195:** 101–106.

Jurcovicova J, Le T & Krulich L (1989a) The paradox of alpha-2 adrenergic regulation of prolactin (prl) secretion. I. The prl-releasing action of the alpha-2 receptor agonists. *Brain Research Bulletin* **23:** 417–424.

Jurcovicova J, Le T & Krulich L (1989b) The paradox of alpha-2 adrenergic regulation of prolactin (prl) secretion. II. The prl-releasing action of the alpha-2 receptor antagonists. *Brain Research Bulletin* **23:** 425–432.

Kabayama Y, Kato Y, Murakami Y, Tanaka H & Imura H (1986) Stimulation by alpha-adrenergic mechanisms of the secretion of growth hormone-releasing factor (GRF) from perifused rat hypothalamus. *Endocrinology* **119:** 432–434.

Kalra SP & Kalra PS (1983) Neural regulation of luteinizing hormone secretion in the rat. *Endocrine Reviews* **4:** 311–351.

Karhuvaara S, Kallio A, Koulu M, Scheinin H & Scheinin M (1990) No involvement of alpha-2 adrenoceptors in the regulation of basal prolactin secretion in healthy men. *Psychoneuroendocrinology* **15:** 125–129.

Kaufman JM & Vermeulen A (1989) Lack of effect of the alpha-adrenergic agonist clonidine on pulsatile luteinizing hormone secretion in a double blind study in men. *Journal of Clinical Endocrinology and Metabolism* **68:** 219–222.

Kaufman JM, Kesner JS, Wilson RC & Knobil E (1985) Electrophysiological manifestation of luteinizing hormone-releasing hormone pulse generator activity in the rhesus monkey: influence of alpha-adrenergic and dopaminergic blocking agents. *Endocrinology* **116:** 1327–1333.

Kelijman M & Frohman LA (1989) Beta-adrenergic modulation of growth hormone (GH) autofeedback on sleep-associated and pharmacologically induced GH secretion. *Journal of Clinical Endocrinology and Metabolism* **69:** 1187–1194.

Khoury SA, Reame NE, Kelch RP & Marshall JC (1987) Diurnal patterns of pulsatile luteinizing hormone secretion in hypothalamic amenorrhea: reproducibility and responses to opiate blockade and an alpha-2 adrenergic agonist. *Journal of Clinical Endocrinology and Metabolism* **64:** 755–762.

Kiss A & Aguilera G (1992) Participation of alpha-1 adrenergic receptors in the secretion of hypothalamic corticotropin-releasing hormone during stress. *Neuroendocrinology* (in press).

Kizer JS, Zivin JA, Jacobowitz DM & Kopin IJ (1975) The nyctohemeral rhythm of plasma prolactin: effects of ganglionectomy, pinealectomy, constant light, constant darkness or 6-OH-dopamine administration. *Endocrinology* **96:** 1230–1240.

Klibanski A, Milbury PE, Chin WW & Ridgway EC (1983) Direct adrenergic stimulation of the release of thyrotropin and its subunits from the thyrotrope in vitro. *Endocrinology* **113:** 1244–1249.

Knobil E (1974) On the control of gonadotropin secretion in the rhesus monkey. *Recent Progress in Hormone Research* **30:** 1–46.

Koch Y, Lu KH & Meites J (1970) Biphasic effects of catecholamines on pituitary prolactin release in vitro. *Endocrinology* **87:** 673–675.

Koshiyama H, Kato Y, Ishikawa Y, Murakami Y, Inoue T & Imura H (1987) Stimulation of prolactin release by L-3,4-dihydroxyphenylserine (L-DOPS) via central norepinephrine in the rat. *Life Sciences* **41:** 983–988.

Koshiyama H, Kato Y, Shimatsu A et al (1989) Possible involvement of endogenous opioid peptides in prolactin secretion induced by alpha-2 adrenergic stimulation in rats. *Proceedings of the Society for Experimental Biology and Medicine* **192:** 105–108.

Krsmanovic LZ, Stojilkovic SS, Merelli F, Dufor S, Virmani MA & Catt KJ (1992) Calcium signalling and pulsatile secretion of GnRH. *Proceedings of the National Academy of Sciences of the USA* (in press).

Krulich L, Mayfield MA, Steele MK, McMillen BA, McCann SM & Koenig JI (1982) Differential effects of pharmacological manipulations of central alpha-1 and alpha-2 adrenergic receptors on the secretion of thyrotropin and growth hormone in male rats. *Endocrinology* **110:** 796–804.

Krulich L, Jurcovicova J & Le T (1989) Prolactin release-inhibiting properties of the alpha-2 adrenergic receptor antagonist idazoxan: comparison with yohimbine. *Life Sciences* **44:** 809–818.

Kvetnansky R, Sun CL, Lake CR, Thoa N, Torda T & Kopin IJ (1978) Effect of handling and forced immobilization on rat plasma levels of epinephrine, norepinephrine, and dopamine-beta-hydroxylase. *Endocrinology* **103:** 1868–1874.

Laakmann G, Zygan K, Schoen HW et al (1986) Effect of receptor blockers (methysergide, propranolol, phentolamine, yohimbine and prazosin) on desipramine-induced pituitary hormone stimulation in humans—I. Growth hormone. *Psychoneuroendocrinology* **11:** 447–461.

Lal S, Tolis G, Martin JB, Brown GM & Guyda H (1975) Effect of clonidine on growth hormone, prolactin, luteinizing hormone, and thyroid-stimulating hormone in the serum of normal men. *Journal of Clinical Endocrinology and Metabolism* **41:** 827–832.

Lancranjan I & Marbach P (1977) New evidence for growth hormone modulation by the alpha-adrenergic system in man. *Metabolism: Clinical and Experimental* **26:** 1225–1230.

Lancranjan I, del Pozo E & Ohnhaus E (1978) Inhibitory effect of guanfacine, a central alpha-adrenoceptor agonist, on prolactin secretion stimulated by insulin-induced hypoglycemia. *Journal of Clinical Endocrinology and Metabolism* **47:** 671–674.

Lantos J, Siegler M & Cuttler L (1989) Ethical issues in growth hormone therapy. *Journal of the American Medical Association* **261:** 1020–1024.

Lauridsen UB, Christensen NJ & Lyngsoe J (1983) Effects of nonselective and beta-1-selective blockade on glucose metabolism and hormone responses during insulin-induced hypoglycemia in normal man. *Journal of Clinical Endocrinology and Metabolism* **56:** 876–882.

Leblanc H, Lachelin GCL, Abu-Fadil S & Yen SSC (1976) Effects of dopamine infusion on pituitary hormone secretion in humans. *Journal of Clinical Endocrinology and Metabolism* **43:** 668–674.

Lechan RM & Jackson IMD (1982) Immunohistochemical localization of thyrotropin-releasing hormone in the rat hypothalamus and pituitary. *Endocrinology* **111:** 55–65.

Leibowitz SF, Jhanwar-Uniyal M, Dvorkin B & Makman MH (1982) Distribution of alpha-adrenergic, beta-adrenergic and dopaminergic receptors in discrete hypothalamic areas of rat. *Brain Research* **233:** 97–114.

Leposavic G, Dashwood MR, Ginsburg J & Buckingham JC (1990) Peripubertal changes in the nature of the GnRH response to alpha-adrenoceptor stimulation in vitro and their modulation by testosterone. *Neuroendocrinology* **52:** 82–89.

Lien EL, Morrison A, Kassarich J & Sullivan D (1986) Alpha-2-adrenergic control of prolactin release. *Neuroendocrinology* **44:** 184–189.

Linton EA, Tilders FJH, Hodgkinson S, Berkenbosch F, Vermes I & Lowry PJ (1985) Stress induced secretion of adrenocorticotropin in rats is inhibited by administration of antisera to corticotropin releasing factor and vasopressin. *Endocrinology* **116:** 966–970.

Liposits Z, Paull WK, Wu P, Jackson IMD & Lechan RM (1987) Hypophysiotrophic thyrotropin releasing hormone (TRH) synthesising neurons. Ultrastructure, adrenergic innervation and putative transmitter action. *Histochemistry* **88:** 1–10.

Liposits Z, Merchenthaler I, Paull WK & Flerko B (1988) Synaptic communication between somatostatinergic axons and growth hormone-releasing factor (GRF) synthesising neurons in the arcuate nucleus of the rat. *Histochemistry* **89:** 247–252.

Liposits Z, Kallo I, Barkovics-Kallo M, Bohn MC & Paull WK (1990) Innervation of somatostatin-synthesising neurons by adrenergic, phenylethanolamine-*N*-methyltransferase (PNMT)-immunoreactive axons in the anterior periventricular nucleus of the rat hypothalamus. *Histochemistry* **94:** 13–20.

Long CNH (1947) The conditions associated with the secretion of the adrenal cortex. *Federation Proceedings* **6:** 461–471.

MacLeod RM (1969) Influence of norepinephrine and catecholamine-depleting agents on the synthesis and release of prolactin and growth hormone. *Endocrinology* **85:** 916–923.

Martha PM, Blizzard RM & Rogol AD (1988) Atenolol enhances growth hormone release to exogenous growth hormone-releasing hormone but fails to alter spontaneous nocturnal growth hormone secretion in boys with constitutional delay of growth. *Pediatric Research* **23:** 393–397.

Martha PM, Blizzard RM, Thorner MO & Rogol AD (1990) Atenolol enhances nocturnal growth hormone (GH) release in GH-deficient children during long term GH-releasing hormone therapy. *Journal of Clinical Endocrinology and Metabolism* **70:** 56–61.

Massara F & Strumia E (1970) Increase in plasma growth hormone concentration in man after infusion of adrenaline-propranolol. *Journal of Endocrinology* **47:** 95–100.

Matta SG & Sharp BM (1992) The role of the fourth cerebroventricle in nicotine-stimulated prolactin release in the rat: involvement of catecholamines. *Journal of Pharmacology and Experimental Therapeutics* **260:** 1285–1291.

Mauras N, Blizzard RM, Thorner MO & Rogol AD (1987) Selective beta-1 adrenergic receptor blockade with atenolol enhances growth hormone releasing hormone and mediated growth hormone release in man. *Metabolism: Clinical and Experimental* **36:** 369–372.

Mefford IN (1987) Are there epinephrine neurons in rat brain? *Brain Research Reviews* **12:** 383–395.

Mellon PK, Windle JJ, Goldsmith PC, Padula CA, Roberts JL & Weiner RI (1990) Immortalization of hypothalamic GnRH neurons by genetically targeted tumorigenesis. *Neuron* **5:** 1–10.

Miki N, Ono M & Shizume K (1984) Evidence that opiatergic and alpha-adrenergic mechanisms stimulate rat growth hormone release via growth hormone-releasing factor (GRF). *Endocrinology* **114:** 1950–1952.

Milsom SR, Donald RA, Espiner EA, Nicholls MG & Livesey JH (1986) The effect of peripheral catecholamine concentrations on the pituitary–adrenal response to corticotrophin releasing factor in man. *Clinical Endocrinology* **25:** 241–246.

Morre MC & Wurtman RJ (1981) Characteristics of synaptosomal tyrosine uptake in various brain regions: effect of other amino acids. *Life Sciences* **28:** 65–75.

Mougey EH, Meyerhoff JL, Pennington LL, Kenion CC & Kant GJ (1986) Pituitary cyclic

AMP and plasma hormone responses to epinephrine administration in vivo. *Life Sciences* **39:** 2305–2313.

Muller EE (1987) Neural control of somatotropic function. *Physiological Reviews* **67:** 962–1053.

Muller EE, Dal Pra P & Pecile A (1968) Influence of brain neurohumors injected into the lateral ventricle of the rat on growth hormone release. *Endocrinology* **83:** 893–896.

Nagatsu T, Levitt M & Udenfriend S (1964) Tyrosine hydroxylase. The initial step in norepinephrine biosynthesis. *Journal of Biological Chemistry* **239:** 2910–2917.

Nakai Y, Imura H, Yoshimi T & Matsukura S (1973) Adrenergic control mechanism for ACTH secretion in man. *Acta Endocrinologica* **74:** 263–270.

Negro-Vilar A, Ojeda SR & McCann SM (1979) Catecholaminergic modulation of luteinizing hormone-releasing hormone release by median eminence terminals in vitro. *Endocrinology* **104:** 1749–1757.

Nicoletti I, Filipponi P, Fedeli L, Santeusanio F & Brunetti P (1981a) Methyl-*p*-tyrosine effect on gonadotropin and prolactin pituitary release in women. *Hormone and Metabolic Research* **13:** 299–300.

Nicoletti I, Filipponi P, Fedeli L et al (1981b) Progesterone positive feedback on gonadotropin release in estrogen-primed postmenopausal women: central nervous system and pituitary as possible sites of action. *Journal of Clinical Endocrinology and Metabolism* **53:** 135–138.

Nicoletti I, Filipponi P, Sfrappini M et al (1984) Catecholamines and pituitary function. *Hormone Research* **19:** 158–170.

Nobin A & Bjorklund A (1973) Topography of the monoamine neuron systems in the human brain as revealed in fetuses. *Acta Physiologica Scandinavica Supplement* **388:** 1–40.

Noel GL, Dimond RC, Wartofsky L, Earll JM & Frantz AG (1974) Studies of prolactin and TSH secretion by continuous infusion of small amounts of thyrotropin-releasing hormone (TRH). *Journal of Clinical Endocrinology and Metabolism* **39:** 6–17.

Oliver C, Mical RS & Porter JC (1977) Hypothalamic–pituitary vasculature: evidence for retrograde blood flow in the pituitary stalk. *Endocrinology* **101:** 598–604.

Paradisi R, Venturoli S, Capelli M et al (1987) Effects of alpha-1 adrenergic blockade on pulsatile luteinizing hormone, follicle-stimulating hormone, and prolactin secretion in polycystic ovary syndrome. *Journal of Clinical Endocrinology and Metabolism* **65:** 841–846.

Paradisi R, Frank G, Grossi G et al (1989) High concentrations of catecholamines in human hypothalamic–hypophysial blood. *Journal of Clinical Investigation* **83:** 2079–2084.

Pardridge WM & Oldendorf WH (1977) Transport of metabolic substrates through the blood–brain barrier. *Journal of Neurochemistry* **28:** 5–12.

Pearson J, Goldstein M, Markey K & Brandeis L (1983) Human brainstem neuronal anatomy as indicated by immunocytochemistry with antibodies to tyrosine hydroxylase. *Neuroscience* **8:** 3–32.

Perkins SN, Evans WS, Thorner MO, Gibbs DM & Cronin MJ (1985) Beta-adrenergic binding and secretory responses of the anterior pituitary. *Endocrinology* **117:** 1818–1825.

Pesce G, Guillaume V, Jezova D, Faudon M, Grino M & Oliver C (1990) Epinephrine in rat hypophysial portal blood is derived mainly from the adrenal medulla. *Neuroendocrinology* **52:** 322–327.

Pescovitz OH & Tan E (1988) Lack of benefit of clonidine treatment for short stature in a double-blind, placebo-controlled trial. *Lancet* **ii:** 874–877.

Peters JR, Foord SM, Dieguez C, Scanlon MF & Hall R (1983) Alpha-1 adrenoceptors on intact rat anterior pituitary cells: correlation with adrenergic stimulation of thyrotropin secretion. *Endocrinology* **113:** 133–140.

Petrovic SL, McDonald JK, Snyder GD & McCann SM (1983) Characterization of beta-adrenergic receptors in rat brain and pituitary using a new high-affinity ligand, (^{125}I)iodocyanopindolol. *Brain Research* **261:** 249–259.

Pintor C, Cella SG, Corda R et al (1985) Clonidine accelerates growth in children with impaired growth hormone secretion. *Lancet* **i:** 1482–1485.

Pintor C, Cella SG, Loche S et al (1987) Clonidine treatment for short stature. *Lancet* **i:** 1226–1230.

Plosker SM, Rabinovic J & Jaffe RB (1991) Inhibition of endogenous catecholamine synthesis augments early follicular phase luteinizing hormone secretion. *Journal of Clinical Endocrinology and Metabolism* **73:** 549–554.

Plotsky PM (1987) Facilitation of immunoreactive corticotropin-releasing factor secretion into the hypophysial–portal circulation after activation of catecholaminergic pathways or central norepinephrine injection. *Endocrinology* **121:** 924–930.

Plotsky PM & Vale W (1985) Patterns of growth hormone-releasing factor and somatostatin secretion into the hypophysial–portal circulation of the rat. *Science* **230:** 461–463.

Plotsky PM, Cunningham ET & Widmaier EP (1989) Catecholaminergic modulation of corticotropin-releasing factor and adrenocorticotropin secretion. *Endocrine Reviews* **10:** 437–458.

Preziosi P, Martire M, Navarra P, Pistritto G & Vacca M (1989) Prolactin-lowering ability of (±)-idazoxan may be linked to a central noradrenergic-serotonergic interplay. *Journal of Pharmacology and Experimental Therapeutics* **249:** 256–263.

Rees L, Butler PWP, Gosling C & Besser GM (1970) Adrenergic blockade and the corticosteroid and growth hormone responses to methylamphetamine. *Nature* **228:** 565–566.

Rivier C & Vale W (1983) Interaction of corticotropin-releasing factor and arginine vasopressin on corticotropin secretion in vivo. *Endocrinology* **113:** 939–942.

Robertson D, Johnson GA, Robertson RM, Nies AS, Shand DG & Oates JA (1979) Comparative assessment of stimuli that release neuronal and adrenomedullary catecholamines in man. *Circulation* **59:** 637–643.

Ross CA, Ruggiero DA, Meeley MP, Park DH, Joh TH & Reis DJ (1984) A new group of neurons in hypothalamus containing phenylethanolamine N-methyltransferase (PNMT) but not tyrosine hydroxylase. *Brain Research* **306:** 349–353.

Rudman D, Kutner MH, Blackston RD, Cushman RA, Bain RP & Patterson JH (1981) Children with normal-variant short stature: treatment with human growth hormone for six months. *New England Journal of Medicine* **305:** 123–131.

Ruffolo RR, DeMarinis R, Wise M & Hieble JP (1988) Structure-activity relationships for alpha-2 adrenergic receptor agonists and antagonists. In Limbird LE (ed.) *The Alpha-2 Adrenergic Receptors*, pp 115–186. Clifton, New Jersey: Humana Press.

Saavedra JM (1985) Central and peripheral catecholamine innervation of the rat intermediate and posterior pituitary lobes. *Neuroendocrinology* **40:** 281–284.

Samorajski T & Marks BH (1962) Localization of tritiated norepinephrine in mouse brain. *Journal of Histochemistry and Cytochemistry* **10:** 392–399.

Santen RJ & Bardin CW (1973) Episodic luteinizing hormone secretion in man. Pulse analysis, clinical interpretation, physiological mechanisms. *Journal of Clinical Investigation* **52:** 2617–2628.

Saxton CA, Faulkner JK & Groom GV (1981) The effect on plasma prolactin, growth hormone and luteinising hormone concentrations of single oral doses of propranolol and tolamolol in normal man. *European Journal of Clinical Pharmacology* **21:** 103–108.

Scanlon MF, Weightman DR, Shale DJ et al (1979) Dopamine is a physiological regulator of thyrotrophin (TSH) secretion in normal man. *Clinical Endocrinology* **10:** 7–15.

Schimchowitsch S & Pelletier G (1988) High-resolution radioautographic localization of beta-adrenergic receptors in the pars intermedia of the rabbit pituitary. *Neuroendocrinology* **47:** 259–262.

Schwanzel-Fukuda M & Pfaff DW (1989) Origin of luteinizing hormone-releasing hormone neurons. *Nature* **338:** 161–164.

Shaar CJ & Clemens JA (1974) The role of catecholamines in the release of anterior pituitary prolactin in vitro. *Endocrinology* **95:** 1202–1212.

Shioda S, Nakai Y, Sato A, Sunayama S & Shimoda Y (1986) Electron-microscopic cytochemistry of the catecholaminergic innervation of TRH neurons in the rat hypothalamus. *Cell and Tissue Research* **245:** 247–252.

Stolk JM, Vantini G, Perry BD, Guchhait RB & U'Prichard DC (1984) Assessment of the functional role of brain adrenergic neurons: chronic effects of phenylethanolamine-N-methyl transferase inhibitor and alpha adrenergic receptor antagonists on brain norepinephrine metabolism. *Journal of Pharmacology and Experimental Therapeutics* **230:** 577–586.

Subramanian MG & Gala RR (1976a) The influence of cholinergic, adrenergic, and serotonergic drugs on the afternoon surge of plasma prolactin in ovariectomized, estrogen-treated rats. *Endocrinology* **98:** 842–848.

Subramanian MG & Gala RR (1976b) Further studies on the effects of adrenergic, serotonergic and cholinergic drugs on the afternoon surge of plasma prolactin in ovariectomized, estrogen-treated rats. *Neuroendocrinology* **22:** 240–249.

Szafarczyk A, Malaval F, Laurent A, Gibaud R & Assenmacher I (1987) Further evidence for a central stimulatory action of catecholamines on adrenocorticotropin release in the rat. *Endocrinology* **121**: 883–892.

Takao T, Hashimoto K & Ota Z (1988) Central catecholaminergic control of ACTH secretion. *Regulatory Peptides* **21**: 301–308.

Tapia-Arancibia L, Arancibia S & Astier H (1985) Evidence for alpha-1 adrenergic stimulatory control of in vitro release of immunoreactive thyrotropin-releasing hormone from rat median eminence: in vivo corroboration. *Endocrinology* **116**: 2314–2319.

Tatar P & Vigas M (1984) Role of alpha$_1$- and alpha$_2$-adrenergic receptors in the growth hormone and prolactin response to insulin-induced hypoglycemia in man. *Neuroendocrinology* **39**: 275–280.

Terasawa E, Krook C, Hei DL, Gearing M, Schultz NJ & Davis GA (1988) Norepinephrine is a possible neurotransmitter stimulating pulsatile release of luteinizing hormone-releasing hormone in the rhesus monkey. *Endocrinology* **123**: 1808–1816.

Terry LC (1986) Regulation of thyrotropin secretion by the central epinephrine system. *Neuroendocrinology* **42**: 102–108.

Terry LC, Crowley WR & Johnson MD (1982) Regulation of episodic growth hormone secretion by the central epinephrine system. Studies in the chronically cannulated rat. *Journal of Clinical Investigation* **69**: 104–112.

Thomas GB, Cummins JT, Smythe GA et al (1989a) Concentrations of dopamine and noradrenaline in hypophysial portal blood in the sheep and in the rat. *Journal of Endocrinology* **121**: 141–147.

Thomas GB, Cummins JT, Doughton BW et al (1989b) Direct pituitary inhibition of prolactin secretion by dopamine and noradrenaline in sheep. *Journal of Endocrinology* **123**: 393–402.

Tsagarakis S, Holly JMP, Rees LH, Besser GM & Grossman A (1988) Acetylcholine and norepinephrine stimulate the release of corticotropin-releasing factor-41 from the rat hypothalamus in vitro. *Endocrinology* **123**: 1962–1969.

Tsagarakis S, Ge F, Rees LH, Besser GM & Grossman A (1989) Stimulation of alpha-adrenoceptors facilitates the release of growth hormone-releasing hormone from rat hypothalamus in vitro. *Journal of Neuroendocrinology* **1**: 129–133.

Tulandi T, Lal S & Kinch RA (1983) Effect of intravenous clonidine on menopausal flushing and luteinizing hormone secretion. *British Journal of Obstetrics and Gynaecology* **90**: 854–857.

Tuomisto J & Mannisto P (1985) Neurotransmitter regulation of anterior pituitary hormones. *Pharmacological Reviews* **37**: 249–332.

Udenfriend S, Zaltzman-Nirenberg P & Nagatsu T (1965) Inhibitors of purified beef adrenal tyrosine hydroxylase. *Biochemical Pharmacology* **14**: 837–845.

Valcavi R, Dieguez C, Azzarito C, Artioli C, Portioli I & Scanlon MF (1987) Alpha-adrenoceptor blockade with thymoxamine reduces basal thyrotrophin levels but does not influence circadian thyrotrophin changes in man. *Journal of Endocrinology* **115**: 187–191.

Valcavi R, Dieguez C, Page MD et al (1988) Alpha-2-adrenergic pathways release growth hormone via a non-GRF-dependent mechanism in normal human subjects. *Clinical Endocrinology* **29**: 309–316.

Vale W, Rivier C, Brazeau P & Guillemin R (1974) Effects of somatostatin on the secretion of thyrotropin and prolactin. *Endocrinology* **95**: 968–977.

Vale W, Vaughan J, Smith M, Yamamoto G, Rivier J & Rivier C (1983) Effects of synthetic ovine corticotropin-releasing factor, glucocorticoids, catecholamines, neurohypophysial peptides, and other substances on cultured corticotropic cells. *Endocrinology* **113**: 1121–1131.

Veldhuis JD, Rogol AD, Williams FA & Johnson ML (1983) Do alpha-adrenergic mechanisms regulate spontaneous or opiate-modulated pulsatile luteinizing hormone secretion in man? *Journal of Clinical Endocrinology and Metabolism* **57**: 1292–1296.

Vogt M (1954) The concentration of sympathin in different parts of the central nervous system under normal conditions and after the administration of drugs. *Journal of Physiology* **123**: 451–481.

Volta C, Ghizzoni L, Muto G, Spaggiari R, Virdis R & Bernasconi S (1991) Effectiveness of growth-promoting therapies. Comparison among growth hormone, clonidine, and levodopa. *American Journal of Diseases of Children* **145**: 168–171.

Westel WC, Valenca MM, Merchenthaler I et al (1992) Intrinsic pulsatile secretory activity of immortalized luteinizing hormone-releasing hormone-secreting neurons. *Proceedings of the National Academy of Sciences of the USA* **89:** 4149–4153.

Whitby LG, Axelrod J & Weil-Malherbe H (1961) The fate of ^{3}H-norepinephrine in animals. *Journal of Pharmacology and Experimental Therapeutics* **132:** 193–201.

Whitnall MH, Smyth D & Gainer H (1987) Vasopressin coexists in half of the corticotropin-releasing factor axons present in the external zone of the median eminence in normal rats. *Neuroendocrinology* **45:** 420–424.

Widmaier EP, Lim AT & Vale W (1989) Secretion of corticotropin-releasing factor from cultured rat hypothalamic cells: effects of catecholamines. *Endocrinology* **124:** 583–590.

Willoughby JO, Day TA, Menadue MF, Jervois PM & Blessing WW (1986) Adrenoceptors in the preoptic-anterior hypothalamic area stimulate secretion of prolactin but not growth hormone in the male rat. *Brain Research Bulletin* **16:** 697–704.

Wray S, Grant P & Gainer H (1989) Evidence that cells expressing luteinizing hormone-releasing hormone mRNA in the mouse are derived from progenitor cells in the olfactory placode. *Proceedings of the National Academy of Sciences of the USA* **86:** 8132–8136.

Wurtman RJ, Larin F, Mostafapour S & Fernstrom JD (1974) Brain catechol synthesis: control by brain tyrosine concentrations. *Science* **185:** 183–184.

Yates FE, Russell SM, Dallman MF, Hedge GA, McCann SM & Dhariwal APS (1971) Potentiation by vasopressin of corticotropin release induced by corticotropin-releasing factor. *Endocrinology* **88:** 3–15.

5

Metabolic actions of catecholamines in man

J. WEBBER
I. A. MACDONALD

The purpose of this chapter is to consider the effects of catecholamines on metabolic processes, and the role of the sympathoadrenal system in the control of metabolic function. It is beyond the scope of this review to cover all aspects of metabolism; attention will be focused on the resting state and clinically related areas such as altered nutritional states, including obesity. The importance of catecholamines in the responses to exercise has been considered in a previous volume in this series (Kjaer et al, 1987) and will not be dealt with here. The majority of the effects described will be derived from studies in humans, both healthy volunteers and patients, with most of the investigations being performed in vivo. The consideration of disordered metabolism will be restricted to altered nutritional states; the role of catecholamines in mediating metabolic responses to acute hypoglycaemia is covered in detail elsewhere (Clutter et al, 1988; Amiel, 1991).

In considering the role of catecholamines in the control of metabolism it is important to distinguish between sympathetic neural effects mediated predominantly through the release of noradrenaline (NA) as the postganglionic neurotransmitter and the influence of circulating catecholamines (mainly adrenaline) acting primarily as hormones. It is now clear from studies in humans and experimental animals that the sympathetic nervous system (SNS) can be activated in a discrete manner, such that systems are selectively stimulated, and that sympathetic responses can occur independently of changes in adrenal medullary secretion (and vice versa). There are major problems in attempting to mimic the effects of sympathetic activation by infusing NA. The plasma NA concentration needed to activate adrenoceptors at sympathetic neuroeffector junctions is so high to enable diffusion from plasma to synapse that stimulation of vascular adrenoceptors is inevitable. Thus, infusion of NA does not provide a useful guide to possible sympathetic nervous influences on metabolism. By contrast, the use of adrenoceptor antagonists, or of clonidine to reduce central sympathetic outflow, can yield useful information.

The influence of catecholamines on metabolism can be considered in two categories; as part of a normally regulated physiological process (e.g. fat mobilization in starvation), or secondary to the catecholamine response to a 'stressful' stimulus. In the latter state the glucose intolerance and fat mobilization produced by sympathoadrenal activation during stress may confer survival value, but this is not always clear. The possible contribution of the sympathoadrenal system to metabolic diseases such as type II diabetes or obesity could result from a disturbance of the normal physiological regulatory role.

FACTORS INFLUENCING CATECHOLAMINE EFFECTS ON METABOLISM

Catecholamines can exert effects on metabolism through direct stimulation of adrenoceptors in the metabolically active tissues, and indirectly through interactions with other endocrine regulators.

Endocrine interactions

The indirect effects of catecholamines are mainly exerted through modulation of pancreatic insulin and glucagon release (see below) but could also involve alterations in the sensitivity to catecholamines. Examples of the latter type of effect are interactions with the glucocorticoids (Harrison et al, 1968) and thyroid hormones (Polikar et al, 1990), both of which appear to enhance the response to exogenous catecholamines.

Adrenoceptors

In many cases the stimulation of α- and β-adrenoceptors have opposite effects on metabolic processes. It is becoming increasingly apparent that α-adrenoceptor stimulation plays an important role in reducing insulin release, modulating pituitary function and inhibiting adipose tissue lipolysis (Ruffolo et al, 1991). As the physiological regulators NA and adrenaline have affinities for both α- and β-receptors, the actual response obtained depends on the balance between these receptors and their affinity for the catecholamines in the tissue of interest. It is clear that the sensitivity of adrenoceptors to stimulation and inhibition varies between tissues, and this needs to be taken into account when considering the overall control of metabolism. For example, sensitivity to β-adrenoceptor stimulation is thought to decrease with age. However, Morrow et al (1991) have shown this is only the case for cardiac and lymphocyte responses to isoprenaline (isoproterenol USP), whereas the β-adrenoceptor-mediated stimulation of insulin release is unchanged with ageing.

CATECHOLAMINES AND INTERMEDIARY METABOLISM

Catecholamines have a wide range of effects on intermediary metabolism which are produced both by activation of the SNS and by stimulation of adrenomedullary secretion. These effects normally result in the rapid mobilization of substrates from the body's fuel stores. The overall result is governed by the extent to which neural and circulating catecholamines

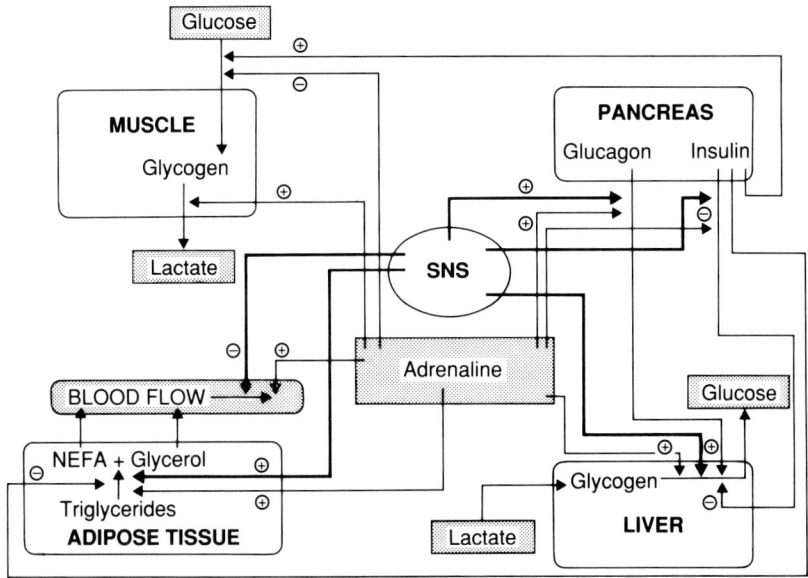

Figure 1. Actions of the sympathetic nervous system and circulating catecholamines on intermediary metabolism. NEFA = non-esterified fatty acids.

operate directly on the tissues involved, their indirect actions on other hormones, and the changes in local blood flow which they cause. The following review will discuss the separate effects of catecholamines on carbohydrate, fat and protein metabolism, with particular reference to the interactions between these and to the major tissues involved, namely, liver, muscle and adipose tissue (Figure 1).

Carbohydrate

Both the direct and indirect effects of catecholamines on carbohydrate metabolism lead to a prompt and sustained rise in plasma glucose. This is due to a combination of enhanced glucose production and decreased peripheral utilization. There is a transient increase in glucose production by the liver which is mediated in humans mainly by β-adrenoceptors. The major component of this increase initially is due to enhanced glycogenolysis and the more sustained elevation is secondary to gluconeogenesis. The regulation of hepatic glucose production appears to be an effect of circulating catecholamines rather than the sympathetic innervation of the liver. Although in rats the neuronal pathways appear to play at least some part in initiating prompt hormonal and metabolic responses (Niijima, 1989), humans receiving liver transplants are not seen to have significant problems with glucose homeostasis despite the inevitable hepatic denervation that occurs with this operation. In humans the predominant effect of catecholamines on the liver is due to the stimulation of β-adrenoceptors. However, an effect of α-adrenoceptor stimulation can be observed in subjects treated with β-adrenoceptor antagonists and somatostatin (to prevent alterations in insulin and glucagon levels) (Rosen et al, 1983).

On binding β-adrenoceptors on the plasma membrane of hepatocytes, catecholamines stimulate adenylate cyclase, so causing the formation of cyclic adenosine monophosphate (cAMP). This in turn activates a protein kinase which phosphorylates both phosphorylase kinase and glycogen synthetase. Phosphorylation activates the former and inactivates the latter, so enhancing glycogen breakdown. However, in muscle the enzyme glucose-6-phosphatase is absent, so glycogen cannot be broken down to provide free glucose, but it can be utilized for energy requirements via the glycogenolytic pathway, the lactate so produced being released into the circulation and acting as a substrate for hepatic gluconeogenesis. The mechanisms by which gluconeogenesis is enhanced are less clear. Studies in dogs indicate that this effect is due to a combination of stimulation of peripheral precursor release, increasing substrate movement into the hepatocyte and by increasing intra-hepatic gluconeogenic efficiency (Connolly et al, 1991; Stevenson et al, 1991). In the longer term, however, it is the sustained effects of the sympathoadrenal system in reducing peripheral utilization of glucose which are the more important direct actions. This process is β-adrenoceptor-mediated and is largely due to the inhibition of skeletal muscle glucose uptake (Sacca et al, 1982).

The indirect actions of catecholamines on carbohydrate metabolism via their inhibition of insulin secretion by the pancreas are perhaps more important quantitatively than their direct effects (Clutter et al, 1988). Inhibition of insulin secretion is mediated by α_2-adrenoceptors on the B cells of the pancreas. The degree of inhibition can be demonstrated by the marked elevation of insulin levels which occurs following the termination of exogenous catecholamine infusions (Clutter et al, 1980).

Further demonstration of the importance of the actions of catecholamines on insulin secretion comes from the use of the pure β-agonist, isoprenaline (Sacca et al, 1980). Despite isoprenaline's direct effects on carbohydrate metabolism, it has little overall effect on plasma glucose since it has no inhibitory effect on the B cells (and does in fact stimulate insulin release) and the consequent rise in insulin counteracts any rise in glucose which would otherwise occur. When there is no insulin response to adrenaline infusion, as in patients with insulin-dependent diabetes mellitus (IDDM), or where somatostatin is infused to prevent a response, the glycaemic response to adrenaline is much more marked (Berk et al, 1985). This is likely to be due to prevention of a secondary rise in insulin subsequent to the raised blood glucose levels. The use of somatostatin to prevent any changes in glucagon levels that might otherwise occur also demonstrates that the effects of adrenaline on glycaemia are independent of β-adrenoceptor-mediated pancreatic glucagon secretion (Berk et al, 1985). The effect of α-adrenoceptor stimulation in reducing pancreatic insulin release has led to the development of α_2-adrenoceptor antagonists to prevent this effect, potentially increasing insulin release as a means of treating type II diabetes mellitus (Ruffolo et al, 1991).

Protein

The effects of catecholamines on protein metabolism are much less clear than for fat and carbohydrate. Infusions of adrenaline lead to a decrease in plasma amino acid levels which is most marked for the branched chain amino acids, but alanine levels remain constant (Shamoon et al, 1980). This action appears to be mediated via β-adrenoceptors since propranolol completely blocks it, and is not related to changes in insulin levels. In contrast to the action of catecholamines being antagonistic to that of insulin on carbohydrate and fat metabolism, the pattern of its effects on protein thus appears to be very similar to that of insulin. This is somewhat surprising given the body of literature devoted to the role catecholamines are likely to play in the hypermetabolism and catabolism associated with injury. More recent studies using tracer methodology have tried to elucidate the underlying changes in protein turnover which contribute to the observed pattern of effects on plasma amino acids (Miles et al, 1984; Castellino et al, 1990; Matthews et al, 1990). These studies provide evidence that adrenaline, like insulin, inhibits proteolysis, although, unlike insulin, there is no stimulation of protein synthesis. Del Prato et al (1990), using arteriovenous techniques in addition to tracers, found that adrenaline augments the splanchnic uptake of gluconeogenic amino acids and there is an increase in the peripheral production of alanine, which biopsy showed to be derived from muscle. Branched chain amino acid levels within muscle fell, indicating reduced synthesis. Two caveats should be mentioned regarding all these studies and their relevance for normal metabolism. Firstly, the plasma levels of catecholamines achieved are normally only seen at times of peak stress and, secondly, although the effects of catecholamines on metabolic rate are prolonged, those on protein metabolism appear minimal beyond the acute changes in plasma amino acids (Matthews et al, 1990).

Fat

The sympathoadrenal system is the main regulator of lipolysis in humans. Human adipocytes possess both stimulatory β-adrenoceptors and inhibitory $α_2$-adrenoceptors, with the activity of the former normally predominating. However, this is not always the case, as samples of adipose tissue removed from obese patients revealed a dominant antilipolytic effect of $α_2$-adrenoceptors in subcutaneous adipose tissue but not in tissue obtained from visceral sites (Richelsen et al, 1991). The rate-limiting step of lipolysis is the initial hydrolysis of stored triglycerides by hormone-sensitive lipase (HSL). The activation of this hormone is via a similar cascade to that involved in glycogenolysis. HSL exists in an active phosphorylated form and an inactive dephosphorylated form. Phosphorylation is catalysed by a protein kinase, whose activity is dependent on intracellular levels of cAMP. Catecholamines act via the β-adrenoceptor to stimulate adenylate cyclase, so producing cAMP and hence activating lipolysis. In the mobilization of lipid there is a close interaction between adrenergic actions on adipose tissue blood flow and those on lipolysis. The sympathetic innervation to white adipose tissue is mainly to the vasculature rather than the fat cells themselves (Fredholm, 1985). Vasoconstrictor effects are mediated by α-adrenoceptors, whereas vasodilatation occurs via β-adrenoceptor mechanisms. From the pattern of innervation and of adrenoceptor subtypes and their distribution, it is presumed that circulating catecholamines act mainly on the fat cells and that neuronal effects on lipolysis are brought about indirectly by changes in blood flow to adipose tissue. This phenomenon means that interpretation of the effects of infused catecholamines on fat metabolism may not represent the normal in vivo effects of sympathoadrenal stimulation. In situations in vivo where there is a reduction in adipose tissue perfusion due to α-adrenergic processes, but concurrent stimulation of lipolysis, there may be local accumulation of fatty acids leading to enhanced re-esterification and low release of fatty acids.

During catecholamine infusions the levels of ketone bodies are also seen to rise (Galster et al, 1981). This appears to be mainly due to a rise in ketone production in the liver secondary to the increased availability of free fatty acids as a substrate for their synthesis (Bahnsen et al, 1984). Ketogenesis is primarily regulated by glucagon (stimulation) and insulin (inhibition), although there may in addition be some direct effects of catecholamines on the stimulation of hepatic ketogenesis since with longer infusions of catecholamines the rates of lipolysis abate but the enhanced ketogenesis persists (Weiss et al, 1984). It has also been proposed that there may be a neural component in the regulation of ketogenesis. Ketogenesis is also stimulated at plasma levels of noradrenaline thought to achieve the synaptic levels of this hormone during increased sympathetic stimulation (Connolly et al, 1991).

Thermogenesis

It is well established that catecholamines are capable of stimulating thermogenesis (metabolic rate) in isolated tissues and the whole body. This is not surprising given the extensive effects of catecholamines in producing mobilization of substrates. Cori and Buchwald (1930) were the first to demonstrate the stimulation of metabolic rate in humans with infusions of relatively small doses of adrenaline. It is now well established that thermogenesis in brown adipose tissue involves stimulation by the sympathetic innervation of that tissue (see below). The stimulation of metabolic rate by adrenaline is a type of non-shivering thermogenesis, as it does not involve any sustained increase in muscle electromyogram (EMG) activity (Gallen et al, 1991), but is unlikely to involve the activation of brown adipose tissue in adult humans. Adrenaline appears to be capable of stimulating splanchnic thermogenesis (Bearn et al, 1951), although the circumstances of these experiments make interpretation rather difficult. There does appear to be substantial stimulation of muscle (non-contractile) oxygen consumption with adrenaline (Lundholm and Svedmyr, 1965) and ephedrine (Astrup, 1986). Although the detailed metabolic processes are not established, Fagher et al (1988) have shown the β$_1$-adrenoceptor antagonist metoprolol reduces muscle thermogenesis measured in vitro in samples taken from surgical patients. In addition, catecholamines produce peripheral tremor through actions on peripheral β-adrenoceptors (Marsden et al, 1967) and so could increase the whole-body metabolic rate as a result.

In animals such as the rat, the stimulation of thermogenesis by catecholamines is mediated via β-adrenoceptor stimulation, with an 'atypical' β₃-receptor being involved. A role for such receptors in the thermogenic response to catecholamines in humans is not proven, although it does seem very likely that catecholamine-induced thermogenesis is due to β-adrenoceptor activation. Furthermore, the stimulation of thermogenesis by adrenaline occurs independently of any changes in insulin or glucagon secretion (Staten et al, 1989). It has been proposed that catecholamine effects on thermogenesis are of physiological significance, as the plasma adrenaline threshold for eliciting a response is well within the physiological range (see below), and there is some evidence for a role of the SNS in mediating part of the thermogenic response to nutrient ingestion (see below).

CATECHOLAMINES AND ELECTROLYTES

Increased plasma adrenaline concentrations are associated with reductions in plasma potassium, and adrenaline infusion reduces plasma potassium via a β₂-adrenoceptor-mediated process (Brown et al, 1983). Studies with β₂-selective and non-selective β-adrenoceptor agonists have shown the effect to be mainly through a β₂-mechanism, presumably via activation of the membrane sodium/potassium adenosine triphosphatase (Na/K-ATPase). This effect of catecholamines on the Na/K-ATPase may contribute to the effect on thermogenesis, as such stimulation of the sodium pump will increase tissue metabolism (Clausen et al, 1991).

Infusion of adrenaline also lowers plasma calcium (Ljunghall et al, 1984), phosphate (Body et al, 1983) and magnesium (Joborn et al, 1985). The effects tend to be less marked than the changes in plasma potassium. For example, the reduction in plasma magnesium in response to adrenaline, or to the β₂-adrenoceptor agonist salbutamol, was less than 0.1 mmol/litre, whilst plasma potassium fell by 0.6 mmol/litre in the same subjects (Whyte et al, 1987). The mechanisms of these electrolyte changes are not established, although in the case of calcium and magnesium the fall in plasma concentration may be secondary to adrenaline-induced adipose tissue lipolysis, with the electrolytes binding to the adipocytes (Akgün and Rudman, 1969; Elliott and Rizack, 1974). These effects of adrenaline on plasma electrolytes may be of clinical importance, as situations such as myocardial infarction are accompanied by increases in plasma adrenaline and disturbances of plasma electrolyte homeostasis.

CATECHOLAMINES AND NUTRITION

The interactions between catecholamines and nutrition can be examined from several standpoints. Thus, the acute effects of ingestion of mixed meals and of the separate dietary constituents on sympathoadrenal activity and the longer term consequences of under- and overnutrition on the sympatho-adrenal system can be measured. The knowledge we have gained about these processes has come from a wide variety of experimental techniques. Much of the early work on animals during dietary manipulation involved the use of radiolabelled NA to measure its turnover in individual tissues, assuming this to be an index of local SNS activity. Later research applied the same methodology to humans, though obviously only whole-body measures can be obtained in human studies. This means that the differential responses of individual organs will be collated, and important tissue differences may be obscured. A simpler technique in humans has been the measurement of plasma and urinary catecholamine levels, the former being used to assess mainly the acute effects of food intake on sympathoadrenal activity, and the latter to look at the longer term correlates of different nutritional states on catecholamines. Again these measurements are plagued by a lack of organ specificity. More recently SNS activity has been monitored with microneu-rography, whereby the firing rates of sympathetic nerves can be measured. This technique is limited to use on superficial nerves supplying the skin or skeletal muscle vasculature. An additional recent advance for in vivo research is the use of microdialysis to measure catecholamine levels in superficial tissues (Gronlund et al, 1991). However, there are substantial methodological problems with this technique and its main contribution at the moment is probably qualitative. When indices of sympathoadrenal activity are being monitored, it should not be overlooked that the end results of this activity in vivo may be negated by changes in adrenoceptor number and sensitivity (Figure 2).

It has long been known that food ingestion causes an increase in metabolic rate (the thermic effect of food; TEF). This effect is primarily due to the energy required for the processing and storage of the different dietary constituents. Several studies in the 1980s showed that food ingestion was associated with increased plasma levels of NA (Welle et al, 1981), with this effect being specific for carbohydrate as opposed to fat or protein. Later work by Astrup and colleagues (1989) showed that meal-induced

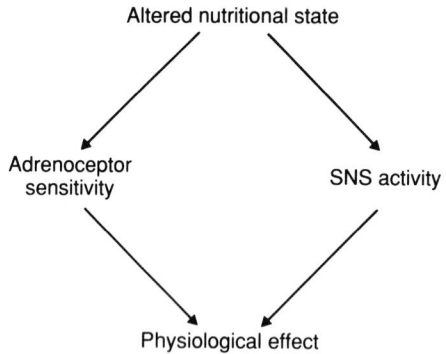

Figure 2. Mechanisms of nutrition-related effects on in vivo physiology.

thermogenesis was reduced from 9.6% of the energy content of the meal to 7.1% by β-blockade and the major site of this effect was skeletal muscle, whose oxygen consumption was decreased by 23%. The role of the SNS in TEF was further confirmed and extended in experiments using the hyperinsulinaemic euglycaemic clamp technique combined with indirect calorimetry, whereby an estimate of both glucose storage and its energy cost can be derived. Again increments in NA were seen (Rowe et al, 1981), and it was further demonstrated that propranolol reduced the rise in metabolic rate seen during the clamp (Acheson et al, 1984). The concept therefore arose of obligatory and facultative thermogenesis, the former representing the obligatory costs of nutrient storage, and the latter a regulatory component, in which the SNS has a major role. Other evidence for SNS involvement in the TEF came in a study using triated NA (^{3}H-NA) where the increment in plasma NA turnover after a meal was correlated to the increment in energy expenditure (Schwartz et al, 1987). In recent studies the activation of the SNS consequent on nutrient ingestion was confirmed using microneurography, with increased firing rates of superficial sympathetic nerves seen following oral carbohydrate administration (Berne et al, 1989).

In a series of animal experiments of NA turnover in a number of tissues, Landsberg and Young (1978) demonstrated that more prolonged overfeeding led to enhanced turnover and underfeeding to a reduction in turnover. Changes in SNS activity were proposed to play a major role in the adaptation to these nutritional stresses. During times of nutritional abundance excess calories could be burnt off via SNS-mediated processes, whilst such regulatory mechanisms could be suppressed during fasting (Landsberg and Young, 1985). This concept was applied to humans by O'Dea et al (1982), who showed that there was an increase in NA spillover rate following 10 days of overfeeding in healthy subjects and a relative decrease after 10 days of underfeeding. The majority of studies in humans on underfeeding have used obese subjects trying to lose weight (Del Rio et al, 1989; Schwartz et al, 1990). In considering such studies and those involving starvation, the obligatory sodium loss and consequent volume depletion leading to reflex SNS activation should be taken into account and prevented with sodium supplementation. These studies have generally shown reduced NA appearance rates or reduced urinary excretion of NA during starvation or underfeeding. Such findings are supported by a recent report of reduced muscle sympathetic nerve activity after chronic underfeeding in obese patients (Andersson et al, 1991).

Although overfeeding has been shown to increase both NA turnover and thermogenesis, the association between these has been called into question. Welle and Campbell (1983) overfed subjects for 20 days causing an increase in the resting metabolic rate (RMR), but intravenous β-blockade did not reduce the elevated RMR nor affect the TEF to a greater extent during overfeeding. A later study from the same group using chronic oral administration of propranolol showed that this did not prevent the increase in RMR secondary to overfeeding (Welle et al, 1989). By contrast, the same group showed that both propranolol, a non-selective β-adrenoceptor antagonist (Welle et al, 1989), and nadolol, a β_1-antagonist (Welle et al,

1991), reduced the fasting RMR in subjects on a normal dietary intake. Further studies arguing against a role for the SNS in the TEF have demonstrated that when physiological levels of insulin are infused during the glucose clamp technique, no changes in plasma NA are seen (Mitrakou et al, 1992). However, plasma NA levels are an insensitive way of studying the subtle changes in the SNS during metabolic stimulation. Even the use of selective adrenergic antagonists is likely to mask underlying tissue differences in sympathetic function.

Table 1. Lipolytic, chronotropic and thermogenic responses to infused catecholamines in acute starvation, underfeeding and chronic undernutrition.

Response	Nutritional state		
	Acute starvation	Underfeeding	Chronic undernutrition
Lipolysis	↑	↑	?
Heart rate	↑	↔	↑
Thermogenesis	↑	↔	↓

Data from Mansell et al (1990), Mansell and Macdonald (1989), Jayarajan and Shetty (1987) and Kurpad et al (1989a).

An alternative to evaluating the sympathoadrenal correlates of changed nutritional circumstances is to examine the sensitivity to exogenous infusions of catecholamines in these states (Table 1 and Figure 3). When adrenaline is infused into healthy young subjects who have been starved for 48 h the thermogenic and heart rate responses are significantly enhanced compared with the control state (Mansell et al, 1990). In addition, the lipolytic response to adrenaline has been shown to be greater after an 84 h fast (Jensen et al, 1987). That adrenergic mechanisms normally play a major role in substrate mobilization during fasting is shown by the demonstration that β-blockade has a greater antilipolytic effect after 84 h of starvation than at 12 h (Klein et al, 1989). Catecholamines also have a minor role to play in the prevention of hypoglycaemia during fasting, and this can become critical when glucagon is deficient (Boyle et al, 1989). In contrast to these effects of acute starvation, Kurpad et al (1989a) saw lower thermogenic responses to infused NA in chronically undernourished labourers, although the same group demonstrated enhanced cardiovascular responses in a similar population (Jayarajan and Shetty, 1987). Whilst underfeeding normal weight subjects for 1 week led to enhanced lipolytic responses to adrenaline, there was no change in its thermogenic or chronotropic effects (Mansell and Macdonald, 1989). In order to explain these results it has been suggested that a 'nutrition-related' reduction in sympathetic activity (as described by Landsberg and Young, 1978) might be accompanied by enhanced adrenoceptor sensitivity. This interpretation is to some extent supported by the finding of increases in β-adrenoceptor number and decreases in α_2-adrenoceptor number in fat cells during fasting (Arner, 1992). In addition, calorie restriction in obesity produces an α-adrenergic supersensitive state (Berlin et al, 1990). However, the disparate effects on individual cell and organ responses compared with the whole body makes it difficult to draw

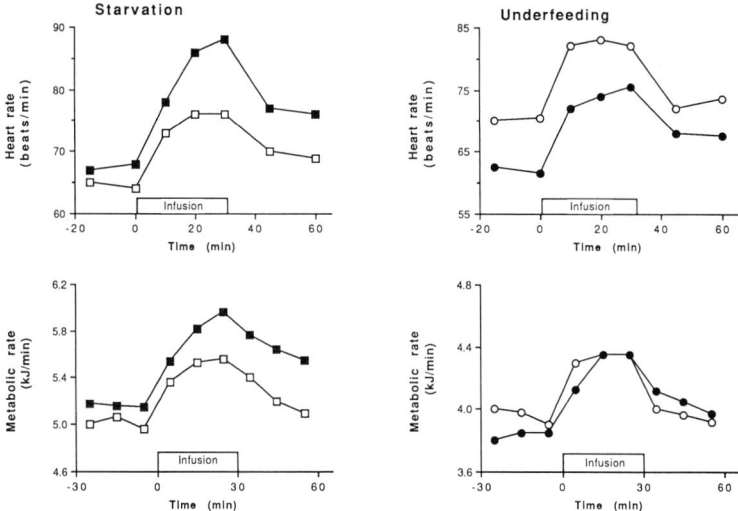

Figure 3. Influences of starvation (left panel) or underfeeding (right panel) on the metabolic rate and heart rate responses to the infusion of adrenaline $(25 \, \text{ng} \cdot \text{kg}^{-1} \cdot \text{min}^{-1})$ for 30 min. Values are means. ■ = starvation; ● = underfeeding; □ and ○ = controls. Adapted from Mansell and Macdonald (1989) and Mansell et al (1990), with permission of the American Physiological Society.

firm conclusions as to the mechanisms underlying the nutritionally induced changes in the whole-body responses to catecholamines.

CATECHOLAMINES AND OBESITY

There is an enormous amount of literature on the metabolic correlates of obesity. The following section restricts itself to discussion of the possible role of altered sympathoadrenal activity and the consequences of this in the obese state. Since the work of Landsberg and Young (1985) demonstrating a major involvement of the sympathoadrenal system in the response to altered nutritional states and their proposition that this is one of the main regulators of changes in energy expenditure, there has been a profusion of studies examining the activity of this system in obese subjects, the underlying hypothesis being that changes in sympathetic function may predispose to the development of the obese state. These studies have been recently reviewed and a heterogeneity of findings reported (Young and Macdonald, 1992). This review suggests that this heterogeneity is not a consequence of the different methods used to measure sympathoadrenal activity, but may reflect real differences in subject populations. Confounding factors in these studies include the effects of age, antecedent diet, blood pressure, physical activity and obesity subtype. In addition, as alluded to above, the results derived from whole-body measurements may hide important regional variations. A further consideration in the study of obesity and its aetiology is whether any abnormalities observed are of primary causal importance or just secondary to the obese state. Much interest has therefore centred on the comparison of the post-obese with both their obese counterparts and normal controls.

If the sympathoadrenal system has a major role in basal energy expenditure, then its underactivity and the consequent lowering of the RMR would predispose to weight gain. However, such a role has proved difficult to demonstrate. Intravenous β-blockade has not been shown to affect the RMR (Vernet et al, 1987), although more recently oral nadolol produced a 7% decrease in the RMR which was not associated with any changes in thyroid function (Welle et al, 1991). Indirect evidence comes from long-term studies of weight change in patients on β-blockers, where some weight gain has been shown (Rossner et al, 1990). Whether or not sympathetic activity has a role in controlling the RMR, the evidence that a low RMR has an aetiological role in obesity remains controversial.

The difficulty in demonstrating a role for impaired sympathoadrenal activity in lowering the RMR in obese subjects has led to a number of studies examining stimulated thermogenesis in such people. These studies have specifically looked for evidence of a reduction in the facultative component of thermogenesis. Several investigators have found a reduced TEF in obesity (Shetty et al, 1981; Astrup et al, 1987); however, the relationship between this impairment and measures of reduced sympathetic activity has not been satisfactorily demonstrated. More recently a lack of glucose-induced sympathetic activation has been shown in the diabetic obese compared with the simple obese. This was teleologically explained by the greater insulin resistance of the diabetics preventing hypothalamic activation of the SNS (Astrup et al, 1991). However, the TEF was not assessed in this study.

At this point the opposite view, namely that of enhanced SNS activity in the obese state, should be mentioned. The association between obesity and hypertension has long been recognized, and it has been proposed that this link is mediated by the hyperinsulinaemia which accompanies obesity (Landsberg, 1986). Hyperinsulinaemia is seen as increasing sympathetic activity as well as having an antinatriuretic effect, both of which may contribute to hypertension. Evidence in favour of this hypothesis comes from epidemiological studies demonstrating the correlation between obesity and hypertension, and from the experimental demonstration of the favourable effect of weight loss on blood pressure and on lowering plasma NA levels (Sowers et al, 1982).

The thermogenic response to infused catecholamines has been extensively studied and, despite initial reports of decreased responsiveness in obesity (Jung et al, 1979), it would appear that there is great heterogeneity in the obese population with regard to this aspect of metabolism. Katzeff and colleagues, amongst others, found no differences between lean and obese subjects in NA-induced thermogenesis (Katzeff et al, 1986; Kush et al, 1986). Thus, although a subgroup of obese subjects may have a blunted thermogenic response to catecholamines, the majority (about 75%) have a normal response (Connacher et al, 1988a). Rather than thermogenesis *per se*, it has been suggested that there may be an abnormality in lipolysis in obese subjects. Studies have demonstrated a decreased palmitate turnover and fatty acid oxidation in response to adrenaline infusion in the obese compared with normal weight controls (Connacher et al, 1991). The authors of this paper suggested that this anomaly might favour fat storage and the development of obesity over long periods of time. The mechanisms underlying such changes remain uncertain, with a recent review commenting that there is no evidence of a major alteration of adipocyte adrenoceptor function in obesity (Arner, 1992).

Due to the unclear situation in obesity *per se*, much recent work has centred on those who have successfully lost weight (the post-obese) to identify any residual impairments in sympathoadrenal activity which might predispose to the development of the obese state. Astrup and Jequiers' groups have contributed much of this research (Jequier, 1990; Astrup and Christensen, 1992). Both groups have shown that defective glucose-induced thermogenesis and blunted increases in plasma NA post-glucose persist after weight reduction, although it should be noted that the subjects remained overweight even after this weight loss. This is of particular relevance since a recent study has shown that depressions in autonomic activity were weakly associated with increasing percentages of body fat (Peterson et al, 1988), thus inferring that unless truly post-obese subjects are studied such abnormalities (although they may contribute to the persistence of the obese state) cannot be said to be causal.

In their review of the literature Young and Macdonald (1992) conclude that the evidence for reduced SNS activity in obesity is inconclusive, but that there is more support for reduced adrenal medullary activity (decreased adrenaline secretion) in this state. The mechanisms by which this might operate to either cause or maintain the obese state are unclear, and indeed this pattern of activity is in contrast to many of the current models of obesity (Bray, 1990) which identify an important contribution from increased adrenocortical function.

BROWN FAT AND NA

Interest in brown adipose tissue (BAT), and specifically the implication of its involvement in human obesity, has multiplied since the demonstration that it is responsible for the elevation in energy expenditure secondary to overfeeding in rats (Rothwell and Stock, 1979). BAT has been described in a wide number of mammalian species and its major role appears to be the generation of heat by the dissipation of energy without the production of adenosine triphosphate (ATP). This is in direct contrast to white adipose tissue (WAT), which has an energy storage function. The mechanism of this process of heat production (thermogenesis) is the mitochondrial proton conductance pathway. A proton gradient is created from the oxidation of substrates, but instead of the protons being used to drive the synthesis of ATP, the gradient is dissipated as heat. Thus, BAT mediates non-shivering thermogenesis and is important in thermoregulation in human neonates and hibernating mammals. The major regulator of BAT thermogenesis is an uncoupling protein situated on the inner mitochondrial membrane. It is the presence of this protein which distinguishes BAT from WAT (Trayhurn, 1990).

BAT is also distinguished from WAT by its rich sympathetic innervation, which appears to be directed to the fat cells much more than to the vasculature. Studies have shown that it is the nerve supply to the tissue rather than circulating catecholamines which activate BAT (Girardier and Seydoux, 1986). NA infusion increases BAT blood flow, despite the fact that mainly vasoconstrictor α-adrenoceptors are present on the blood vessels in BAT (in contrast to WAT). This in vivo vasodilatation may be due to local metabolite changes subsequent to the activation of BAT thermogenesis. The activation of this thermogenesis seems to occur via a novel subtype of β-adrenoceptor, β_3 (Arch et al, 1984). Activation of this both stimulates lipolysis and activates the proton conductance pathway. Apart from this acute effect on BAT metabolism, chronic sympathetic stimulation leads to increases in cell number, mitochondrial content and uncoupling protein concentration (Trayhurn, 1990). These longer term effects are particularly important in the adaptation to cold and overnutrition.

Rothwell and Stock (1986) demonstrated that young rats fed a palatable diet had a marked increase in food intake, but despite this did not put on weight. This was explained by a concomitant hypertrophy of BAT and an increase in its thermogenic capacity. A similar response is seen during the adaptation to cold exposure in these animals, and in both conditions there is an enhanced whole-body thermogenic response to NA infusion, whilst the enhanced RMR can be reduced by β-adrenoceptor blockade with propranolol. By contrast, underfeeding is accompanied by reduced BAT mass and thermogenic responsiveness.

Although the contribution of BAT to non-shivering and diet-induced thermogenesis in rats has been demonstrated conclusively, its role in adult humans is less certain (Astrup et al, 1984). The presence of BAT in significant amounts has been shown in neonates and infants and in adults with phaeochromocytomas (Lean and James, 1986). Studies in mammalian neonates (summarized by Nedergaard et al, 1986) have shown a close relationship between the presence of uncoupling protein and the capacity for non-shivering thermogenesis. In humans, BAT is present at birth and variations in its presence and activity may cause either impaired heat production or hyperthermia and hence may account for some cot deaths (Lean and James, 1986). Although in adult humans only small amounts of BAT are present, the potential for hypertrophy of this tissue, as seen in patients with phaeochromocytomas, and the dramatic effects of BAT shown in animals have led to the development of drugs targeted at the β_3-adrenoceptor. Agonists of this adrenoceptor have been shown to increase energy expenditure without causing intolerable cardiovascular side-effects and so may have a part to play as antiobesity drugs (Connacher et al, 1988b).

CATECHOLAMINES AND METABOLISM—PHYSIOLOGICAL RELEVANCE AND OVERALL SUMMARY

The preceding sections have outlined the potential effects of circulating catecholamines and the SNS in the control of metabolism. The general effects are mobilization of substrates for energy metabolism, with direct stimulation of thermogenesis in some tissues. Some of these metabolic effects are likely to be secondary to changes in tissue perfusion, whereas others are primary and give rise to secondary blood flow responses. However, the effects of catecholamines on metabolism described above are not all activated by the same level of stimulus. It is obviously difficult to quantify or manipulate sympathetic nervous stimuli, so the information available on the sensitivity of the various responses in humans relates exclusively to plasma concentrations. The major drawback of infusing catecholamines intravenously is the inability to mimic the normal route of delivery. The adrenal medulla does not release just catecholamines into the circulation, but also a series of peptides including some endorphins. Thus, the following information relates strictly to plasma concentrations of the catecholamines without any possible modulating effect of some of the other products of the adrenal medulla. In addition, there is some evidence of increased thermogenic sensitivity to NA during stepwise infusion (Kurpad et al, 1989b); thus the plasma thresholds determined with such infusion regimens may be different from those determined with different infusion rates on different occasions.

Other chapters in this volume have dealt with normal resting plasma catecholamine concentrations, and the exchange which occurs in the peripheral tissues. For the purposes of this discussion, we will assume normal resting arterial adrenaline levels are 0.1–0.5 nmol/litre, with corresponding NA levels of 0.5–2.5 nmol/litre. Unfortunately, there are very few publications which have measured arterial catecholamines during infusion studies assessing metabolic responses. Thus, we will have to assume that during adrenaline infusion the arterialized venous (heated hand) samples usually obtained are within 10% of arterial levels (which seems true up to arterial adrenaline levels of 2 nmol/litre; Liu et al, 1992) and that levels in antecubital venous samples are approximately 50% of arterial levels. Similar assumptions are difficult to make during NA infusions as there are few data to base them on.

The plasma adrenaline thresholds for metabolic and cardiovascular effects were first described by Clutter et al (1980) using antecubital venous blood samples in healthy men. This study showed effects on heart rate, systolic blood pressure and plasma glycerol at *venous* adrenaline levels of 0.5 nmol/litre or less, whilst increases in plasma glucose and lactate, and reductions in diastolic blood pressure, occurred at approximately 1 nmol/ litre. Subsequent observations by Sjostrom et al (1983) of the plasma adrenaline thresholds for metabolic and cardiovascular effects in healthy women utilized arterialized venous blood sampling, which would be expected to yield apparently higher 'plasma thresholds' than venous samples because of the peripheral extraction of adrenaline. However, the effectiveness of the arterialization was not quantified by Sjostrom et al (1983). The plasma thresholds observed by Sjostrom et al (1983) were consistent with previous results, except that the women studied showed a greater sensitivity with respect to changes in diastolic blood pressure and plasma lactate and glucose, and a reduced sensitivity to the effects on heart rate. These differences were relatively minor and probably due to differences in experimental design, as we have recently observed similar thresholds and sensitivities to the effects of adrenaline in men and women (J. Webber and I.A. Macdonald, unpublished observation). Sjostrom et al (1983) observed that the threshold for the stimulation of thermogenesis was similar to that for lipolysis (a plasma adrenaline of 0.6 nmol/litre). This is consistent with our own observations in healthy men (Fellows et al, 1985), where a *venous* adrenaline of 0.7 nmol/litre was accompanied by a 10% increase in metabolic rate. The actual adrenaline threshold for a decrease in plasma potasssium has not been determined, but it is likely to be similar to that for a change in plasma glucose, as there was no change in either glucose or potassium at a venous adrenaline level of 0.7 nmol/litre, which produced significant increases in plasma glycerol and thermogenesis (Fellows et al, 1985). The likely plasma adrenaline thresholds for eliciting metabolic effects are listed in Table 2, and it is apparent that many of these responses are activated by modest elevations in adrenaline.

Table 2. Plasma adrenaline thresholds for metabolic and cardio-vascular effects. Values are estimated as arterial levels. Baseline levels are 0.1–0.5 nmol/litre.

Variable	Plasma adrenaline threshold (nmol/litre)
Systolic blood pressure	0.55
Plasma NEFA/glycerol	0.60
Thermogenesis	0.65
Heart rate	0.80
Plasma glucose/lactate	0.90
Limb blood flow	Less than 1.0
Plasma potassium	Approx. 1.0

NEFA = non-esterified fatty acids. Data from Clutter et al (1980), Sjostrom et al (1983) and Fellows et al (1985).

The plasma thresholds for the effects of NA on metabolism are less clear. The early studies of Silverberg et al (1978) showed no effects of infused NA until venous plasma levels exceeded 10 nmol/litre. However, Izzo (1983) and Hjemdahl et al (1983) observed effects at lower venous plasma levels (approximately 5 nmol/litre), although in both cases the protocols involved stepwise infusion and the early, low rates of infusion may have increased the sensitivity to the subsequent doses. Nevertheless, the plasma levels of NA needed to elicit metabolic responses are in excess of those seen in the resting state, although such levels are seen during moderate to severe exercise.

Thus, the SNS and adrenal medulla have important roles in the control of metabolism, not only in emergency 'fight and flight' responses, but also in the normal state. Disturbances of these effects may contribute to several endocrine/metabolic diseases (e.g. obesity, type II diabetes), but further work is needed to distinguish between situations in which catecholamines are primary, causative factors and those in which they change secondary to pathophysiological influences.

REFERENCES

Acheson K, Jéquier E & Wahren J (1983) Influence of β-adrenergic blockade on glucose-induced thermogenesis in man. *Journal of Clinical Investigation* **72**: 981–986.
Acheson KJ, Ravussin E, Wahren J & Jéquier E (1984) Thermic effect of glucose in man. Obligatory and facultative thermogenesis. *Journal of Clinical Investigation* **74**: 1572–1580.
Akgün S & Rudman D (1969) Relationships between mobilization of free fatty acids from adipose tissue, and the concentration of calcium in the extracellular fluid and in the tissue. *Endocrinology* **84**: 926–930.
Amiel S (1991) Glucose counter-regulation in health and disease—current concepts in hypoglycaemia recognition and response. *Quarterly Journal of Medicine* **80**: 707–727.
Andersson B, Elam M, Wallin BG, Bjorntorp P & Andersson OK (1991) Effect of energy-restricted diet on sympathetic muscle nerve activity in obese women. *Hypertension* **18**: 783–789.
Arch JRS, Ainsworth AT, Cawthorne MA et al (1984) Atypical β-adrenoceptors on brown adipocytes as target of antiobesity drugs. *Nature* **309**: 163–165.
Arner P (1992) Adrenergic receptor function in fat cells. *American Journal of Clinical Nutrition* **55**: 228S–236S.
Astrup A (1986) Thermogenesis in human brown adipose tissue and skeletal muscle induced by sympathomimetic stimulation. *Acta Endocrinologica* **12**: 1–30.
Astrup A & Christersen NJ (1992) Role of the sympathetic nervous system in obese and postobese subjects. In Kinney JM & Tucker HN (eds) *Energy Metabolism: Tissue Determinants and Cellular Corollaries*, pp 299–309. Raven Press: New York.
Astrup A, Bulow J, Christensen NJ & Madsen J (1984) Ephedrine-induced thermogenesis in man: no role for interscapular brown adipose tissue. *Clinical Science* **66**: 179–186.
Astrup A, Anderson T, Henriksen O et al (1987) Impaired glucose-induced thermogenesis in skeletal muscle in obesity. The role of the sympathoadrenal system. *International Journal of Obesity* **11**: 51–66.
Astrup A, Simonsen L, Bülow J, Madsen J & Christensen NJ (1989) Epinephrine mediates facultative carbohydrate-induced thermogenesis in human skeletal muscle. *American Journal of Physiology* **257**: E340–E345.
Astrup A, Christensen NJ & Breum L (1991) Reduced activity of the sympathetic nervous system in obese patients with and without NIDDM. *Clinical Science* **80**: 53–58.
Bahnsen M, Burrin JM, Johnston DG, Pernet A, Walker M & Alberti KGMM (1984) Mechanisms of catecholamine effects on ketogenesis. *American Journal of Physiology* **247**: E173–E180.
Bazelmans J, Nestel PJ, O'Dea K & Esler MD (1985) Blunted norepinephrine responsiveness to changing energy states in obese subjects. *Metabolism: Clinical and Experimental* **34**: 154–160.
Bearn AG, Billing B & Sherlock S (1951) The effect of adrenaline and noradrenaline on hepatic blood flow and splanchnic carbohydrate metabolism in man. *Journal of Physiology* **115**: 430–441.
Berk MA, Clutter WE, Skor DA, Gingerich RP, Parvin CA & Cryer PE (1985) Enhanced glycaemic responsiveness to epinephrine in insulin dependent diabetes mellitus is the result of the inability to secrete insulin. *Journal of Clinical Investigation* **75**: 1842–1851.
Berlin I, Berlan M, Crespo-Laumonnier B et al (1990) Alterations in β-adrenergic sensitivity and platelet α₂-adrenoceptors in obese women: Effect of exercise and caloric restriction. *Clinical Science* **78**: 81–87.

Berne C, Fagius J & Niklasson F (1989) Sympathetic response to oral carbohydrate administration. Evidence from microelectrode nerve recordings. *Journal of Clinical Investigation* **84:** 1403–1409.

Body JJ, Cryer PE, Offord KP & Health H III (1983) Epinephrine is a hypophosphataemic hormone in man. *Journal of Clinical Investigation* **71:** 572–578.

Boyle PJ, Shah SD & Cryer PE (1989) Insulin, glucagon, and catecholamines in prevention of hypoglycaemia during fasting. *American Journal of Physiology* **256:** E651–E661.

Bray GA (1990) Obesity—a state of reduced sympathetic activity and normal or high adrenal activity (the autonomic and adrenal hypothesis revisited). *International Journal of Obesity* **14(supplement 3):** 77–92.

Brown MJ, Brown DC & Murphy MB (1983) Hypokalaemia from beta$_2$-receptor stimulation by circulating epinephrine. *New England Journal of Medicine* **309:** 1414–1419.

Castellino P, Luzi L, Del Prato S & DeFronzo RA (1990) Dissociation of the effects of epinephrine and insulin on glucose and protein metabolism. *American Journal of Physiology* **258:** E117–E125.

Clausen T, Van Hardeveld C & Everts ME (1991) Significance of cation transport in control of energy metabolism and thermogenesis. *Physiological Reviews* **71:** 733–774.

Clutter WE, Bier DM, Shah SD & Cryer PE (1980) Epinephrine plasma metabolic clearance rates and physiological thresholds for metabolic and hemodynamic actions in man. *Journal of Clinical Investigation* **66:** 94–101.

Clutter WE, Rizza RA, Gerich JE & Cryer PE (1988) Regulation of glucose metabolism by sympathochromaffin catecholamines. *Diabetes/Metabolism Reviews* **4:** 1–15.

Connacher AA, Jung RT, Mitchell PEG et al (1988a) Heterogeneity of noradrenergic thermic responses in obese and lean humans. *International Journal of Obesity* **12:** 267–276.

Connacher AA, Jung RT & Mitchell PEG (1988b) Weight loss in obese subjects on a restricted diet given BRL 26830A, a new atypical β-adrenoceptor agonist. *British Medical Journal* **296:** 1217–1220.

Connacher AA, Bennet WM, Jung RT et al (1991) Effect of adrenaline infusion on fatty acid and glucose turnover in lean and obese human subjects in the post-absorptive and fed states. *Clinical Science* **81:** 635–644.

Connolly CC, Steiner KE, Stevenson RW et al (1991) Regulation of glucose metabolism by norepinephrine in conscious dogs. *American Journal of Physiology* **261:** E764–E772.

Cori CF & Buchwald KW (1930) Effect of continuous injection of epinephrine on the carbohydrate metabolism, basal metabolism and vascular system of normal man. *American Journal of Physiology* **95:** 71–78.

Deibert DC & DeFronzo RA (1980) Epinephrine-induced insulin resistance in man. *Journal of Clinical Investigation* **65:** 717–721.

Del Prato S, DeFronzo RA, Castellino P, Wahren J & Alvestrand A (1990) Regulation of amino acid metabolism by epinephrine. *American Journal of Physiology* **258:** E878–E887.

Del Rio G, Marrama P, Fiorani P & Della Casa L (1989) Very low calorie diet induces opposite effects on sympathetic nervous system and adrenomedullary responses. *International Journal of Obesity* **13(supplement 2):** 173–175.

Elliott DA & Rizack MA (1974) Epinephrine and adrenocorticotrophic-hormone stimulated magnesium accumulation in adipocytes and their plasma membranes. *Journal of Biological Chemistry* **249:** 3985–3990.

Fagher B, Monti M & Thulin T (1988) Selective β$_1$-adrenoceptor blockade and muscle thermogenesis. *Acta Medica Scandinavica* **223:** 139–145.

Fellows IW, Bennett T & Macdonald IA (1985) The effect of adrenaline upon cardiovascular and metabolic functions in man. *Clinical Science* **69:** 215–222.

Fredholm BB (1985) Nervous control of circulation and metabolism in white adipose tissue. In Cryer A & Van RLR (eds) *New Perspectives in Adipose Tissue: Structure, Function and Development*, pp 45–64. London: Butterworths.

Gallen IW, Macdonald IA, Fone KCF & Maggs DG (1991) The effect of a graded infusion of adrenaline on metabolic rate, forearm electromyographic activity and oxygen consumption. *Proceedings of the Nutrition Society* **50:** 29A.

Galster AD, Clutter WE, Cryer PE, Collins JA & Bier DM (1981) Epinephrine plasma thresholds for lipolytic effects in man: Measurements of fatty acid transport with [1-^{13}C] palmitic acid. *Journal of Clinical Investigation* **67:** 1729–1738.

Girardier L & Seydoux J (1986) Neural control of brown adipose tissue. In Trayhurn P & Nicholls DG (eds) *Brown Adipose Tissue*, pp 122–151. London: Arnold.

Gronlund B, Astrup A, Bie P & Christensen NJ (1991) Noradrenaline release in skeletal muscle and in adipose tissue studied by microdialysis. *Clinical Science* **80:** 595–598.

Harrison TS, Chawla R & Wojtalik RS (1968) Steroidal influences on catecholamines. *New England Journal of Medicine* **279:** 136–143.

Hjemdahl P, Akerstedt T, Pollare T & Gillberg M (1983) Influence of β-adrenoceptor blockade by metoprolol and propranolol on plasma concentrations and effects of noradrenaline and adrenaline during i.v. infusion. *Acta Physiologica Scandinavica Supplement* **515:** 43–53.

Izzo J (1983) Cardiovascular hormonal effects of circulating norepinephine. *Hypertension* **5:** 787–789.

Jayarajan MP & Shetty PS (1987) Cardiovascular β-adrenoceptor sensitivity of undernourished subjects. *British Journal of Nutrition* **58:** 5–11.

Jensen MD, Haymond MW, Gerich JE, Cryer PE & Miles JM (1987) Lipolysis during fasting. Decreased suppression by insulin and increased stimulation by epinephrine. *Journal of Clinical Investigation* **79:** 207–213.

Jequier E (1990) Energy metabolism in obese patients before and after weight loss, and in patients who have relapsed. *International Journal of Obesity* **14(supplement 1):** 59–67.

Joborn H, Akerström G & Ljunghall S (1985) Effects of exogenous catecholamines and exercise on plasma magnesium concentrations. *Clinical Endocrinology* **23:** 219–226.

Jung RT, Shetty PS, James WPT, Barrand MA & Callingham BA (1979) Reduced thermogenesis in obesity. *Nature* **279:** 322–323.

Katzeff HL, O'Connell M, Horton ES et al (1986) Metabolic studies in human obesity during overnutrition and undernutrition: Thermogenic and hormonal responses to norepinephrine. *Metabolism: Clinical and Experimental* **35:** 166–175.

Kjaer M, Secher NH & Galbo H (1987) Physical stress and catecholamine release. *Baillière's Clinical Endocrinology and Metabolism* **1:** 279–298.

Klein S, Peters EJ, Holland OB & Wolfe RR (1989) Effect of short- and long-term β-adrenergic blockade on lipolysis during fasting in humans. *American Journal of Physiology* **257:** E65–E73.

Kurpad AV, Kulkarni RN, Sheela ML & Shetty PS (1989a) Thermogenic responses to graded doses of noradrenaline in undernourished Indian male subjects. *British Journal of Nutrition* **61:** 201–208.

Kurpad AV, Kulkarni RN, Vaz M & Shetty PS (1989b) Repeated infusions of identical doses of norepinephrine show potentiation of metabolic responses in human subjects. *Metabolism: Clinical and Experimental* **38:** 979–982.

Kush RD, Young JB, Katzeff HL et al (1986) Effect of diet on energy expenditure and plasma norepinephrine in lean and obese Pima Indians. *Metabolism: Clinical and Experimental* **35:** 1110–1120.

Landsberg L (1986) Diet, obesity and hypertension: An hypothesis involving insulin, the sympathetic nervous system, and adaptive thermogenesis. *Quarterly Journal of Medicine* **236:** 1081–1090.

Landsberg L & Young JB (1978) Fasting, feeding and regulation of the sympathetic nervous system. *New England Journal of Medicine* **298:** 1295–1301.

Landsberg L & Young JB (1985) The influence of diet on the sympathetic nervous system. *Neuroendocrine Perspectives* **4:** 191–218.

Lean MEJ & James WPT (1986) Brown adipose tissue in man. In Trayhurn P & Nicholls DG (eds) *Brown Adipose Tissue*, pp 339–365. London: Arnold.

Leibel RL, Berry EM & Hirsh J (1991) Metabolic and hemodynamic responses to endogenous and exogenous catecholamines in formerly obese subjects. *American Journal of Physiology* **260:** R785–R791.

Liu D, Andreasson K, Lins PE et al (1992) Adrenaline and noradrenaline responses during insulin-induced hypoglycaemia in man: should the hormone levels be measured in arterialized venous blood? *Acta Endocrinologica* (in press).

Ljunghall S, Akerström G, Benson L, Hetta J, Rudberg C & Wide L (1984) Effects of epinephrine and norepinephrine on serum parathyroid hormone and calcium in normal subjects. *Experimental and Clinical Endocrinology* **84:** 313–318.

Lundholm L & Svedmyr N (1965) Influence of adrenaline on blood flow and metabolism in the human forearm. *Acta Physiologica Scandinavica* **65:** 344–351.

Mansell PI & Macdonald IA (1989) Underfeeding and the physiological responses to infused epinephrine in lean women. *American Journal of Physiology* **256:** R583–R589.

Mansell PI, Macdonald IA & Fellows IW (1990) 48 h starvation enhances the thermogenic response to infused epinephrine. *American Journal of Physiology* **258:** R87–R93.

Marsden CD, Foley TH, Owen DAL & McAllister RG (1967) Peripheral β-adrenergic receptors concerned with tremor. *Clinical Science* **33:** 53–65.

Matthews DE, Pesola G & Campbell RG (1990) Effect of epinephrine on amino acid and energy metabolism in humans. *American Journal of Physiology* **258:** E948–E956.

Miles JM, Nissen SL, Gerich JE & Haymond ML (1984) Effect of epinephrine infusion on leucine and alanine kinetics in humans. *American Journal of Physiology* **247:** E166–E172.

Mitrakou A, Mokan M, Bolli G et al (1992) Evidence against the hypothesis that hyperinsuli-naemia increases sympathetic nervous system activity in man. *Metabolism: Clinical and Experimental* **41:** 198–200.

Morrow LA, Rosen SG & Halter JB (1991) Beta-adrenergic regulation of insulin secretion: evidence of tissue heterogeneity of beta-adrenergic responsiveness in the elderly. *Journal of Gerontology* **46:** M108–M113.

Nedergaard J, Connolly E & Cannon B (1986) Brown adipose tissue in the mammalian neonate. In Trayhurn P & Nicholls DG (eds) *Brown Adipose Tissue*, pp 152–213. London: Arnold.

Niijima A (1989) Nervous regulation of metabolism. *Progress in Neurobiology* **33:** 135–147.

O'Dea K, Esler M, Leonard P, Stockigt JR & Nestel P (1982) Noradrenaline turnover during under- and over-eating in normal weight subjects. *Metabolism: Clinical and Experimental* **31:** 896–899.

Peterson HR, Rothschild M, Weinberg CR et al (1988) Body fat and the activity of the autonomic nervous system. *New England Journal of Medicine* **318:** 1077–1083.

Polikar R, Kennedy B, Maisel A et al (1990) Decreased adrenergic sensitivity in patients with hypothyroidism. *Journal of the American College of Cardiology* **15:** 94–98.

Richelsen B, Pedersen SB, Møller-Pedersen T & Bak JF (1991) Regional differences in triglyceride breakdown in human adipose tissue: effects of catecholamines, insulin and prostaglandin E_2. *Metabolism: Clinical and Experimental* **40:** 990–996.

Rizza RA, Haymond MW, Cryer PE & Gerich JE (1979) Differential effects of epinephrine on glucose production and disposal in man. *American Journal of Physiology* **237:** E356–E362.

Rizza RA, Cryer PE, Haymond MW & Gerich JE (1980) Adrenergic mechanisms of catechol-amine action on glucose homeostasis in man. *Metabolism: Clinical and Experimental* **29(supplement 1):** 1155–1163.

Rosen SG, Clutter WE, Shah SD, Miller JP, Bier DM & Cryer PG (1983) Direct α-adrenergic stimulation of hepatic glucose production in human subjects. *American Journal of Physiology* **245:** E616–E626.

Rossner S, Taylor CL, Byington RP et al (1990) Long term propranolol treatment and changes in body weight after myocardial infarction. *British Medical Journal* **300:** 902–903.

Rothwell NJ & Stock MJ (1979) A role for brown adipose tissue in diet-induced thermogenesis. *Nature* **281:** 31–35.

Rothwell NJ & Stock MJ (1986) Brown adipose tissue and diet-induced thermogenesis. In Trayhurn P & Nicholls DG (eds) *Brown Adipose Tissue*, pp 269–298. London: Arnold.

Rowe JW, Young JB, Minaker KL, Stevens AL, Pallotta J & Landsberg L (1981) Effect of insulin and glucose infusions on sympathetic nervous system activity in normal man. *Diabetes* **30:** 219–225.

Ruffolo RR, Nichols AJ & Hieble JP (1991) Metabolic regulation by α_1- and α_2-adrenoceptors. *Life Sciences* **49:** 171–183.

Sacca L, Morrone G, Cicala M, Corso G & Ungaro B (1980) Influence of epinephrine, norepinephrine and isoproterenol on glucose homeostasis in normal man. *Journal of Clinical Endocrinology and Metabolism* **50:** 680–684.

Sacca L, Vigorito C, Cicala M, Ungaro B & Sherwin RS (1982) Mechanisms of epinephrine-induced glucose intolerance in normal humans: Role of the splanchnic bed. *Journal of Clinical Investigation* **69:** 284–293.

Schwartz RS, Halter JB & Bierman EL (1983) Reduced thermic effect of feeding in obesity: Role of norepinephrine. *Metabolism: Clinical and Experimental* **32:** 114–117.

Schwartz RS, Jaeger LF, Silberstein S & Veith RC (1987) Sympathetic nervous system activity and the thermic effect of feeding in man. *International Journal of Obesity* **11:** 141–149.

Schwartz RS, Jaeger LF, Veith RC et al (1990) The effect of diet or exercise on plasma norepinephrine kinetics in moderately obese young men. *International Journal of Obesity* **14**: 1–11.

Shamoon H, Jacob R & Sherwin RS (1980) Epinephrine-induced hypoaminoacidemia in normal and diabetic human subjects. Effect of beta blockade. *Diabetes* **29**: 875–881.

Sherwin RS & Sacca L (1984) Effect of epinephrine on glucose metabolism in humans: contribution of the liver. *American Journal of Physiology* **247**: E157–E165.

Shetty PS, Jung RT, James WPT, Barrand MA & Callingham BA (1981) Postprandial thermogenesis in obesity. *Clinical Science* **60**: 519–525.

Silverberg AB, Shah SD, Haymond MW & Cryer PE (1978) Norepinephrine: hormone and neurotransmitter. *American Journal of Physiology* **234**: E252–E256.

Sjostrom L, Schutz Y, Gudinchet F, Hegnell L, Pittet PhG & Jéquier E (1983) Adrenaline sensitivity with respect to metabolic rate and other variables in women. *American Journal of Physiology* **245**: E431–E442.

Sowers JR, Nyby M, Stern N et al (1982) Blood pressure and hormone changes associated with weight reduction in the obese. *Hypertension* **4**: 686–691.

Staten MA, Matthews DE, Cryer PE & Bier DM (1989) Epinephrine's effect on metabolic rate is independent of changes in plasma insulin or glucagon. *American Journal of Physiology* **257**: E185–E192.

Stevenson RW, Steiner KE, Connolly CC et al (1991) Dose-related effects of epinephrine on glucose production in conscious dogs. *American Journal of Physiology* **260**: E363–E370.

Trayhurn P (1990) Energy expenditure and thermogenesis: Animal studies on brown adipose tissue. *International Journal of Obesity* **14(supplement 1)**: 17–29.

Vernet O, Nacht C-A, Christin L et al (1987) β-Adrenergic blockade and intravenous nutrient-induced thermogenesis in lean and obese women. *American Journal of Physiology* **253**: E65–E71.

Weiss M, Keller U & Stauffacher W (1984) Effect of epinephrine and somatostatin-induced insulin deficiency on ketone body kinetics and lipolysis in man. *Diabetes* **33**: 738–744.

Welle SL & Campbell RG (1983) Stimulation of thermogenesis by carbohydrate overfeeding. Evidence against sympathetic nervous system mediation. *Journal of Clinical Investigation* **71**: 916–925.

Welle SL, Lilavivat U & Campbell RG (1981) Thermic effect of feeding in man: Increased plasma norepinephrine levels following glucose but not protein or fat consumption. *Metabolism: Clinical and Experimental* **30**: 953–958.

Welle SL, Nair KS & Campbell RG (1989) Failure of chronic β-adrenergic blockade to inhibit overfeeding-induced thermogenesis in humans. *American Journal of Physiology* **256**: R653–R658.

Welle S, Schwartz RG & Statt M (1991) Reduced metabolic rate during β-adrenergic blockade in humans. *Metabolism: Clinical and Experimental* **40**: 619–622.

Whyte KF, Addis GJ, Whitesmith R & Reid JL (1987) Adrenergic control of plasma magnesium in man. *Clinical Science* **72**: 135–138.

Young JB & Macdonald IA (1992) Sympathoadrenal activity in human obesity: Heterogeneity of findings since 1980. *International Journal of Obesity* **16**: 959–967.

6

Catecholamines and essential hypertension

MURRAY DAVID ESLER

The present story of catecholamines and essential hypertension begins with the description of the vasomotor nerves (Bernard, 1851), the isolation and synthesis of an adrenal medullary pressor principle, adrenaline (Elliot, 1905), and the characterization of the neurotransmitter of the vasomotor (sympathetic) nerves as noradrenaline (von Euler, 1946).

By the turn of the century the origin of circulating adrenaline from the adrenal gland and many of its actions as a hormone, including its blood pressure raising properties, were clearly established. The pressor action of injected adrenaline resembled that produced by electrical stimulation of vasomotor nerves, leading for a time to the incorrect conclusion that adrenaline was the neurotransmitter. Soon after he had demonstrated that the sympathetic transmitter was, in fact, noradrenaline, von Euler introduced biochemical methods to the clinical study of sympathetic nervous system function in human hypertension by measuring the urinary excretion of noradrenaline in patients, to gauge the level of sympathetic nervous activity (von Euler et al, 1954).

From this seminal study, for more than 40 years research on catecholamines and essential hypertension has primarily involved the biochemical quantification of sympathetic nervous function by the measurement of noradrenaline in a range of body fluids. However, the subject of catecholamines and hypertension has a broader context (Table 1). This chapter will consider these further matters, such as the likely involvement in hypertension pathogenesis of central nervous system (CNS) catecholaminergic neurones, the possible pathogenetic significance of adrenaline released as a cotransmitter in sympathetic nerves, and the role of renal tubular dopamine mechanisms in regulating body sodium balance, in addition to the important issue of the causes and consequences of sympathetic nervous overactivity in essential hypertension.

Table 1. Catecholamines and essential hypertension: the issues.

Regulation of sympathetic nervous outflow by brain catecholamines
Sympathetic nerve activity and noradrenaline release
Adrenal medullary release of adrenaline
Release of adrenaline from sympathetic nerves
Thr renal tubule dopaminergic natriuretic system

Baillière's Clinical Endocrinology and Metabolism—
Vol. 7, No. 2, April 1993
ISBN 0–7020–1698–5

SYMPATHETIC NERVOUS FUNCTION IN ESSENTIAL HYPERTENSION

From the time of von Euler's demonstration that the sympathetic neuro-transmitter was noradrenaline, the potential value of measurements of the noradrenaline release rate as an index of nerve firing was seen. Peart (1949) described noradrenaline overflow into the venous effluent of an organ (the cat spleen) on electrical stimulation of its nerve supply, followed soon after by the demonstration of Brown and Gillespie (1957) that the wash-out of noradrenaline was proportional to the rate of sympathetic nerve stimulation. This relationship, which as a general principle has been amply confirmed (Esler et al, 1990a), provides the foundation for the use of measurements of noradrenaline release as an index of sympathetic nervous system activity in clinical research.

Subsequent to the development of sensitive radioenzymatic assays for catecholamines, elevated plasma noradrenaline levels were soon reported in patients with essential hypertension. Many similar studies followed, often with very conflicting results. The influential reviews of Goldstein (1981, 1983) on the subject now appear to have settled the matter: the plasma concentration of noradrenaline is elevated in a proportion (perhaps 40%) of resting patients with essential hypertension, principally younger ones. Plasma adrenaline values have been found to be elevated less consistently than plasma noradrenaline values (Goldstein, 1983). The reported plasma concentrations of adrenaline, if elevated, have in most instances been less than the threshold concentration for direct stimulation of the cardiovascular system (Clutter et al, 1980).

Clinical methods for assessing sympathetic nervous system function

Plasma noradrenaline measurements, although providing a useful guide to sympathetic nervous system function, have substantial limitations (Esler et al, 1990a):

1. Only a small, and usually indeterminate, fraction of the total released noradrenaline diffuses to plasma where it can be measured.
2. The plasma concentration of noradrenaline is dependent on the rate at which noradrenaline is removed from the circulation, and not just sympathetic tone and noradrenaline release. In a given context, 20 to 50% of the variance in plasma concentration values will be attributable to differences in noradrenaline plasma clearance.
3. The sources of the noradrenaline in plasma are not identified, and regional patterns of sympathetic response cannot be delineated.

This latter limitation is a serious deficiency of plasma noradrenaline concentration measurements. Responses of the sympathetic nervous system typically show regional differentiation. With certain reflex responses and disease states, some sympathetic outflows may be activated but others unchanged or inhibited (Esler et al, 1990a). For a comprehensive analysis of sympathetic nervous dysfunction in human hypertension, the regional pattern of sympathetic activation needs to be investigated.

A number of clinical tests of regional sympathetic nervous activity have been developed (Figure 1). Of these the most powerful are clinical microneurography, an electrophysiological technique for studying sympathetic nerve firing rates (Hagbarth and Vallbo, 1968), biochemical techniques based on radiotracer methodology for measuring rates of organ-specific noradrenaline spillover to plasma (Esler et al, 1979), and power spectral analysis, which allows biological interpretation of spontaneous, superimposed circulatory rhythms (Guzzetti et al, 1988). These tests are complementary, rather than competing, methodologies and measure different aspects of sympathetic nervous function.

Clinical microneurography

Developed by Hagbarth and Vallbo (1968), clinical microneurography provides a method for studying nerve firing rates in subcutaneous sympathetic nerves distributed to skin and skeletal muscle. The technique involves the

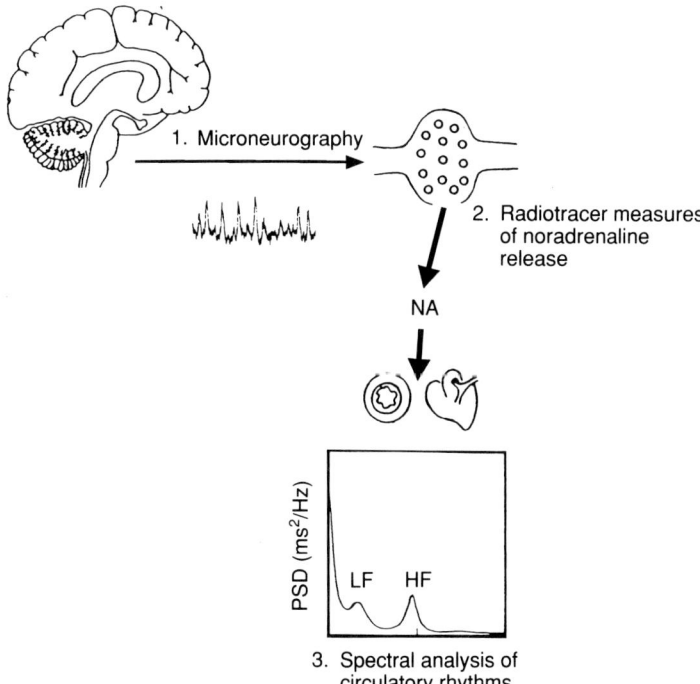

Figure 1. Individual elements in the sympathetic nervous control of the cardiovascular system: 1. Sympathetic nerve traffic measured by microneurography; 2. transmitter release estimated from radiotracer-derived measurement of noradrenaline spillover to plasma; 3. cardiovascular rhythms studied by spectral analysis. LF = low frequency; HF = high frequency; PSD = power spectral density.

insertion of fine tungsten electrodes through the skin, with careful positioning of the electrode tip in sympathetic fibres of, most commonly, the common peroneal or median nerves. Multifibre recordings of 'bursts' of nerve activity, synchronous with the heart beat, are generated. The method has been used extensively in the study of sympathetic nervous control of the cardiovascular system (Wallin et al, 1973).

Power spectral analysis of circulatory rhythms

This technique uses sophisticated mathematical partitioning to dissect out individual, superimposed rhythms producing cyclical variation in heart rate and arterial pressure (Guzzetti et al, 1988). Heart rate variability is largely attributable to the influence of the autonomic nervous system. High frequency (approximately 0.3 Hz) and low frequency (approximately 0.1 Hz) components of heart rate variability can be delineated (Figure 1). The high frequency component is linked to respiration, associated in particular with vagal function and abolished by atropinization. Low frequency variability derives in part from the influence of the cardiac sympathetic nerves, and is reduced by β-adrenergic blockade.

Noradrenaline spillover rate measurements

Noradrenaline spillover measurements give the appearance rate of the sympathetic neurotransmitter in plasma from individual organs or for the body as a whole (Esler et al, 1979, 1982). With microneurographic methods for studying sympathetic nerve firing rates, only the nerves to skeletal muscle and skin can be studied. An important limitation in hypertension research is the inaccessibility to testing of the sympathetic nerves to internal organs. Noradrenaline spillover measurements are more helpful in this regard. The relationship which exists between the rate of sympathetic nerve firing in an organ and the overflow of noradrenaline into its venous drainage provides the experimental justification for the use of transmitter spillover measurements in the study of sympathetic nervous function (Esler et al, 1990a). Rather than the rate of release of noradrenaline from sympathetic nerve varicosities, which is unmeasurable clinically, the noradrenaline spillover rate gives the rate at which released noradrenaline enters plasma; in humans this is approximately 10–20% of the noradrenaline synthesis rate (Hoeldtke et al, 1983).

The total noradrenaline spillover rate to plasma is measured by isotope dilution. Tritiated L-noradrenaline (^{3}H-NA) is infused into an antecubital vein to reach a steady state in plasma (invariably reached within 60 min), and the appearance rate of noradrenaline (NA) in plasma, with arterial sampling, is calculated from the equation (Esler et al, 1979, 1990a):

$$\text{Total NA spillover rate} = \frac{{}^3\text{H-NA infusion rate}}{\text{Plasma NA specific radioactivity}}$$

Regional noradrenaline spillover rates can be calculated from the equation (Esler et al, 1982):

$$\text{Organ NA spillover rate} = [(C_V - C_A) + C_A (E)] \times PF$$

where C_A and C_V are the plasma noradrenaline concentrations in arterial and regional venous plasma, E is the fractional extraction of tritiated noradrenaline in transit through the organ vascular bed, and PF is the organ plasma flow. Renal, cardiac, hepatomesenteric, skeletal muscle and pulmonary noradrenaline spillover rates can be derived from appropriate organ plasma flow and plasma tritiated noradrenaline and endogenous noradrenaline measurements, using regional venous catheterization for plasma sampling (Esler et al, 1984).

Increased sympathetic nervous activity in essential hypertension

The application of these methods provides compelling evidence for the existence of sympathetic nervous activation in a substantial proportion of patients with essential hypertension (Esler et al, 1990b). The sympathetic stimulation involves the neural outflows to the kidneys, heart and skeletal muscle (Table 2), but is present only in young and not elderly patients, as

Table 2. Independent indices of sympathetic nerve firing in primary human hypertension.

Method	Sympathetic outflow activated	Reference
Clinical microneurography	Skeletal muscle	Anderson et al (1989) Yamada et al (1989)
Measurement of regional noradrenaline spillover	Heart, kidneys	Esler et al (1985)
Spectral analysis of variation in heart rate	Heart	Guzzetti et al (1988)

From Esler et al (1990) with permission.

exemplified by the noradrenaline spillover rate measurements shown in Figure 2.

When clinical microneurography was first applied to the investigation of sympathetic nervous function in essential hypertension, early reports suggested that muscle sympathetic nerve firing was normal (Wallin et al, 1973). More recently two large scale studies of borderline hypertension (Anderson et al, 1989) and established hypertension (Yamada et al, 1989) have documented the presence of increased muscle sympathetic nerve firing (Table 2). With spectral analysis measurements in untreated patients with essential hypertension, the low frequency element in heart rate variability is enhanced and the high frequency component is reduced or absent (Guzzetti et al, 1988), consistent with the presence of cardiac sympathetic stimulation and parasympathetic withdrawal.

Measurements of regional noradrenaline release to plasma suggest that a selective activation of the sympathetic nervous system, involving the outflows to the heart and kidneys (Figure 2) but sparing the lungs and hepatomesenteric circulation, is present in essential hypertension, but only in

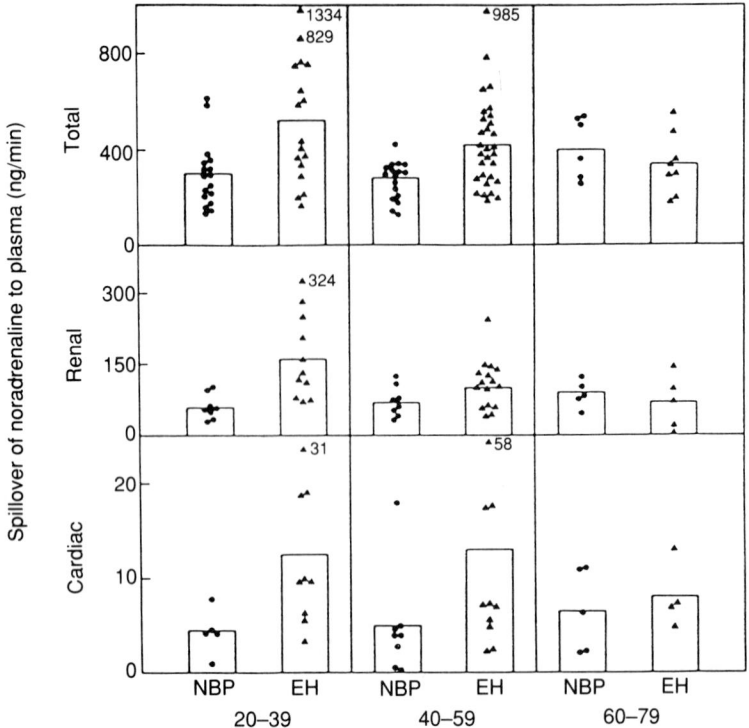

Figure 2. Total, renal and cardiac noradrenaline (norepinephrine) spillover to plasma in patients with essential hypertension (EH) and healthy subjects with normal blood pressure (NBP) according to age. Increased noradrenaline release was present particularly in young patients. From Esler et al (1989) with permission.

younger patients (Esler et al, 1985). The elevated cardiorenal noradrenaline spillover is not readily attributable to causes other than increased nerve firing rates such as facilitated wash-out with higher blood flows, as renal and coronary sinus plasma flows are not increased in essential hypertension, or faulty noradrenaline reuptake, since extraction of radiolabelled noradrenaline across the heart and kidneys, which is dependent on neuronal uptake, is not reduced (Esler et al, 1988). As discussed below, this increased renal and cardiac sympathetic firing provides a plausible mechanism for the development of hypertension.

Causes of sympathetic overactivity in essential hypertension

The possible causes of the increased sympathetic activity in essential hypertension, listed in Table 3, remain largely conjectural. Lifestyle factors, specifically physical inactivity and overeating (with or without obesity), may possibly be involved.

Table 3. Possible causes of sympathetic nervous overactivity in essential hypertension.

Obesity and increased dietary energy intake
Sedentary lifestyle
Stress and behavioural factors
CNS catecholamines
Insulin resistance and hyperinsulinaemia

Obesity and increased dietary energy intake

Patients with primary hypertension are commonly overweight. Since positive energy balance initiates thermogenesis by stimulation of the sympathetic nervous system, and this sympathetic activation is regionalized, involving the heart, for example (Landsberg and Young, 1978), the sympathetic activation seen in essential hypertension could perhaps represent an adaptive response to overeating. An excessive dietary calorie load is known to stimulate the sympathetic nervous system and elevate arterial pressure, while calorie restriction reduces both sympathetic activity and blood pressure (Jung et al, 1979; O'Dea et al, 1982). In an experimental canine model of obesity produced by overfeeding, weight gain, sympathetic nervous activity and blood pressure increased in parallel (Rocchini et al, 1989). Evidence supporting the presence of sympathetic activation in human obesity and in obesity-related essential hypertension, however, is inconclusive (Sowers et al, 1982; Peterson et al, 1988).

Physical inactivity

An additional, but at present unproven factor possibly contributing to sympathetic nervous overactivity in hypertensive patients is a sedentary lifestyle. If a programme of repetitive aerobic exercise is applied in sedentary subjects, inhibition of sympathetic nervous system activity results (Jennings et al, 1986). Epidemiological studies have demonstrated a direct relationship between low habitual level of physical activity and prevailing blood pressure, and isotonic exercise is a proven non-pharmacological antihypertensive measure (Nelson et al, 1986). Sympathetic nervous system inhibition appears to be the mechanism of blood pressure reduction with exercise training (Jennings et al, 1986; Nelson et al, 1986). The dose-response relationship of exercise level to sympathetic inhibition and to blood pressure reduction is steep, that is the maximum effect of exercise on both is seen with rather low levels of physical training.

Stress

Also unsettled is the role of stress in the sympathetic activation of hypertensive patients and in hypertension pathogenesis in general. Clinical, epidemiological and experimental laboratory research provides some support for the notion that behavioural and psychological factors are of importance in the pathogenesis of hypertension (Folkow, 1982). As a group, hypertensive patients consistently exhibit a behavioural pattern (suppression of hostility) that is particularly associated with activation of the sympathetic nervous system (Esler et al, 1977). The concept that essential hypertension may be a psychosomatic illness is provocative, but as yet unproven.

CNS catecholamines

Since CNS noradrenergic mechanisms are of importance in the regulation of sympathetic nervous system responses, including those accompanying stress reactions, a direct experimental approach to investigating the cause of the sympathetic overactivity in essential hypertension might be to attempt to study noradrenaline release within the brain. Noradrenaline is widely distributed in the brain and in the grey matter of the spinal cord. In subcortical areas of the brain noradrenaline-containing cells are assorted into nuclei and located in different areas classified as A1 to A7 (Dahlstrom and Fuxe, 1964). The largest group of noradrenaline-containing neurones, estimated to account for not less than 50% of the noradrenaline in the brain, is the locus coeruleus (A6), located in the pons near the wall of the fourth ventricle (Foote et al, 1983). Electrophysiological and anatomical studies carried out in animals provide evidence of a connection between pressor hypothalamic and bulbar noradrenergic nuclei involved in cardiovascular regulation and sympathetic preganglionic neurones in the thoracolumbar cord, relayed in part via the rostral ventral medulla (Blessing et al, 1981; Fleetwood-Walker and Coote, 1981; Nakata et al, 1991).

Given the importance of central noradrenergic neurotransmission in influencing sympathetic nervous outflow from the brain, noradrenaline spillover from the brain has been measured using samples from the internal jugular vein, analogous to the measurement of noradrenaline spillover from peripheral organs, in order to seek underlying abnormalities in CNS noradrenergic cardiovascular control in primary hypertension. Reports of an elevated noradrenaline concentration in cerebrospinal fluid in essential hypertension (Eide et al, 1979) provided an additional impetus to do this. The existence of a blood-brain barrier to monoamines, blocking the passage of neurotransmitters between the bloodstream and brain, would invalidate any efforts to assess CNS noradrenaline release using measurements of noradrenaline spillover to plasma, but evidence suggests that, while there are strong grounds for believing that an impediment to noradrenaline passage from the bloodstream to the brain exists, the barrier to movement in the reverse direction, from the brain to the circulation, is much less complete (Glowinski et al, 1965; Hardebo and Owman, 1980).

Noradrenaline is released into the cerebrovascular circulation in both hypertensive patients and healthy subjects (Ferrier et al, 1992) (Figure 3). This release is present after administration of the ganglion blocker trimetaphan (trimethaphan USP), indicating that brain neurones and not cerebrovascular sympathetic nerves are the probable source. Although differing among hypertensive patients, noradrenaline spillover on average is higher than in healthy subjects. CNS noradrenaline spillover was found to

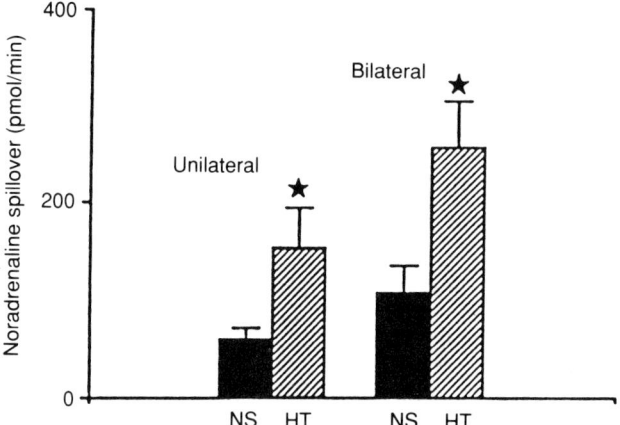

Figure 3. Spillover of noradrenaline (norepinephrine) into the cerebrovascular circulation in hypertensive patients and healthy volunteers. Measurements of noradrenaline spillover into one internal jugular vein, 'unilateral spillover', were obtained with sampling from either left ($n = 4$), right ($n = 7$), or both ($n = 5$) internal jugular veins in normal subjects, and from right ($n = 11$) or both ($n = 6$) internal jugular veins in hypertensive patients. Bilateral noradrenaline spillover measurements (sum of right plus left) were obtained in five normal and six hypertensive subjects. There was a significant difference in unilateral and bilateral noradrenaline spillover between normal and hypertensive subjects ($P < 0.05$). NS = normal subjects; HT = hypertensive patients. From Ferrier et al (1992) with permission.

be elevated in six of 17 patients tested (Figure 3), in whom the accompanying whole-body noradrenaline spillover rate (an index of peripheral sympathetic activity) was also higher than in the remaining patients. Additional clinical studies with the tricyclic antidepressant desipramine, which inhibits noradrenergic neurones within the CNS (Svenssen and Usdin, 1978; Engberg and Eriksson, 1991), have demonstrated a direct relation between brain neuronal noradrenaline release, noradrenaline spillover from the brain, and rates of peripheral sympathetic nerve firing (Esler et al, 1990a).

The biological basis of the increased sympathetic nerve firing present in some patients with essential hypertension, particularly in the early developmental phase, is obscure. These findings provide evidence of a possible link between human cerebral noradrenergic activity and the prevailing level of sympathetic nervous outflow, and suggests that increased sympathetic nerve firing rates present in a proportion of patients with essential hypertension, whatever the initiating mechanism, may possibly derive from increased noradrenaline release in the brain.

Consequences of the sympathetic nervous activation

At one time the view was held that increased sympathetic nervous activity could not cause sustained elevation of blood pressure and could not be of importance in the pathogenesis of essential hypertension. The regulatory effects of sympathetic nerves on renin release, glomerular filtration rate and renal tubular reabsorption of sodium, and their influence on both cardiac performance and cardiovascular cell growth, are now seen to provide a range of potential hypertension-producing mechanisms.

It is possible that the clinical relevance of sympathetic nervous activation in essential hypertension goes beyond that of hypertension pathogenesis. The contribution made by increased sympathetic activity to hyperlipidaemia and atherosclerosis development, to arteriolar and ventricular hypertrophy, to ventricular arrhythmias in hypertensive patients, and to insulin resistance and hyperinsulinaemia is under active investigation.

Haemodynamics of early hypertension

The changes which occur in the haemodynamics of hypertension as the disease develops and evolves are probably dictated in part by progressive changes in the level of cardiac sympathetic stimulation. As elegantly demonstrated by the longitudinal studies of Lund-Johansen (1989) (Table 4), the

Table 4. Progression of haemodynamics in primary human hypertension.

	Initial	After 10 years	After 20 years
Mean blood pressure (mmHg)	114	115	122
Cardiac index (litre·min^{-1}·m^{-2})	3.72	3.22	2.48
Total peripheral resistance (dynes·cm^{-5}·m^{-2})	2499	2971	4031
Heart rate (beats/min)	81	77	71

From Lund-Johansen (1989) with permission.

high heart rate and cardiac output common at the initiation of the hypertensive process give way over the years to normal or reduced values and an arterial pressure elevation based on increased total peripheral vascular resistance. Although this progressive reduction in cardiac output is no doubt due in part to the gradual development of secondary cardiovascular hypertrophy, it is paralleled by, and perhaps jointly caused by, the fall in cardiac sympathetic nervous stimulation with age in hypertensive patients (Figure 2) (Esler et al, 1985).

Renal renin release and 'renin status' in essential hypertension

Release of renin from the juxtaglomerular cells of the kidney is, importantly, under neural control, with the renal sympathetic nerves stimulating renin release by a β-adrenergic mechanism. Plasma renin activity in essential hypertensive patients differs widely, with patients having values both above and below the normal range. In young patients with 'high renin' essential hypertension, indirect evidence has previously pointed to the presence of increased sympathetic activity as the underlying mechanism of elevated plasma renin activity (Esler et al, 1977). Strong and direct supporting evidence is now available to indicate that elevated rates of release of

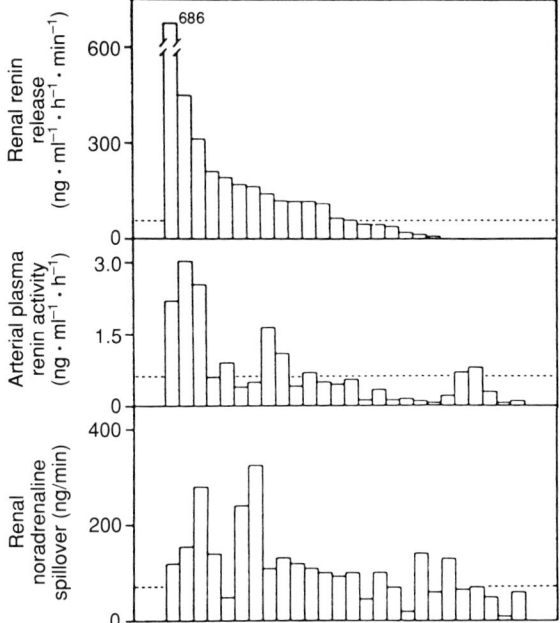

Figure 4. Renal renin release measurements are shown rank-ordered for 26 patients with essential hypertension in whom renal noradrenaline (norepinephrine) spillover was measured concurrently. Mean values in the healthy subjects are shown by the broken lines. Overall, a significant relationship existed between renin secretion and renal noradrenaline spillover ($r_s = 0.60$; $P < 0.01$, Spearman's rank correlation). Elevated renin release and high plasma renin activity, present in some patients, are attributable to increased renal sympathetic nervous activity, indicated by increased renal noradrenaline spillover to plasma (lower panel). From Esler et al (1989) with permission.

renin from the kidneys and high plasma renin activity in essential hypertensive patients is, in fact, a result of increased renal sympathetic nervous activity (Figure 4).

Insulin resistance and hyperinsulinaemia in essential hypertension: cause or consequence?

Non-obese patients with essential hypertension characteristically have insulin resistance and mildly elevated serum insulin values (Modan et al, 1985). The biological significance of this abnormality is uncertain, and whether the peripheral insulin resistance is a cause or a consequence of the hypertension is debated. The most commonly held view is that the insulin resistance is the primary abnormality, which, by the hyperinsulinaemia it causes, results in facilitated renal tubular reabsorption of sodium, sympathetic nervous system activation, and ultimately hypertension (Ferrari and Weidmann, 1990). High serum insulin values, substantially greater than those present in hypertensive patients, have been shown to promote renal tubular sodium reabsorption and to stimulate sympathetic nervous activity (De Fronzo, 1981). Contrary to this thesis of the hypertension-provoking tendency of insulin, however, is experimental evidence that chronic infusion of insulin in dogs does not raise the blood pressure (Hall et al, 1990).

An alternative viewpoint which is gaining favour is that the hyperinsulinaemia of essential hypertension is a secondary phenomenon, resulting from the underlying haemodynamic abnormalities present. Glucose utilization by skeletal muscle under the influence of insulin, which is the process largely determining measured insulin resistance, is dictated by muscle blood flow (Baron et al, 1990). Reduced skeletal muscle blood flow in hypertension, resulting either from neural vasoconstriction or from vascular rarefaction, may possibly be the primary cause of the insulin resistance and the attendant hyperinsulinaemia.

Cardiovascular hypertrophy

While cardiac and arteriolar smooth muscle hypertrophy in essential hypertension undoubtedly represent in part a reaction to increased work load, there is a commonly held view that increased sympathetic activity might have a cardiovascular growth-promoting effect. Growth of cardiac myocytes in cell culture is stimulated by catecholamines (Simpson and McGrath, 1983). Despite this expectation, our early experience in a continuing study is that left ventricular mass, measured by echocardiography, and cardiac sympathetic activity, estimated from measurements of noradrenaline spillover, are unrelated in untreated hypertensive patients (Esler et al, 1990b). Perhaps the level and duration of the blood pressure elevation are of overriding importance.

Hyperlipidaemia and atherosclerosis development

The failure of antihypertensive therapy to reduce the incidence of coronary artery disease in patients with essential hypertension, despite blood pressure reduction, has suggested that hypertension and atherogenesis might share a common mechanism. This could possibly be overactivity of the sympathetic nervous system, since in non-human primate models of stress-induced atherosclerosis, for example, activation of the sympathetic nervous system has been demonstrated to be the major atherogenic mechanism (Clarkson et al, 1987). However, it is not clear at present whether increased sympathetic nervous activity in hypertensive patients contributes materially to atherogenesis.

Although hyperlipidaemia is common in patients with essential hypertension, often accompanied by hyperinsulinaemia, the cause of the coexistence of these metabolic characteristics with elevated blood pressure has not been established. One possible mediating mechanism involves sympathetic nervous activation and plasma catecholamine excess, which have complex but potentially important effects on blood lipids. A range of possibly atherogenic lipid changes have been demonstrated (Landsberg and Young, 1992). Clearance of chylomicrons in the periphery and chylomicron remnants by the liver is slowed, leading to prolongation of the postabsorptive phase of chylomicronaemia. This change has been attributed to adrenergic vaso-constriction reducing regional blood flows and consequently chylomicron clearance. Catecholamine-induced hypercholesterolaemia also reflects, in part, enhanced cholesterol biosynthesis. Lipolysis in adipose tissue is activated due to stimulation of hormone-sensitive lipase. The released free fatty acids serve as a substrate for hepatic lipogenesis.

The chronic effects of antiadrenergic antihypertensives on plasma lipids is complex and not readily predicted from the known effects of infused cate-cholamines. Most striking, and potentially adverse in terms of atherosclero-sis development, is the effect of β-adrenergic blocking drugs, which consistently reduce plasma high density lipoprotein levels, and rather more variably elevate plasma low density and very low density lipoproteins (Tanaka et al, 1976; Wallace et al, 1980).

Cardiac arrhythmias

Patients with essential hypertension are prone to cardiac arrhythmias and sudden death. The importance of neural mechanisms in arrhythmogenesis is well established, with stimulation of the cardiac sympathetic outflow predis-posing to ventricular tachycardia and fibrillation in a variety of experimental models of arrhythmia development, including those due to myocardial ischaemia (Verrier and Lown, 1984). Increased cardiac sympathetic nerve firing, as measured by cardiac noradrenaline spillover, has also been demon-strated to commonly underly clinical ventricular arrhythmias (Meredith et al, 1991a). The relative contributions of left ventricular hypertrophy, which promotes re-entrant arrhythmias, increased cardiac sympathetic activity and coronary atherosclerosis to arrhythmia development in hypertensive patients is unclear at this stage.

Effects of antihypertensive therapy on sympathetic nervous system activity and plasma noradrenaline concentration

Changes commonly occur in sympathetic nervous system function with drug administration. These have recently been reviewed by Esler et al (1990a). With antihypertensive drug therapy, in some instances these changes repre-sent the therapeutic sympathoinhibitory action of the drug (Table 5), and in others the changes are homeostatic adaptations which oppose the mechan-isms of action of the drug, undermining its efficacy as an antihypertensive. Examples of the former are the reduction in sympathetic nerve firing with clonidine, while the reflex sympathetic activation produced by vasodilators (Keeton and Biediger, 1988) and the selective activation of the renal sym-pathetic outflow with diuretics (Esler et al, 1984) are examples of the latter (Table 5).

Non-pharmacological antihypertensive measures in some instances also modify sympathetic nervous function. Restriction of dietary energy intake by a reducing diet is sympathoinhibitory (Jung et al, 1979; O'Dea et al, 1982). A low salt diet selectively activates the renal sympathetic outflow

Table 5. Effects of treatment of hypertension on sympathetic nervous system function and noradrenaline release.

Treatment	Effects
Drugs	
Diuretics	Selective activation of renal sympathetic outflow
Hydralazine, minoxidil, nitroprusside, vasodilator calcium antagonists	Reflex sympathetic stimulation
Clonidine, methyldopa, ganglion blockers	Reduced sympathetic nerve firing
β-Adrenergic blockers	Reduced noradrenaline plasma clearance
ACE inhibitors	Minimal effects
Non-pharmacological treatment	
Reduced dietary energy intake	Sympathetic nervous system inhibition
Low salt diet	Selective activation of renal sympathetic outflow
Exercise training	Selective renal sympathetic nervous inhibition

ACE = angiotensin-converting enzyme.

(Friberg et al, 1990), much as diuretics do, while exercise training selectively inhibits renal sympathetic nerve firing (Meredith et al, 1991b) (Table 5).

An elevated noradrenaline plasma concentration or urinary excretion in hypertensive patients, either from the sympathetic nervous activation intrinsic to their disease or due to their therapy, may suggest a possible diagnosis of phaeochromocytoma. Biochemical testing for phaeochromocytoma is described in Chapters 10 and 11.

THE POSSIBLE ROLE OF ADRENALINE IN ESSENTIAL HYPERTENSION

Adrenaline, the principal hormone of the adrenal medulla, is also present in low concentrations in extra-adrenal tissues (Caramona and Soares-da-Silva, 1985). In certain regions of the CNS, in adrenergic nuclei and their projections, adrenaline has a well-established role as a neurotransmitter. Although brain stem adrenaline-containing neurones are of importance in the CNS regulation of sympathetic outflow to the cardiovascular system, having a documented pressor function in some instances and projecting directly to the preganglionic sympathetic neurones of the spinal cord, we will review only adrenaline in the periphery in considering the role of adrenaline in hypertension pathogenesis.

Adrenaline is found in peripheral organs. In the heart and kidneys, for example, the adrenaline to noradrenaline tissue concentration ratio is approximately 1 : 50, most of the adrenaline being contained within sympathetic nerves (Caramona and Soares-da-Silva, 1985). The functional significance of tissue adrenaline in peripheral organs is uncertain. Adrenaline in peripheral tissues appears to have been largely derived from hormone circulating in plasma rather than synthesis in situ (Majewski et al, 1982).

Evidence exists that adrenaline within sympathetic nerves, derived from this source, may be released with noradrenaline, and act as a cotransmitter facilitating the release of the major neurotransmitter (Adler-Graschinsky and Langer, 1975; Majewski et al, 1980). There are grounds for thinking that adrenaline may stimulate presynaptic β-receptors on sympathetic nerves in this way, increasing the amount of noradrenaline released per nerve impulse.

One theory of the pathogenesis of essential hypertension draws on these concepts, envisaging that stress-induced elevations in the plasma concentration of adrenaline may enlarge the neuronal adrenaline pool and increase neuronal adrenaline release, facilitating noradrenaline release, cardiovascular stimulation and the development of arterial hypertension (Brown and Macquin, 1981; Majewski et al, 1981). The plasma concentration of adrenaline has, however, been less consistently found to be elevated in patients with essential hypertension than the plasma concentration of the sympathetic neurotransmitter noradrenaline (Goldstein, 1983). Further, the reported plasma concentrations of adrenaline, if elevated, have in most instances been less than the threshold concentration for direct stimulation of the cardiovascular system (Clutter et al, 1980). Special significance is given within this conceptual framework to minimally elevated plasma adrenaline values in hypertension pathogenesis (Brown and Macquin, 1981; Majewski et al, 1981). The central questions of the neuronal adrenaline/cotransmitter/ neuromodulator hypothesis of essential hypertension pathogenesis are:

1. Is adrenaline released from sympathetic nerves, and is it released to an increased degree in patients with essential hypertension?
2. Is plasma adrenaline the source of neuronal adrenaline, and is an elevated plasma adrenaline concentration in hypertensive patients the basis for an enlarged neuronal adrenaline pool?
3. Does adrenaline released as a cotransmitter enhance noradrenaline release?
4. Is such facilitation of noradrenaline release a cause of essential hypertension?

Although it has not been easy to test all the elements of this hypothesis in human subjects, the findings are consistent with the view that under certain conditions adrenaline is released by human sympathetic nerves.

Release of adrenaline from human sympathetic nerves

To detect outward flux of adrenaline to plasma, indicative of release of adrenaline from neuronal (and perhaps extraneuronal) stores, in the face of the net extraction of plasma adrenaline which occurs across all organs except the adrenal medulla, radiotracer methodology is needed. The principle applied is that the outward flux of adrenaline can be measured from the reduction in the ratio of plasma radiolabelled to unlabelled adrenaline concentrations (the isotope dilution) occurring in the passage of blood through an organ. Techniques of this type, initially developed for measuring noradrenaline release from sympathetic nerves, have recently been

A

HEALTHY SUBJECTS : Plasma Adrenaline
                              Specific Radioactivity (dpm/pg)

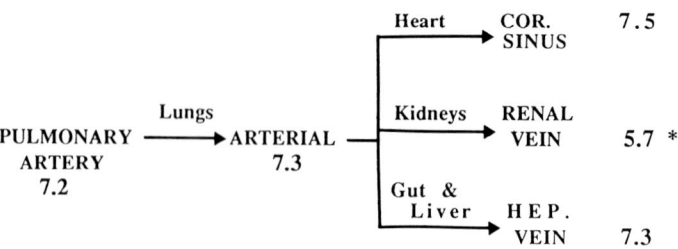

Mean Tritiated Adrenaline Infusion Rate 1.44 x 10⁶ dpm/min

B

CARDIAC ADRENALINE KINETICS : EXERCISE

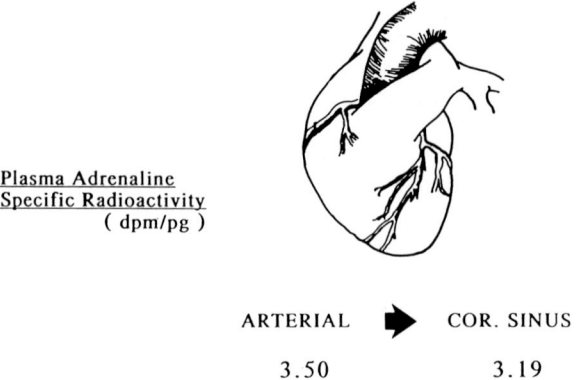

Cardiac Adrenaline Spillover = 1.63 ng/min

Figure 5. (A) Plasma adrenaline specific radioactivity (plasma tritiated/endogenous adrenaline) (in dpm/pg) at steady-state for a range of sampling points in the circulation during a constant rate infusion of tritiated adrenaline in healthy subjects at rest. There was no detectable regional adrenaline overflow for the lungs, heart or hepatomesenteric circulation, as indicated by the absence of material plasma adrenaline isotope dilution across the respective vascular beds. Isotope dilution was evident in the right renal vein ($*P<0.05$, paired t-test), but an adrenal medullary source of this adrenaline release is suspected. *(B)* Transcardiac plasma adrenaline specific radioactivity shown in healthy subjects during aerobic exercise, a strong stimulus to cardiac neuronal firing. During the exercise adrenaline overflow from the heart was detectable ($*P<0.05$, paired t-test). From Esler et al (1991) with permission.

modified to enable simultaneous measurement of adrenaline and nor-adrenaline release.

Under certain circumstances adrenaline is, in fact, released from human sympathetic nerves. We have been able to demonstrate release of adrenaline from the heart in healthy subjects, but only with the extreme level of stimulation of the cardiac sympathetic nerves which accompanies aerobic exercise (Esler et al, 1991) (Figure 5). No release of adrenaline is evident from the resting heart or during the less extreme activation of the cardiac sympathetic outflow which accompanies isometric exercise and mental challenge. Presumably adrenaline is released from the cardiac sympathetic nerves at a low, undetectable rate at rest, and it is only with the 10- to 30-fold increase in nerve firing occurring with aerobic exercise that this adrenaline release becomes measurable. During aerobic exercise, we found adrenaline spillover to plasma to be approximately 1–2% of the associated noradrenaline spillover rate, this representing the relative proportions of the two catecholamines in the heart (Esler et al, 1991). Release of adrenaline has also been reported from the dog heart with electrical stimulation of the cardiac sympathetic nerves (Peronnet et al, 1988).

In healthy resting subjects there is no detectable release of adrenaline into the hepatomesenteric circulation or from the lungs. Overflow of adrenaline does occur, however, into the right renal vein. We found the rate of spillover of adrenaline into the right renal vein to be equivalent to approximately 8% of the associated noradrenaline overflow. This is much greater than the adrenaline/noradrenaline tissue concentration ratio in the kidney. Although adrenal medullary venous drainage occurs directly into the left but not the right renal vein, some contamination of the renal vein sample by adrenal venous effluent must be suspected.

Source of adrenaline in human sympathetic nerves

The source of the adrenaline released from the heart is most likely circulating adrenaline secreted by the adrenal medulla and extracted from plasma by the cardiac sympathetic nerves. Findings with the neuronal noradrenaline uptake blocker desipramine demonstrate the capacity of the human heart to extract adrenaline from plasma by a process of neuronal uptake (Eisenhofer et al, 1990) (Figure 6). A report that cardiac tissue contains enzymes capable of synthesizing adrenaline, however, does raise the possibility that some cardiac adrenaline may be synthesized locally (Elayan et al, 1990). In the presence of a high prevailing plasma adrenaline level, in a patient with an adrenaline-secreting phaeochromocytoma, neuronal release of adrenaline was markedly increased (Figure 7), being equivalent to fully 12% of the total plasma adrenaline appearance rate (Esler et al, 1991).

Does neuronal adrenaline facilitate release of noradrenaline from human sympathetic nerves such as to cause essential hypertension?

It has been envisaged that chronic stress may elevate plasma adrenaline concentration and load the sympathetic neuronal adrenaline pool, thereby

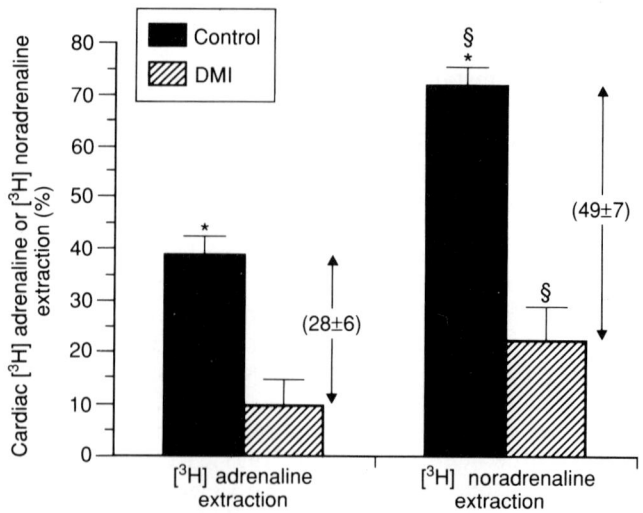

Figure 6. Cardiac extraction of tritiated plasma adrenaline and noradrenaline in human subjects at steady-state during infusion of the radiotracers. Cardiac extraction of adrenaline from plasma was dependent on uptake into sympathetic nerves, as demonstrated by the inhibition of extraction after administration of the selective neuronal uptake blocker, desipramine (DMI). $* = P < 0.05$, significant difference between ^{3}H norepinephrine and ^{3}H epinephrine extractions (by paired t-test); $\S = P < 0.05$, significant difference in ^{3}H norepinephrine and ^{3}H epinephrine extractions before and after desipramine (by paired t-test). From Eisenhofer et al (1990) with permission.

facilitating release of noradrenaline, amplifying sympathetic nervous signals and causing hypertension (Majewski et al, 1981). The first step in the testing of this hypothesis in humans has involved studying the effects of infusion of adrenaline on the release of noradrenaline. Adrenaline infusions typically, but not invariably, elevate the plasma concentration of noradrenaline (Floras, 1992). However, this does not necessarily represent a presynaptic effect of neuronally released adrenaline on noradrenaline release. Sympathetic nerve firing increases during an adrenaline infusion, possibly due to its vasodilator actions (Persson et al, 1989).

Perhaps more interesting are the sustained after-effects of adrenaline on noradrenaline release and sympathetic nervous cardiovascular responses. Prolonged increases in heart rate and reflexly induced vasoconstrictor responses have been noted after infusions of adrenaline (Floras, 1992). But again, increased sympathetic nerve firing also occurs, perhaps attributable to an accompanying, long-lasting reduction in central venous pressure (Persson et al, 1989).

In short, it is now clear that under certain circumstances adrenaline is released from human sympathetic nerves, and that extraction of circulating adrenaline from plasma is the source of at least some of this neuronally released adrenaline, but the causal chain linking a stress-related elevation of plasma adrenaline concentration to a neurogenic pathogenesis of essential hypertension still remains very incomplete.

PHAEOCHROMOCYTOMA : Plasma Adrenaline
Specific Radioactivity (dpm/pg)

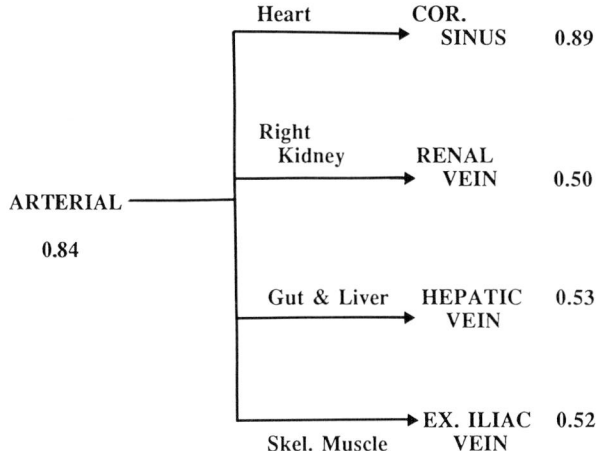

Tritiated Adrenaline Infusion Rate 1.39 x 10^6 dpm/min

Figure 7. Regional release of adrenaline in a patient with an adrenaline-secreting phaeochromocytoma. Adrenaline spillover from the right kidney, skeletal muscle and gut and liver, signified by the presence of plasma adrenaline isotope dilution (values in dpm/pg). From Esler et al (1991) with permission.

THE POSSIBLE ROLE OF DOPAMINE IN ESSENTIAL HYPERTENSION

The catecholamines noradrenaline, adrenaline and dopamine are widely distributed in mammalian species. Dopamine is a precursor of noradrenaline and adrenaline and is found with them in tissues. It is also an important CNS transmitter, and perhaps a transmitter within the peripheral nervous system. It is within the kidney that the case for such 'dopaminergic nerves' is strongest (Bell, 1987).

It has been difficult to definitively demonstrate renal dopaminergic nerves in which the principal neurotransmitter is dopamine. Continuing uncertainty rests on whether renal dopamine/noradrenaline tissue concentration ratios in excess of 1 : 10 can be explained by the presence of dopamine as a noradrenaline precursor in sympathetic nerves, or whether a subset of dopaminergic fibres must exist. A substantial fraction of the dopamine found in the kidney, in fact, is extraneuronal, formed in the proximal renal tubules by decarboxylation of dihydroxyphenylalanine (dopa) extracted from plasma. The urinary excretion of dopamine greatly exceeds that attributable to filtration from plasma at the glomerulus (Lee, 1982; Bradley and Hjemdahl, 1986). The excess largely derives from this tubular decarboxylation of dopa (Lee, 1982; Baines et al, 1985). The urinary excretion of dopamine is determined by a variety of influences, the most striking effect being the very marked increase in urinary dopamine excretion occurring with sodium loading (Oates et al, 1979). It now seems probable that renal tubular generation of dopamine is important in the regulation of urinary sodium excretion, representing a natriuretic mechanism (Lee, 1982; Williams et al, 1986). The interest in dopamine as being possibly causally involved in the pathogenesis of essential hypertension centres on this natriuretic action and evidence that renal dopaminergic natriuretic processes may possibly be defective in patients with essential hypertension (Perkins et al, 1980; Shikuma et al, 1986).

The first report of decreased urinary excretion of dopamine in patients with essential hypertension was by Kuchel et al (1979). Subsequent studies have demonstrated reduced urinary dopamine excretion, or reduced dopamine/dopa urinary excretion ratios, in hypertensive patients on a high salt diet, 'salt-sensitive hypertensives' who show an above normal blood pressure rise on a high salt diet, and subjects with normal blood pressure who are genetically predisposed to essential hypertension (Weinberger et al, 1982; Saito et al, 1984).

These results suggest that there is deficient renal uptake or decarboxylation of dopa in at least a subset of essential hypertensives—those showing undue sensitivity to the pressor effects of dietary sodium. Although there is as yet no proof that this is a causal mechanism of their hypertension, the evidence is very provocative.

SUMMARY

Given the ubiquitous distribution of catecholamines in mammals, and their importance in a range of physiological processes pivotal to blood pressure regulation, the subject of catecholamines and essential hypertension has a broader context than simply consideration of sympathetic nervous system and adrenal medullary dysfunction. These further matters are the likely involvement in hypertension pathogenesis of the CNS catecholaminergic neurones influencing peripheral sympathetic outflow, the possible pathogenetic significance of adrenaline released as a cotransmitter in sympathetic nerves, and the natriuretic renal tubular dopamine mechanisms for regulating body sodium balance which appear to be impaired in patients with essential hypertension. The central consideration, however, remains the important issue of the causes and consequences of the now well-documented sympathetic nervous overactivity which characterizes the early developmental phases of essential hypertension.

REFERENCES

Adler-Graschinsky E & Langer SZ (1975) Possible role of a β-adrenoceptor in the regulation of noradrenaline release by nerve stimulation through a positive feedback mechanism. *British Journal of Pharmacology* **53**: 43–50.

Anderson EA, Sinkey CA, Lawton WJ et al (1989) Elevated sympathetic nerve activity in borderline hypertensive humans: evidence from direct intraneural recordings. *Hypertension* **14**: 177–183.

Baines AD, Drangova R & Hatcher C (1985) Dopamine production by isolated glomeruli and tubules from rat kidneys. *Canadian Journal of Physiology and Pharmacology* **63**: 155–158.

Baron AD, Laakso M, Brechtel G et al (1990) Reduced postprandial skeletal muscle blood flow contributes to glucose intolerance in human obesity. *Journal of Clinical Endocrinology and Metabolism* **70**: 1525–1533.

Bell C (1987) Endogenous renal dopamine and control of blood pressure. *Clinical and Experimental Hypertension* **9**: 955–975.

Bernard C (1851) Influence du grand Sympathique sur la sensibilité et sur la calorification. *Compte Rendu de la Societé de Biologie* **3**: 163.

Blessing WW, Goodchild AK, Dampney RAL et al (1981) Cell groups in the lower brainstem of the rabbit projecting to the spinal cord with special reference to catecholamine-containing neurones. *Brain Research* **221**: 35–55.

Bradley T & Hjemdahl P (1986) Renal extraction of endogenous and radiolabelled catecholamines in the dog. *Acta Physiologica Scandinavica* **122**: 369–379.

Brown GL & Gillespie JS (1957) The output of sympathetic transmitter from the spleen of the cat. *Journal of Physiology* **138**: 81–102.

Brown MJ & Macquin N (1981) Is adrenaline the cause of essential hypertension? *Lancet* **ii**: 1079–1082.

Caramona MM & Soares-da-Silva P (1985) The effects of chemical sympathectomy on dopamine, noradrenaline and adrenaline content in some peripheral tissues. *British Journal of Pharmacology* **86**: 351–356.

Clarkson TB, Kaplan JR & Adams MR (1987) Psychological influences on the pathogenesis of atherosclerosis among nonhuman primates. *Circulation* **76**: I-29–I-40.

Clutter W, Bier D, Shah S et al (1980) Epinephrine: plasma metabolic clearance rates and physiological thresholds for metabolic and hemodynamic actions in man. *Journal of Clinical Investigation* **66**: 94–101.

Dahlstrom A & Fuxe K (1964) Evidence for existence of monoamine-containing neurones in the central nervous system. I. Demonstration of monoamines in the cell bodies of brainstem neurones. *Acta Physiologica Scandinavica Supplement* **232**: 1–55.

De Fronzo RA (1981) The effect of insulin on renal sodium metabolism. *Diabetologia* **21**: 165–171.

Eide I, Kolloch R, De Quattro V et al (1979) Raised cerebrospinal fluid norepinephrine in some patients with primary hypertension. *Hypertension* **1**: 255–260.

Eisenhofer G, Esler MD, Cox HS et al (1990) Differences in the neuronal removal of circulating epinephrine and norepinephrine. *Journal of Clinical Endocrinology and Metabolism* **70**: 1710–1720.

Elayan HH, Kennedy BP & Ziegler MG (1990) Cardiac atria and ventricles contain different inducible adrenaline synthesizing enzymes. *Cardiovascular Research* **24**: 53–56.

Elliot TR (1905) The action of adrenaline. *Journal of Physiology* **32**: 401–467.

Engberg G & Eriksson E (1991) Effects of α₂-adrenoceptor agonists on locus coeruleus firing rate and brain noradrenaline turnover in N-ethoxycarbonyl-2-ethoxy-1,2-dihydro-quinilone (EEDQ)-treated rats. *Naunyn-Schmiedeberg's Archives of Pharmacology* **343**: 472–477.

Esler M, Julius S, Zweifler A et al (1977) Mild high-renin essential hypertension: a neurogenic human hypertension? *New England Journal of Medicine* **296**: 405–411.

Esler M, Jackman G, Bobik A et al (1979) Determination of norepinephrine apparent release rate and clearance in humans. *Life Sciences* **25**: 1461–1470.

Esler M, Blombery P, Leonard P et al (1982) Radiotracer methodology for the simultaneous estimation of total, and renal, sympathetic nervous system activity in humans. *Clinical Science* **63(supplement 8)**: 285S–287S.

M. D. ESLER

Esler M, Jennings G, Korner P et al (1984) Measurement of total and organ-specific norepinephrine kinetics in humans. *American Journal of Physiology* **247**: E21–E28.

Esler M, Jennings G, Biviano B et al (1985) Mechanism of elevated plasma noradrenaline in the course of essential hypertension. *Journal of Cardiovascular Pharmacology* **8(supplement 5)**: 539–544.

Esler M, Jennings G, Korner P et al (1988) Assessment of human sympathetic nervous system activity from measurements of norepinephrine turnover. *Hypertension* **11**: 3–20.

Esler M, Lambert G & Jennings G (1989) Regional norepinephrine turnover in human hypertension. *Clinical and Experimental Hypertension* **11(supplement 1)**: 75–89.

Esler M, Jennings G, Lambert G et al (1990a) Overflow of catecholamine neurotransmitters to the circulation: source, fate, and functions. *Physiological Reviews* **70**: 963–985.

Esler M, Lambert G & Jennings G (1990b) Increased regional sympathetic nervous activity in human hypertension: Causes and consequences. *Journal of Hypertension* **8(supplement 7)**: S53–S57.

Esler M, Eisenhofer G, Chin J et al (1991) Is adrenaline released by sympathetic nerves in man? *Clinical Autonomic Research* **1**: 103–108.

Ferrari P & Weidmann P (1990) Insulin, insulin sensitivity and hypertension. *Journal of Hypertension* **8**: 491–500.

Ferrier C, Esler M, Eisenhofer G et al (1992) Increased norepinephrine spillover into the cerebrovascular circulation in essential hypertension: Evidence of high central nervous system norepinephrine turnover? *Hypertension* **19**: 62–69.

Fleetwood-Walker SM & Coote JH (1981) The contribution of brain stem catecholamine cell groups to the innervation of the lateral cell column. *Brain Research* **205**: 141–155.

Floras JS (1992) Epinephrine and the genesis of hypertension. *Hypertension* **19**: 1–18.

Folkow B (1982) Physiological aspects of primary hypertension. *Physiological Reviews* **62**: 347–504.

Foote SL, Bloom FE & Aston-Jones G (1983) Nucleus coeruleus: New evidence of anatomical and physiological specificity. *Physiological Reviews* **63**: 844–914.

Friberg P, Meredith I, Jennings G et al (1990) Evidence of increased renal noradrenaline spillover rate during sodium restriction in man. *Hypertension* **16**: 121–130.

Glowinski J, Kopin IJ & Axelrod J (1965) Metabolism of [^{3}H] norepinephrine in the rat brain. *Journal of Neurochemistry* **12**: 25–30.

Goldstein DS (1981) Plasma norepinephrine in essential hypertension: a study of the studies. *Hypertension* **3**: 48–52.

Goldstein DS (1983) Plasma catecholamines and essential hypertension: an analytical review. *Hypertension* **5**: 86–99.

Guzzetti S, Piccaluga E, Casati R et al (1988) Sympathetic predominance in essential hypertension: a study employing spectral analysis of heart rate variability. *Journal of Hypertension* **6**: 711–717.

Hagbarth K-E & Vallbo AB (1968) Pulse and respiratory grouping of sympathetic impulses in human muscle nerves. *Acta Physiologica Scandinavica* **74**: 96–108.

Hall JE, Brands MW, Kivlighn SD et al (1990) Chronic hyperinsulinemia and blood pressure. Interactions with catecholamines. *Hypertension* **15**: 519–527.

Hardebo JE & Owman CH (1980) Barrier mechanisms for neurotransmitter monoamines and their precursors at the blood-brain barrier interface. *Annals of Neurology* **8**: 1–11.

Hoeldtke RD, Cilmi KM, Reichard GA Jr et al (1983) Assessment of norepinephrine secretion and production. *Journal of Laboratory and Clinical Medicine* **101**: 772–782.

Jennings G, Nelson L, Nestel P et al (1986) The effects of changes in physical activity on major cardiovascular risk factors, hemodynamics, sympathetic function, and glucose utilization in man: a controlled study of four levels of activity. *Circulation* **73**: 30–40.

Jung RT, Shetty PS, Barrand M et al (1979) Role of catecholamines in hypotensive response to dieting. *British Medical Journal* **i**: 12–13.

Keeton TK & Biediger AM (1988) The measurement of norepinephrine clearance and spillover rate into plasma in spontaneously hypertensive rats. *Naunyn-Schmiedeberg's Archives of Pharmacology* **338**: 350–360.

Kuchel O, Buu NT, Unger T et al (1979) Free and conjugated plasma and urinary dopamine in human hypertension. *Journal of Clinical Endocrinology and Metabolism* **48**: 425–429.

Landsberg L & Young JB (1978) Fasting, feeding and regulation of the sympathetic nervous system. *New England Journal of Medicine* **298**: 1295–1301.

Landsberg L & Young JB (1992) Catecholamines and the adrenal medulla. In Wilson JD & Foster DW (eds) *Williams Textbook of Endocrinology*, pp 621–705. Philadelphia: WB Saunders.

Lee MR (1982) Dopamine and the kidney. *Clinical Science* **62:** 439–448.

Lund-Johansen P (1989) Central haemodynamics is essential hypertension at rest and during exercise: a 20-year follow-up study. *Journal of Hypertension* **7(supplement 6):** S52–S55.

Majewski H, McCulloch M, Rand MJ et al (1980) Adrenaline activation of prejunctional β-adrenoceptors in guinea pig atria. *British Journal of Pharmacology* **71:** 435–444.

Majewski H, Tung LH & Rand MJ (1981) Adrenaline-induced hypertension in rats. *Journal of Cardiovascular Pharmacology* **3:** 179–185.

Majewski H, Hedler L & Starke K (1982) The noradrenaline release rate in the anaesthetized rabbit: Facilitation by adrenaline. *Naunyn-Schmiedeberg's Archives of Pharmacology* **321:** 20–27.

Meredith IT, Broughton A, Jennings GL et al (1991a) Evidence for a selective increase in resting cardiac sympathetic activity in some patients suffering sustained out of hospital ventricular arrhythmias. *New England Journal of Medicine* **325:** 618–624.

Meredith IT, Friberg P, Jennings GL et al (1991b) Regular exercise lowers renal but not cardiac sympathetic activity in man. *Hypertension* **18:** 575–582.

Modan M, Halkin H, Almog S et al (1985) Hyperinsulinaemia. A link between hypertension, obesity and glucose tolerance. *Journal of Clinical Investigation* **75:** 809–817.

Nakata T, Berard W, Kogosov E & Alexander N (1991) Effect of environmental stress on release of norepinephrine in the posterior nucleus of the hypothalamus in awake rats: Role of sinoaortic nerves. *Life Sciences* **48:** 2021–2026.

Nelson L, Jennings G, Esler M et al (1986) Effect of changing levels of physical activity on blood pressure and haemodynamics in essential hypertension. *Lancet* **ii:** 473–476.

Oates NS, Ball SG, Perkins CM & Lee MR (1979) Plasma and urine dopamine in man given sodium chloride in the diet. *Clinical Science* **56:** 261–264.

O'Dea K, Esler M, Leonard P et al (1982) Noradrenaline turnover during under- and over-eating in normal weight subjects. *Metabolism: Clinical and Experimental* **31:** 896–899.

Peart WS (1949) The nature of splenic sympathin. *Journal of Physiology* **108:** 491–501.

Perkins CM, Casson IF, Cope GF et al (1980) Failure of salt to mobilize renal dopamine in human hypertension. *Lancet* **ii:** 1370.

Peronnet F, Nadeau R, Boudreau G et al (1988) Epinephrine release from the heart during left stellate ganglion stimulation in dogs. *American Journal of Physiology* **254:** R659–R662.

Persson B, Andersson OK & Hjemdahl P (1989) Adrenaline infusion in man increases muscle sympathetic nerve activity and noradrenaline overflow to plasma. *Journal of Hypertension* **7:** 747–756.

Peterson HR, Rothschild M, Weinberg CR et al (1988) Body fat and the activity of the autonomic nervous system. *New England Journal of Medicine* **318:** 1077–1083.

Rocchini AP, Moorehead C, DeRemer S et al (1989) Pathogenesis of weight-related changes in blood pressure in dogs. *Hypertension* **13:** 922–928.

Saito I, Takeshita E, Saruta T et al (1984) Plasma prolactin, renin and catecholamines in young normotensive and borderline hypertensive subjects. *Journal of Hypertension* **2:** 61–64.

Shikuma R, Yoshimura M, Kambara S et al (1986) Dopaminergic modulation of salt sensitivity in patients with essential hypertension. *Life Sciences* **38:** 915–921.

Simpson P & McGrath A (1983) Norepinephrine-stimulated hypertrophy of cultured rat myocardial cells is an α_1-adrenergic response. *Journal of Clinical Investigation* **72:** 732–738.

Sowers JR, Whitfield LA, Catania RA et al (1982) Role of the sympathetic nervous system in blood pressure maintenance in obesity. *Journal of Clinical Endocrinology and Metabolism* **54:** 1181–1186.

Svensson TH & Usdin T (1978) Feedback inhibition of brain noradrenaline neurons by tricyclic antidepressant: α-receptor mediation. *Science* **8:** 1089–1091.

Tanaka N, Sagaguchi K, Oshige K et al (1976) Effect of chronic administration of propranolol on lipoprotein composition. *Metabolism: Clinical and Experimental* **25:** 1071–1075.

Verrier RL & Lown B (1984) Behavioral stress and cardiac arrhythmias. *Annual Review of Physiology* **46:** 155–176.

von Euler US (1946) A specific sympathetic ergone in adrenergic nerve fibres (sympathin) and its relation to adrenaline and noradrenaline. *Acta Physiologica Scandinavica* **12:** 73–97.

von Euler US, Hellner S & Purkhold A (1954) Excretion of noradrenaline in the urine in hypertension. *Scandinavian Journal of Clinical and Laboratory Investigation* **6:** 54–59.

Wallace RB, Hunninghake DB & Reiland S (1980) Alteration of plasma high-density lipoprotein cholesterol levels associated with consumption of selected medications: the Lipid Research Clinics Program Prevalence Study. *Circulation* **62(supplement 4):** IV77–IV82.

Wallin BG, Delius W & Hagbarth K-E (1973) Comparison of sympathetic nerve activity in normotensive and hypertensive subjects. *Circulation Research* **33:** 9–21.

Weinberger MH, Luft FC & Henry DP (1982) The role of the sympathetic nervous system in the modulation of sodium excretion. *Clinical and Experimental Hypertension, Part A: Theory and Practice* **4:** 719–735.

Williams M, Young JB, Rosa RM et al (1986) Effect of protein ingestion on urinary dopamine excretion. Evidence for the functional importance of renal decarboxylation of circulatory 3,4-dihydroxyphenylalanine in man. *Journal of Clinical Investigation* **78:** 1687–1693.

Yamada Y, Miyajima E, Tochikubo O et al (1989) Age-related changes in muscle sympathetic nerve activity in essential hypertension. *Hypertension* **13:** 870–877.

7

Sympathetic dysfunction in heart failure

KAZUMASA SHIMIZU
BARRY P. McGRATH

Congestive heart failure (CHF) is a complex and life-threatening clinical syndrome which affects 2–4% of the population aged 45–75 years in Western societies (Smith, 1985). It is widely accepted that enhanced peripheral vascular tone plays a major role in the pathophysiology of CHF, and there is now good evidence that increased activity of the sympathetic nervous system is one of the most important factors responsible for the increased afterload in CHF. Dysfunction of the sympathetic nervous system in CHF involves not only the heart but also many other organs, particularly the kidney. In addition, other humoral factors closely interrelated with the sympathetic nervous system have an important role in the pathophysiology of CHF.

This chapter focuses on sympathetic dysfunction in heart failure, with particular emphasis on the pathophysiology of the syndrome of CHF and the recent advances of research in this field.

NERVOUS CONTROL OF THE CIRCULATION

Sympathetic and parasympathetic neurones in the medulla and spinal cord regulate the circulation through changes in cardiac output and vascular tone in the following way. Afferent signals from various sensors, which detect changes of homeostasis in organs or tissues, terminate at central neurones in the vasomotor centre of the medulla. Central neurones connect to the efferent cardiovascular neurones and are also connected to other central nervous system (CNS) neurones through long and short reflex arcs. Efferent signals generated in the CNS are distributed to the heart and vascular beds and control vascular tone (Abboud and Thames, 1983).

The cardiac atria are well supplied with both sympathetic and para-sympathetic nerves; the ventricles are mainly supplied by sympathetic nerves. These efferent cardiac nerves mediate inotropic and chronotropic responses of the pump to a variety of stimuli. Blood vessels, both arteries and veins, are also regulated by the sympathetic nervous system. The innervation of the large vessels, in particular the central veins, make it possible for sympathetic stimulation to change the volume of the peripheral circulatory system, with resultant translocation of blood into the heart and significant changes in circulatory homeostasis. Although both vasocon-strictor and vasodilator fibres are carried in sympathetic nerves, it is the sympathetic vasoconstrictor fibres which are most important in the control of arteriolar tone. These fibres are distributed to essentially all segments of the circulation, but there are significant variations among different tissues. Moreover, there is increasing evidence for a significant degree of selectivity in the organization of sympathetic pathways going to different organs. There are vasoconstrictor signals continuously, even in the resting condition. On the other hand, parasympathetic stimulation has no effect on blood vessels.

Both baroreceptor and chemoreceptor reflexes are important in the rapid adaptation of the circulation via neural activity. Baroreceptor reflexes are initiated by stretch receptors (baroreceptors, mechanoreceptors or pressor receptors) located in the aorta and carotid sinus which respond to acute changes in arterial pressure. Other stretch receptors, called 'low pressure' cardiopulmonary receptors, exist in both atria and in the pulmonary arteries. There are also cardiac sensory receptors in the ventricles of the heart. Chemoreceptor reflexes are closely allied to baroreceptor reflexes: chemoreceptors located in the carotid and aortic areas detect falls in oxygen, carbon dioxide excess, or hydrogen ion excess. When the blood pressure falls, impulses from the chemoreceptors excite the vasomotor centre, result-ing in elevation of the blood pressure.

Cardiac afferent impulses are transmitted via both the vagus and sympathetic nerves. Cardiac afferents respond to both mechanical stimuli and chemical substances. Excitation of vagal cardiac afferents causes a reflex bradycardia through increasing vagal drive to the sinoatrial pacemaker, and a fall in blood pressure due to withdrawal of sympathetic vasoconstrictor drive to the major vascular beds. Sympathetic afferents transmit the sensation of cardiac pain, but innocuous stimuli may cause a reflex tachy-cardia and a rise in blood pressure (Ludbrook, 1990).

Somatic afferent nerve impulses from skeletal muscle and abdominal viscera also impinge on the pressor and depressor centres in the medulla. There is also significant interaction between the afferents from skeletal muscle and afferents from arterial and/or cardiopulmonary receptors. This skeletal muscle reflex may have an important role, especially in exercise (Mitchell and Schmidt, 1983).

PLASMA CATECHOLAMINES IN CHF AND THEIR SIGNIFICANCE

Plasma catecholamine levels and sympathetic activity

A rise in circulating noradrenaline levels generally reflects increased sympathetic nervous activity, since most of the noradrenaline in plasma arises from peripheral nerve endings rather than from the adrenal gland, and a positive correlation is usually assumed between sympathetic activity and plasma noradrenaline levels (Lake et al, 1976). However, there are important limitations in the use of plasma noradrenaline as an index of sympathetic nervous activity. Plasma noradrenaline is determined not only by the rate of spillover to plasma after release but also by the rate of clearance from plasma, which includes uptake 1 (neuronal uptake) and uptake 2 (metabolism in non-neuronal tissue). Circulating noradrenaline represents less than 22% of the noradrenaline released from nerve endings (Hoeldtke et al, 1983). Also, a decrease in noradrenaline clearance has been reported in heart failure patients (Hasking et al, 1986; Davis et al, 1988). Other confounding influences on plasma catecholamine levels include collection techniques and reduced cutaneous blood flow in conditions such as CHF. Despite these objections, venous noradrenaline provides a reasonable indirect index of sympathetic neural activity and can be used to evaluate average sympathetic tone in disease states in humans (Goldstein et al, 1983).

Plasma catecholamine levels and severity of CHF

Several studies have shown that the plasma concentration of noradrenaline and the urinary excretion of catecholamines are increased in patients with CHF compared with normal subjects, and that the more severe grades of CHF are associated with the highest levels (Chidsey et al, 1965; Thomas and Marks, 1978; Levine et al, 1982). In most of these studies it has been difficult to exclude treatment effects resulting from the use of diuretics or vasodilator drugs. However, increased levels of circulating noradrenaline have also been reported in animal models of heart failure when there are no drugs involved (Riegger and Liebau, 1982; McGrath, 1987).

Francis et al (1982) reported that supine resting plasma noradrenaline levels were related to the severity of the CHF as assessed by resting haemodynamic measurements, especially stroke volume, stroke work index, and right atrial pressure. In addition, they showed that plasma noradrenaline levels were more closely correlated with exercise capacity (as measured by peak oxygen consumption) than were tests of left ventricular performance at rest. On the other hand, Levine et al (1982) reported that correlations between objective measurements of heart failure severity and plasma noradrenaline concentration were not very strong. Lehmann et al (1990) concluded that the level of noradrenaline in the plasma was not particularly helpful as a marker of cardiac function.

Dopamine-β-hydroxylase (DBH) is the enzyme which converts dopamine to noradrenaline and is located in sympathetic nerve endings. Plasma DBH activity has been reported to be reduced in patients with CHF compared with normal controls (Minami et al, 1983).

Plasma catecholamines and arrhythmias in CHF

Catecholamines may potentiate the arrhythmic substrate through an increase in myocardial ischaemia and a decrease in the threshold for ventricular fibrillation. Meredith et al (1991) reported increases in arterial noradrenaline concentration and total and cardiac noradrenaline spillover in a group of patients with ventricular arrhythmias. Moreover, there was an exponential inverse relation between cardiac sympathetic activation and left ventricular ejection fraction. It was suggested that ventricular dysfunction results in reflex cardiac sympathetic activation and this contributes to the genesis of arrhythmia in patients with CHF.

Plasma catecholamine levels and prognosis in CHF

It has been shown that resting supine plasma noradrenaline levels are related to prognosis, those patients having the highest concentrations showing the greatest increase in mortality (Cohn et al, 1984; Rector et al, 1987). This is depicted in Figure 1. Olivari et al (1983) also reported that the

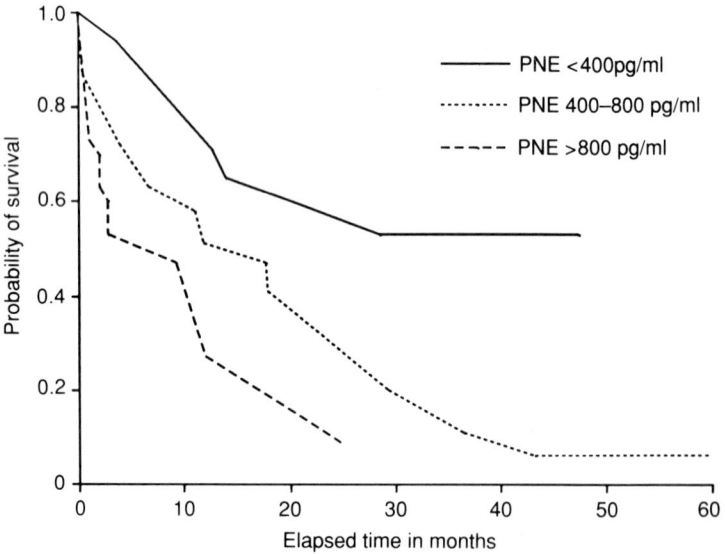

Figure 1. Survival in relation to resting plasma noradrenaline (PNE) levels in patients with CHF. From Cohn et al (1984) with permission.

prognosis was considerably poorer in patients in whom the neurohumoral response to nitroprusside was attenuated than in those with preserved noradrenaline responses to nitroprusside.

DIRECT RECORDING OF SYMPATHETIC ACTIVITY IN CHF

Direct recording from sympathetic nerves in the peroneal or brachial nerves has shown that the number of sympathetic bursts per minute was greater in patients with moderate to severe grades of CHF when compared with normal controls (Leimbach et al, 1986).

SYMPATHETIC ACTIVATION DURING THE DEVELOPMENT OF CHF

Recent evidence from animal studies suggests that the sympathetic nervous system is activated early during the course of CHF. In rabbits treated chronically with doxorubicin, which produces a slowly progressive form of CHF, resting levels of plasma renin activity and noradrenaline concentration were increased after 4 weeks of doxorubicin treatment, a stage when resting haemodynamic measurements did not differ from controls (McGrath et al, 1987). Ganguly and Scherwood (1991) showed that noradrenaline turnover and metabolism in the myocardium were altered soon after imposing an increased workload in rats with heart failure following aorta ligation.

Activation of the sympathetic nervous system may also occur early in the course of human CHF. Recently it was shown as part of the Studies of Left Ventricular Dysfunction (SOLVD) that plasma noradrenaline, plasma renin activity, plasma atrial natriuretic peptide and plasma vasopressin were all elevated in asymptomatic and mildly symptomatic patients with left ventricular dysfunction compared with normal subjects (Francis et al, 1990).

The mechanism(s) of the increased sympathetic nerve activity in CHF have not been defined. Baroreflex dysfunction, alteration in the function of cardiac afferents, and positive interaction of the sympathetic nervous system and the renin–angiotensin system may all play a role. Whatever the mechanism, this increase in sympathetic activity is part of the vicious cycle of CHF and results in excessive vasoconstriction and sodium and water retention.

REFLEX SYMPATHETIC ACTIVITY IN CHF

In normal humans and animals, baroreceptors in the heart, lungs and great vessels contribute to the distribution of cardiac output by regulating regional vascular resistances. In CHF, in humans and in animal models, there is compelling evidence that both the arterial baroreceptor reflex function and the cardiopulmonary reflex function are impaired.

Several methods have been used to assess the function of the arterial and cardiopulmonary baroreflexes. Injection of phenylephrine and nitroprusside, which result in loading and unloading of the baroreceptors respectively, are used to evaluate reflex heart rate responses. This method offers a physiological stimulus to all arterial baroreceptors, but measurement is limited to heart rate changes and important changes in baroreflex control of vascular resistance cannot be determined (Kassis, 1989). It should be noted that nitroprusside has both venodilator and arterial dilator effects which influence cardiopulmonary as well as aortic baroreceptors.

Eckberg et al (1971) reported that the sensitivity of the baroreflex-heart rate reflex was reduced in patients with CHF. Higgins et al (1972) showed that phenylephrine-induced bradycardia is inhibited in conscious dogs with heart failure. They also showed that the pressor response to carotid occlusion is attenuated in this model. The reflex sympathetic responses to sodium nitroprusside, including changes in plasma noradrenaline and heart rate, were shown to be blunted in patients with CHF compared with normal subjects (Olivari et al, 1983).

Head-up tilting or lower body negative pressure (LBNP) have also been utilized for unloading baroreceptors. Upright tilt normally leads to tachycardia, an increase in systemic vascular resistance, and increases in plasma noradrenaline and plasma renin activity. In patients with CHF these responses are impaired. Goldstein et al (1975) showed that the tachycardia response to baroreceptor deactivation caused by tilt or by glyceryl trinitrate infusion was reduced in heart failure. Kubo and Cody (1983) reported that an impairment of the heart rate reflex during tilt was more apparent in patients with more severe cardiac dysfunction. Renal and hepatic blood flow and neurohormonal responses were reported to be greatly attenuated during head-up tilt in patients with severe CHF (Lilly et al, 1984). In the patients with CHF studied by Davis et al (1987), a paradoxical fall in noradrenaline spillover was observed during tilt, in contrast to the increase in noradrenaline spillover seen in normal subjects.

In normal subjects, modest degrees of LBNP cause a decrease in central venous pressure and forearm blood flow but have no effect on aortic mean pressure and heart rate. More intense LBNP results in unloading of arterial baroreceptors, leading to an increase in heart rate and vasoconstriction. In patients with ventricular dysfunction, the responses of plasma noradrenaline and plasma renin activity to a modest degree of LBNP were found to be attenuated, consistent with an abnormality of low pressure mechanoreceptors (Ferguson et al, 1984).

The sensitivity of atrial receptors and renal responses to increases in central venous and left atrial pressures during volume expansion were found to be impaired in the experimental dog model of low output heart failure studied by Greenberg et al (1974) and the high output dog model of CHF studied by Zucker et al (1979, 1985). The reported effects of diminished activity of cardiac sensory afferents in heart failure include tachycardia, vasoconstriction, increased sympathetic efferent activity and increased renin and vasopressin levels (Abboud and Thames, 1983).

These results clearly point to a reduction in the sensitivity of arterial and cardiopulmonary reflexes in heart failure. Although the mechanism of this impairment is not clear, it may be due to a functional derangement because it can be at least partially reversed by medical treatment. The effects of medical treatment on reflex function is discussed later in this chapter.

REGIONAL SYMPATHETIC ACTIVITY IN CHF

Regional blood redistribution and sympathetic activity in CHF

The distribution of the cardiac output is altered in patients with CHF. Resting blood flows to skin, splanchnic, limb and renal vascular beds are reduced, whereas coronary and cerebral blood flow are usually preserved (Zelis and Flaim, 1982). Figure 2a summarizes the distribution of resting blood flow to

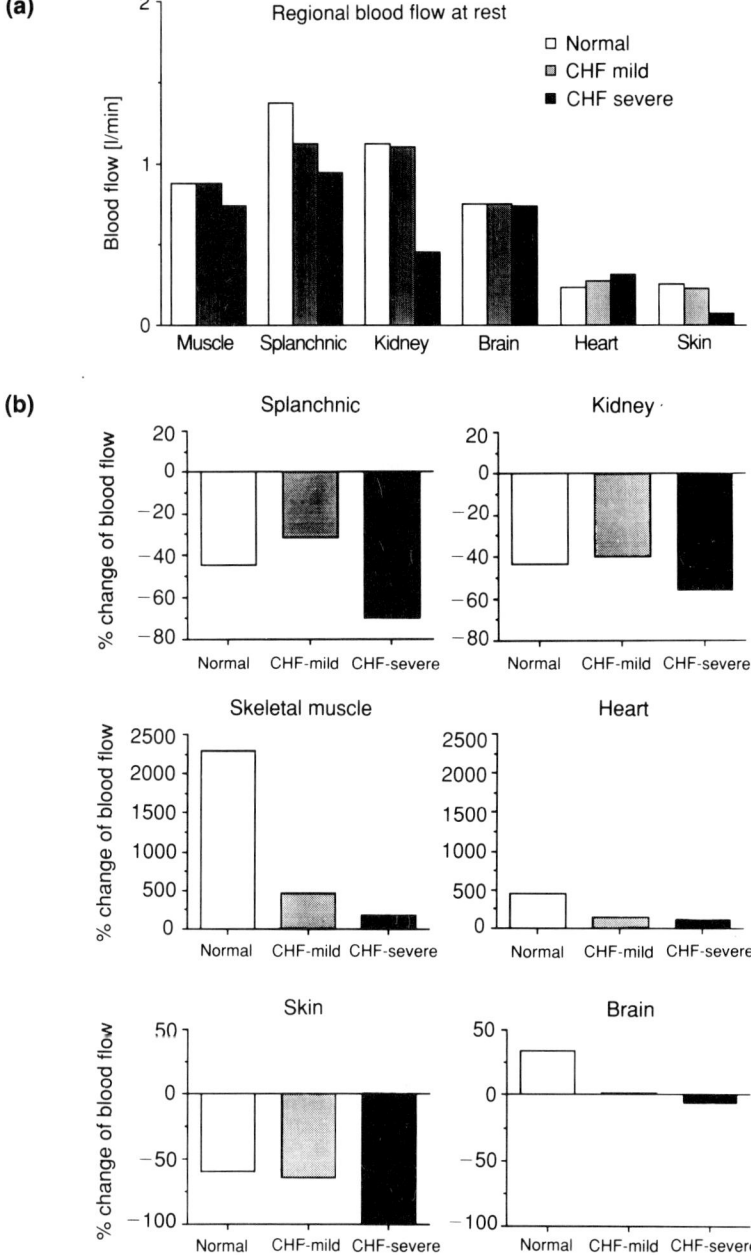

Figure 2. (a) Regional blood distribution at rest in control subjects and patients with CHF. At rest, patients with CHF exhibit decreased blood flow to splanchnic, kidney and muscle beds, whereas blood flows to brain and heart are preserved. (b) Changes of blood flow during exercise shown as a percentage change from resting values. The increase in blood flow to exercising muscle beds is reduced in CHF and there are greater falls in splanchnic, renal and skin blood flows during exercise in patients with CHF compared with control subjects. Data derived from the review by Zelis and Flaim (1982).

different organs in CHF. In normal subjects, there is a marked increase in blood flow to exercising skeletal muscle beds. This response is significantly blunted in CHF. The redistribution of blood flow during exercise in severe CHF is also altered with greater percentage falls observed in splanchnic, renal and cutaneous vascular beds, whereas blood flow to the brain is preserved (Figure 2b). Vasoconstriction mediated by the sympathetic nervous system, may be primarily responsible for this redistribution of peripheral blood flow. Regional differences in the distribution of noradrenaline spillover, as an index of sympathetic activity, were observed in human CHF by Esler et al

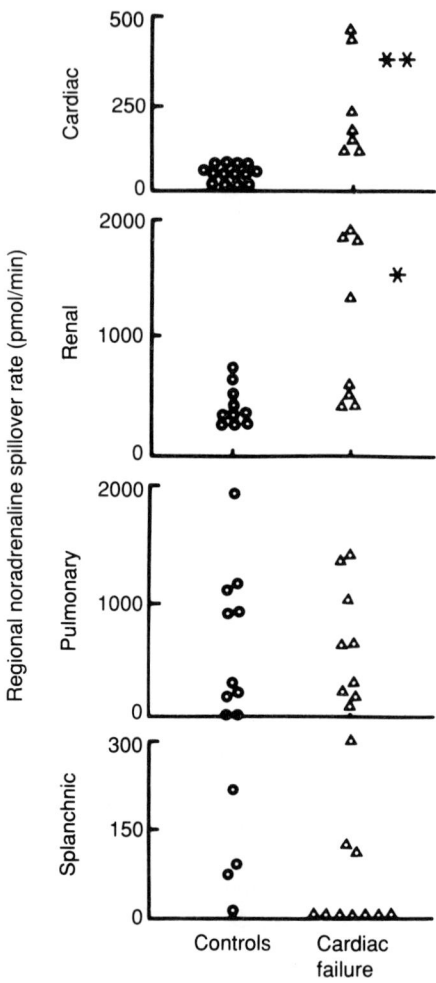

Figure 3. Regional noradrenaline spillover rates under resting conditions in patients with CHF and control subjects. Noradrenaline spillover is significantly increased in the heart and kidneys but not changed in the lung and splanchnic region in patients with CHF compared with control subjects. From Esler et al (1985) with permission.

(1985). This data is summarized in Figure 3. Compared with control subjects, patients with CHF exhibited greater resting noradrenaline spillover in the heart and kidneys, but normal spillover to lungs and hepatomesenteric beds.

Physiological stress results in more pronounced maldistribution of regional blood flow in CHF. Langton and colleagues (1990b) showed that the reduction of renal blood flow during exercise was exaggerated in rabbits with doxorubicin-induced cardiomyopathic heart failure compared with normal control rabbits. Renal sympathectomy abolished the renal vaso-constrictor responses to exercise in heart failure animals. These results were similar to those reported 20 years ago by Millard et al (1972) in an elegant study of exercise responses in dogs with chronic right heart failure induced by pulmonary stenosis and tricuspid incompetence.

Baroreceptor reflex control of regional circulation is non-uniform and this is particularly evident in CHF. Creager et al (1990) showed that LBNP induced a decrease in splanchnic and renal blood flow, but not in forearm blood flow, in heart failure patients. On the other hand, low levels of LBNP caused forearm vasoconstriction and only more negative levels of LBNP caused the vasoconstriction of renal and splanchnic vascular beds in normal subjects. These results indicate that there is baroreceptor regulation of splanchnic and renal vascular resistance, but not limb vascular resistance, in patients with CHF. Attenuation or absence of forearm vasoconstriction during orthostasis or LBNP is a consistent finding and a marker of baroreflex dysfunction in CHF (Goldsmith et al, 1983; Ferguson et al, 1984). The forearm vasodilatation induced by captopril during tilt was only seen after α-blockade in heart failure patients (Creager et al, 1985).

The splanchnic circulation appears to be regulated by carotid baro-receptors, while the subcutaneous vascular beds are controlled by the cardiopulmonary reflex during orthostasis. Both types of receptor partici-pate in the regulation of skeletal muscle blood flow in humans (Kassis, 1989).

The heart and coronary artery

Cardiac noradrenaline content may be depleted in heart failure, despite the increased circulating noradrenaline concentrations. In the Syrian hamster, an animal which exhibits a congenital form of cardiomyopathy, sympathetic stimulation results in a decrease in noradrenaline and an increase in dopamine in cardiac sympathetic nerve terminals (Sole et al, 1977). Reduction of tyrosine hydroxylase activity was observed in an earlier study (Pool et al, 1967). In the Syrian hamster, Sole et al (1982) found an increase in tyrosine hydroxylase activity and showed a reduction in the transport of dopamine into noradrenergic vesicles. Pierpont et al (1987) also reported decreased noradrenaline and increased dopamine levels in cardiac biopsies from humans with cardiomyopathy. Howes et al (1989) reported that, in hearts from rats with cardiac failure resulting from myocardial infarction, the ratio of 3,4-dihydroxyphenylethylene glycol (DHPG) to noradrenaline was higher than in controls, consistent with increased noradrenaline turnover. Anderson et al (1992) showed that neuropeptide Y, a cotransmitter of noradrenaline, was depleted in the human ventricular myocardium in patients with CHF. They also showed that the ratio of dopamine to noradrenaline was decreased compared with normal hearts. Merlet et al (1992) showed that there was impaired neuronal noradrenaline uptake in patients with idiopathic dilated cardiomyopathy using metaiodobenzylguanidine (MIBG) scintigraphy. In contrast, Hasking et al (1986) showed normal noradrenaline extraction, implying normal neuronal noradrenaline uptake, in CHF.

A number of studies have shown reduced cardiac responsiveness to catecholamines and a decreased ventricular β-adrenergic receptor density in human CHF (Fowler et al, 1986; Glison et al, 1990). Calderone et al (1991) reported decreased β-adrenergic receptor density, decreased adenylate cyclase reactivity and blunting of β-adrenergic responses in a CHF-rapid ventricular pacing model in dogs. They also showed that the α_1-adrenergic responses were decreased despite normal α_1-adrenergic receptor density. The downregulation of β adrenergic receptors may be different in ischaemic heart disease and idiopathic cardiomyopathy (Bristow et al, 1991). In our previous study in rabbits with doxorubicin-treated cardiomyopathy, the cardiac β-receptor density was not altered and receptor interaction with the adenylate cyclase stimulatory coupling factor was unimpaired (Woodcock et al, 1988). Prolonged stimulation of sympathetic nerves may exhaust noradrenaline stores, although it remains a controversial issue whether there is any alteration in noradrenaline synthesis. This noradrenaline loss in myocardium is also known to be heterogeneous (Pierpont et al, 1987). This heterogeneous sympathetic innervation in CHF may contribute to the haemodynamic dysfunction through asynchronous myocardial contractions and to arrhythmias as a result of electrical heterogeneity.

The kidney

The kidney has an important role in the pathophysiology of CHF as well as being a major target organ in this complex syndrome. A number of factors may influence the behaviour of the kidney in CHF, including the sympathetic nervous system, the renin–angiotensin–aldosterone system, vasopressin, atrial natriuretic peptide and renal prostaglandins. There is now good evidence that resting renal sympathetic nerve activity is increased in CHF (Esler et al, 1985). This increases markedly in exercise (Langton et al, 1990b). Increased renal sympathetic nervous activity in CHF contributes to altered renal haemodynamics, sodium and water retention, increased renin secretion, and modulation of the intrarenal action of a number of hormones.

In dogs with right heart failure, a marked fall in renal blood flow was observed during exercise and this could be almost abolished by renal denervation (Millard et al, 1972). This has recently been confirmed in another model of CHF, doxorubicin-induced cardiomyopathic heart failure in the rabbit (Langton et al, 1990b). In a dog model of CHF, Zucker et al (1979) reported a blunted fall in renal nerve activity in response to volume expansion. DiBona et al (1988) recorded renal nerve activity directly and noted that the fall in renal sympathetic nerve activity after an acute saline load was less in rats with myocardial infarction than in controls. Bilateral renal denervation restored the renal excretory responses to those of the control rats. In humans, the basal sympathetic outflow to the kidney is significantly increased in patients with heart failure as determined by the renal noradrenaline spillover method (Hasking et al, 1986). These results clearly show that the kidney is an important site of increased sympathetic nerve activity and that this has important functional consequences.

In a study conducted in our laboratories the renal noradrenaline spillover technique was used to assess renal sympathetic activity in rabbits at different stages of CHF as a result of doxorubicin-induced cardiomyopathy and in matching controls (Sano et al, 1990; Noshiro et al, 1991b). Renal spillover was shown to reflect the alteration in renal sympathetic activity (Noshiro et al, 1991a). Renal noradrenaline spillover at rest was found to be increased at an early stage of heart failure and rose further as CHF developed in treated rabbits compared with controls. In this model, the baroreflex-renal noradrenaline spillover response to hypotension was shifted upwards at an early

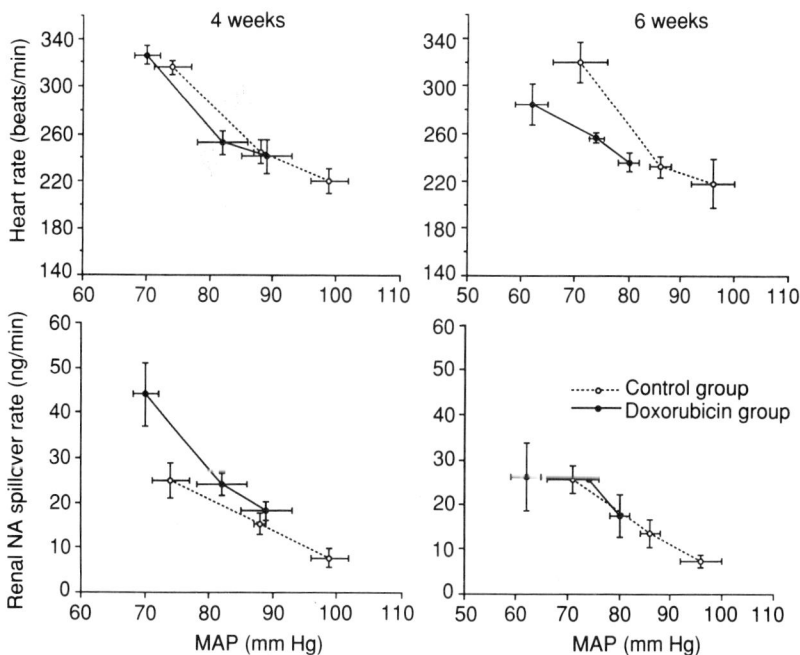

Figure 4. Heart rate and renal noradrenaline (NA) spillover responses in control and heart failure rabbits. The baroreflex-renal noradrenaline spillover response to hypotension induced by nitroprusside is shifted upwards at 4 weeks' treatment with doxorubicin, whereas baroreflex-heart rate responses are maintained. After 6 weeks of doxorubicin treatment (established CHF), both responses are blunted. MAP = mean arterial pressure. From McGrath et al (1990), with permission.

stage of heart failure (4 weeks' treatment), whereas the baroreflex-heart rate response was maintained. In the established stage of CHF (6 weeks' treatment), both the heart rate and the renal noradrenaline spillover responses were blunted (Sano et al, 1990). These results are summarized in Figure 4. It was suggested that there was an early increase in resting renal sympathetic activity in this model of heart failure and that different mechanisms may be operative in the increase in renal sympathetic activity at different stages of CHF.

EXERCISE TOLERANCE IN CHF

The cardinal feature of CHF is limitation of exercise capacity, even when patients are asymptomatic at rest. Exercise capacity is known to be related to cardiac function and the level of plasma noradrenaline (Francis et al, 1982). Szlachcic et al (1985) reported a significant correlation between prognosis and exercise capacity.

A major factor implicated in the genesis of exercise fatigue is an inadequate blood flow to working skeletal muscle relative to the metabolic demands of this active tissue. The increase in muscle blood flow during exercise is up to 75% of the total cardiac output in normal humans (Dargie, 1990). As shown in Figure 2b, reported changes from resting levels in blood flows to exercising skeletal muscle were mean increases of 2300%, 460% and 170% in control subjects, mild CHF and severe CHF, respectively (Zelis and Flaim, 1982). Redistribution of the blood flow during exercise is, at least in part, regulated by the sympathetic nervous system through baroreflex mechanisms.

In the rabbit model of doxorubicin-induced cardiomyopathy, Langton et al (1990b) found that there was an exaggerated diversion of blood flow from the kidney during exercise which was abolished by renal denervation. A paradoxical increase in systemic vascular resistance was observed in rabbits with CHF towards the end of exercise, suggesting that sympathetic vasoconstrictor drive was greatly exaggerated and affected even the exercising muscle vascular beds (Langton et al, 1990a). It was postulated that this abnormal vasoconstrictor response to exercise may result from a combination of the failure of the arterial pressure to reach the elevated set point of the arterial baroreflex which occurs during exercise, increased afferent input from exercising muscle, and increases in central command.

Impaired vasodilatation during exercise in patients with CHF may not be restored by α-blockers or angiotensin-converting enzyme (ACE) inhibition, so that mechanisms other than those mediated by sympathetic activity and angiotensin II (AngII) are also proposed, such as metabolic factors, vasoconstriction by endothelin, blunted release of endothelium-derived relaxing factors (EDRF), and vascular structural changes. Sterns et al (1991) reported that, in patients with CHF, skeletal muscle metaboreceptor responses were impaired, which suggested the central command was activated.

INTERACTION BETWEEN SYMPATHETIC ACTIVITY AND OTHER NEUROENDOCRINE MECHANISMS IN CHF

The autonomic nervous system and various circulating hormones interact closely. Firstly, release of some hormones depends on afferent sensory input from the heart and/or efferent sympathetic nerve activity: for example, vasopressin release is modulated by cardiac afferent receptors and renin release is regulated by efferent renal sympathetic nerves. Secondly, hormones may modify neuronal reflex responses through an influence on the sensory input, the autonomic neurones themselves, or the neuroeffector junction. The interaction of AngII and the sympathetic nervous system is the best example of this. AngII facilitates noradrenaline release during sympathetic stimulation and reduces the reflex bradycardia during blood pressure elevation by interrupting vagal efferent activity. Interactions between other hormonal systems and the autonomic nervous system have also been defined: for example, prostaglandins reduce noradrenaline release during sympathetic stimulation, vasopressin enhances the reflex bradycardia during elevation of arterial pressure, and atrial natriuretic peptide inhibits renal sympathetic activity.

Renin–angiotensin system

The sympathetic nervous system and the renin–angiotensin system regulate blood pressure, body fluid and electrolyte homeostasis in a highly inter-dependent way. Plasma renin activity is often increased in heart failure patients. This rise in renin activity may be a response to increased sympathetic nervous activity. In heart failure, cardiac and arterial baroreflex dysfunction may reduce inhibitory afferent stimuli, leading to increased renal sympathetic efferent activity and increased renin release. Conversely, AngII facilitates the release of noradrenaline from nerve endings through presynaptic AngII receptors (Zimmerman et al, 1972), blocks neuronal uptake of noradrenaline (Palaic and Khairallah, 1967), accelerates noradrenaline biosynthesis (Boadle et al, 1969) and increases vascular responsiveness to noradrenaline. The efficacy of ACE inhibitors in the treatment of CHF may therefore reflect not only interruption of the renin–angiotensin–aldosterone pathways, but also indirect inhibition of sympathetic activity.

Atrial natriuretic peptide

Atrial natriuretic peptide (ANP) is a peptide of cardiac origin which is a potent natriuretic and vasodilator hormone. It also inhibits renin production and aldosterone secretion and therefore appears to be well positioned to counteract the influences of the vasoconstrictor and antinatriuretic systems operative in CHF. Plasma ANP concentration is found to be increased, due to increased cardiac release of the peptide, in patients with CHF and in some animal models of heart failure. In the conscious rat, ANP has an inhibitory influence on renal sympathetic activity which appears to be mediated through vagal afferents (Imaizumi et al, 1987). On the other hand, Genovesi et al

(1990) showed in the cat that renal efferent nerve activity increased after ANP infusion and also that renal nerve activity attenuated renal natriuretic and diuretic responses to ANP. Cody et al (1986) showed that, in CHF, the kidney is relatively unresponsive, not only to increased endogenous ANP concentrations, but also to infusions of ANP. This was also observed in a rabbit model of CHF (Langton et al, 1989). Petterson et al (1989) showed that renal denervation reversed the blunted excretory response to ANP in rats with chronic ischaemic heart failure. Feng et al (1990) reported that the α_2-adrenergic agonist clonidine reversed the blunted renal response to ANP in rats following myocardial infarction.

Vasopressin

The circulating levels of arginine vasopressin (AVP) are elevated in many patients with more advanced stages of CHF and in some experimental models of CHF. This increase in AVP results in vasoconstriction as well as having important effects on water retention. As AVP release is modulated by afferent sensory input from the heart, it is likely that the decreased sensitivity of atrial stretch receptors contributes to this increase in circulating AVP. Increased AngII may also be implicated in the increased release of AVP in CHF. A vasoconstrictor role for AVP in CHF was reported by Arnolda et al (1986, 1991); in their study in rabbits with CHF, the resting AVP level was not elevated but there was a significant haemodynamic response to a selective AVP V1 antagonist and also increased pressor sensitivity to exogenous AVP.

This increased sensitivity to AVP in heart failure may be due to impaired baroreflex activity. AVP has specific effects on baroreflex mechanisms that tend to buffer its pressor actions, and AVP infusion was shown to cause greater decreases in lumbar and renal sympathetic nerve activity than equipressor doses of phenylephrine in rabbits (Guo et al, 1982; Undresser et al, 1985).

Endothelin

McMurray et al (1992) recently showed that plasma levels of endothelin were elevated in patients with CHF. This increase in plasma endothelin has also been reported in animal models of heart failure (Cavero et al, 1990). Although the meaning of this increase in heart failure is unclear, such a potent vasoactive hormone may well have an important role in CHF. It has been reported that catecholamines, AngII and AVP all increase endothelin production (Emori et al, 1989). It has also been reported that vasoconstrictor responses to noradrenaline are augmented by subthreshold doses of endothelin (Yang et al, 1990). The interactions of endothelin, the sympathetic nervous system and other humoral factors may prove to be an important area for further investigations into the pathophysiology of CHF.

Dopamine system

Circulating dopamine (DA) levels may be increased in patients with heart failure (Viquerat et al, 1985). Increased circulating levels of dihydroxy-phenylacetic acid (DOPAC) but not DA have also been reported (Mercuro et al, 1984). These changes in DA may be a consequence of sympathetic activation. Urinary excretion of DA was also reported to be increased in CHF (Asakura et al, 1989), but this has not been confirmed (Lehmann et al, 1990). DA has been used for the treatment of CHF since it can increase renal blood flow and glomerular filtration rate and cause natriuresis (Goldberg et al, 1963; McDonald et al, 1964). These effects are promoted by DA_1 receptor activation, which results in vasodilatation in a number of vascular beds including the coronary, renal, cerebral and mesenteric circulations. Also, prejunctional DA_2 receptor activation may contribute to this effect in part, since DA_2 stimulation results in inhibition of noradrenaline release from sympathetic nerve endings. Although the beneficial effects of DA or DA analogues in heart failure have been reported, not much is known of the endogenous renal DA system.

EFFECTS OF MEDICAL TREATMENT ON SYMPATHETIC ACTIVITY

Digitalis

Digitalis is widely used for the treatment of CHF. Digitalis may reduce the sympathetic outflow from the CNS by exerting α_2-agonist effects or via improvement of baroreceptor reflex activity (Ferrari et al, 1981). Imamura et al (1985) showed the cardiopulmonary receptor reflex was enhanced after administration of digitalis. The blunted forearm vasoconstrictive response to LBNP in CHF was normalized after administration of digitalis (Ferguson et al, 1984). Thus, the beneficial effects of digitalis in CHF have been shown to be accompanied by an improvement in the impaired cardiovascular reflex.

ACE inhibitors

ACE inhibition has become the gold standard of therapy for CHF in the past 10 years. The effects of ACE inhibition on plasma catecholamine levels in CHF have varied. In some cases, after acute or chronic ACE inhibition, a decrease in plasma noradrenaline was observed, whereas other studies revealed no significant change in this parameter (Cody et al, 1982; Kluger et al, 1982).

ACE inhibition has been shown to attenuate pressor but not heart rate responses to sympathetic activation. It was reported that captopril augmented baroreflex control of the heart rate in patients with hypertension or CHF (Mancia et al, 1982; Osterziel et al, 1988). Stead and Bloor (1990) showed that captopril reduced the catecholamine response to sodium nitroprusside in rats. Recently, Noshiro et al (1991b) have reported that endogenous AngII augments baroreflex responses to sodium nitroprusside-induced hypotension in normal rabbits. Zucker et al (1991) showed in the dog that captopril reduced renal sympathetic nerve activity despite a fall in blood pressure. This effect was reversed by a cyclo-oxygenase inhibitor. These results suggests ACE inhibition attenuates efferent sympathetic responses.

McGrath and Arnolda (1986) reported that chronic enalapril treatment reduced the noradrenaline response to exercise in patients with CHF. Riegger (1991) reported that chronic quinapril treatment improved the exercise tolerance in patients with mild to moderate CHF.

Diuretics

Diuretics have long been used for the treatment of heart failure. Lake et al (1979) showed that sympathetic nervous activation occurred during thiazide therapy in hypertensive patients. It was suggested that increased plasma noradrenaline during diuretic therapy may be secondary to baroreflex activation. Ito et al (1988) reported that diuretic treatment decreased the pressor response to infused noradrenaline in borderline hypertensive patients and in normal subjects. There is little data available on the effects of diuretic therapy on sympathetic activity in CHF.

β-Adrenergic receptor blocking drugs

β-Blockers and sympathetic antagonists may have beneficial effects on vascular tone and improve cardiac function. Short-term administration of β-blockers increases peripheral vascular resistance because of the activation of α-receptors. However, long-term treatment with a β-blocker may produce regression of vascular smooth muscle hypertrophy and may also suppress the renin–angiotensin system and secretion of vasopressin. A number of clinical studies have reported the potential benefits of chronic administration of β-blocker therapy in patients with heart failure (Waagstein et al, 1975; Swedberg et al, 1980; Engelmeier et al, 1985; Eichhorn et al, 1990). These beneficial effects may be due to a restoring of the downregulated β-adrenergic pathway leading to improved catecholamine responsiveness (Heilbrunn et al, 1989).

α-Adrenergic antagonists

α-Receptor responsiveness may be blunted in heart failure patients, as the effects of noradrenaline on blood pressure and vascular resistance were reported to be reduced in heart failure patients (Goldsmith et al, 1983). It was reported that α_2-adrenoreceptor density in platelets was decreased in heart failure (Weiss et al, 1983).

α_1-Antagonist therapy would be expected to decrease vascular resistance and to have beneficial effects in CHF. Several α_1-adrenergic antagonists have been shown to produce favourable haemodynamic effects in patients with CHF in short-term studies. In the long-term Veterans Administration Cooperative Study (VHeFT) I study, however, no favourable effects of prazocin on mortality were demonstrated and this was thought to be due to the development of tolerance (Cohn et al, 1986).

The α_2-agonist clonidine acts primarily on the CNS and also inhibits the release of noradrenaline peripherally through a presynaptic α_2-receptor mechanism. Clonidine decreases resting noradrenaline levels and also attenuates the rise of noradrenaline during exercise (Pernow et al, 1988). Garty et al (1990) showed that clonidine decreased renal noradrenaline spillover by inhibition of renal sympathetic nervous activity. Although there are very few studies which have evaluated the effects of clonidine used as treatment in CHF, beneficial effects have been reported (Giles et al, 1987).

DA agonists

DA has been introduced for the management of several cardiovascular disorders following the pioneering work of Goldberg and his colleagues. Beneficial effects have been shown in the treatment of CHF (Goldberg et al, 1963; McDonald et al, 1964). Recently, new DA relatives which selectively stimulate subclassed DA receptors have been developed. Dopexamine is a DA receptor agonist which also has β_2-agonist action. It has no α-adrenergic activity and inhibits the neural uptake of noradrenaline. Ibopamine is an orally active DA_1 agonist with β_2-adrenoceptor agonist properties. A fall in plasma noradrenaline levels after administration of ibopamine was reported, in contrast to an elevation after levodopa administration (Rajfer et al, 1986, 1987). Further studies of DA agonists and prodrugs in CHF are currently in progress.

EFFECTS OF CARDIAC TRANSPLANTATION ON SYMPATHETIC ACTIVITY

Olivari et al (1987) showed that within 2 weeks of successful heart trans-plantation plasma noradrenaline fell to nearly normal levels and remained at these levels throughout follow-up. Levine et al (1986) showed that sympa-thetic responses to the stresses of orthostatic tilt and nitroprusside infusion normalized within 6 months after heart transplantation and exercise tolerance also improved. These data suggest that the abnormal neuro-humoral state in heart failure is reversible after heart transplantation.

There have been some studies of the catecholamine content of trans-planted hearts. Myocardial catecholamines are markedly reduced after transplantation because of interruption of the postganglionic cardiac sympathetic nerves. Myocardial noradrenaline levels in autotransplanted canine hearts are strikingly depleted in the short term, and depleted by about half in the long term, after transplantation compared with control hearts (Mohanty et al, 1986). Regitz et al (1990) reported that, in humans, myocardial catecholamines were undetectable up to 5 years after trans-plantation.

In a recent study using positron emission tomography, Schwainger et al (1991) showed that sympathetic reinnervation of the transplanted heart occurred in patients who underwent transplantation more than 2 years previously (see Figure 5). Although the time course is not known for

(a)
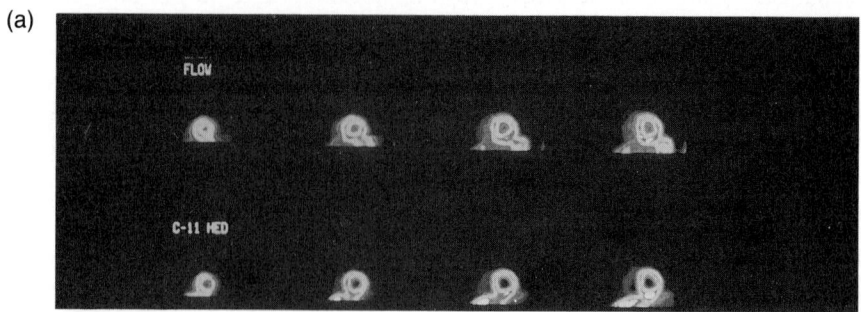

(b)
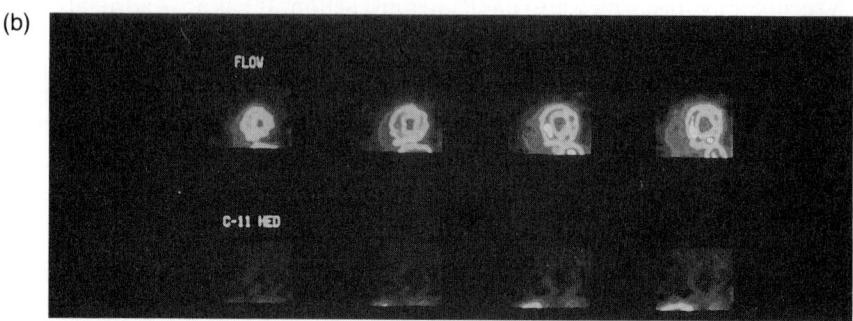

(c)
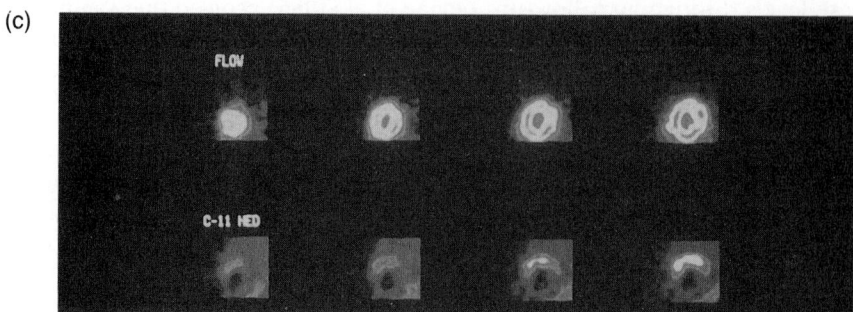

Figure 5. Regional sympathetic reinnervation of the heart after cardiac transplantation. Rubidium-82 images indicating blood flow are shown in the upper panel and [¹¹C]hydroxy-ephedrine images indicating sympathetic innervation are shown in the lower panel. (a) Normal volunteer. (b) Three months after cardiac transplantation. (c) Fifty-five months after cardiac transplantation. From Schwainger et al (1991), by copyright permission of the American Society for Clinical Investigation.

reinnervation of the human heart, reinnervation appears to be prolonged compared with animals.

Cyclosporin is widely used after organ transplantation and has been a major advance in this area. However, it has been shown that cyclosporin produces hypertension in more than 90% of these patients (Cohen et al, 1984). Sympathetic activation is thought to be implicated in the pathogenesis of the hypertension. Scherrer et al (1990) reported a higher rate of sympathetic nerve firing in heart transplant recipients receiving cyclosporin than in those not receiving cyclosporin. Plasma noradrenaline levels in recipients with cyclosporin were within the normal range but higher than those without cyclosporin. It was also suggested that cardiac denervation may facilitate the sympathoexcitatory effect of cyclosporin because similar doses of cyclosporin were associated with larger increases in sympathetic activity and blood pressure in heart transplant recipients than in patients with myasthenia gravis. Morgan et al (1991) showed, in the anaesthetized rat, that acute cyclosporin administration caused increased renal and lumbar sympathetic nervous activity, resulting in increased regional vascular resistances and raised blood pressure. These effects were attenuated or abolished by ganglionic blockade or clonidine, but not by converting enzyme inhibition. The precise mechanism whereby cyclosporin exerts its effects on sympathetic activity have yet to be defined.

SUMMARY

CHF is a common, complex and life-threatening clinical syndrome. It is widely accepted that enhanced peripheral vascular tone plays a major role in the pathophysiology of CHF. Increased activity of the sympathetic nervous system is one of the most important factors responsible for the increased afterload in CHF. This increase in sympathetic activity occurs early in the course of development of CHF. Efferent sympathetic activity is distributed in a non-uniform way in CHF, with significant increases to the heart and kidney but normal activity to some other organs such as the lung. Increased renal sympathetic activity contributes significantly to altered neural haemodynamics, sodium and water retention, and modulation of the actions of other vasoactive hormones. The regional alteration in sympathetic activity may be largely responsible for the changes in resting regional blood flow to different organs in CHF and the maldistribution of blood flow that occurs during the stress of exercise. Disordered function of cardiovascular reflexes is observed in CHF and may contribute to disordered sympathetic function. In CHF there are significant interactions between the sympathetic nervous system and other humoral systems such as the renin–angiotensin system, AVP, ANP, endothelin and renal DA. The various drugs used in the treatment of CHF have different effects on sympathetic activity: digitalis and ACE inhibitors tend to suppress activity while diuretics may have the opposite effect. Following cardiac transplantation, there is a prompt return of sympathetic function towards normal, although the heart may remain significantly denervated for a long time, with gradual reinnervation. Cyclosporin therapy tends to increase sympathetic activity and this may contribute to post-transplant hypertension.

REFERENCES

Abboud FM & Thames MD (1983) Interaction of cardiovascular reflexes in circulatory control. In Shepherd JT, Abboud FM & Bethesda SRG (eds) *Handbook of Physiology: The Cardiovascular System III*, pp 675–753. Bethesda, Maryland: The American Physiological Society.

Anderson FL, Port JD, Reid BB et al (1992) Myocardial catecholamine and neuropeptide Y depletion in failing ventricles of patients with idiopathic dilated cardiomyopathy: correlation with β-adrenergic receptor downregulation. *Circulation* **85:** 46–53.

Arnolda L, McGrath BP, Cocks M et al (1986) Vasoconstrictor role for vasopressin in experimental heart failure in the rabbit. *Journal of Clinical Investigation* **78:** 674–679.

Arnolda L, McGrath BP & Johnston CI (1991) Vasopressin and angiotensin II contribute equally to the increased afterload in rabbits with heart failure. *Cardiovascular Research* **25:** 68–72.

Asakura S, Tabei K, Muto S et al (1989) The role of endogenous dopamine in congestive heart failure. *Japanese Heart Journal* **30:** 115–127.

Boadle MC, Hughes J & Roth RH (1969) Angiotensin accelerates catecholamine biosynthesis in sympathetically innervated tissues. *Nature* **222:** 987–988.

Bristow MR, Anderson FL, Port JD et al (1991) Differences in β-adrenergic neuroeffector mechanisms in ischemic versus idiopathic dilated cardiomyopathy. *Circulation* **84:** 1024–1039.

Calderone A, Bouvier M, Li K et al (1991) Dysfunction of the β- and α-adrenergic systems in a model of congestive heart failure: The pacing-overdrive dog. *Circulation Research* **69:** 332–343.

Cavero PG, Miller WL, Heublein DM et al (1990) Endothelin in experimental congestive heart failure in the anesthetized dog. *American Journal of Physiology* **259:** F312–317.

Chidsey CA, Braunwald E & Morrow AG (1965) Catecholamine excretion and cardiac stores of norepinephrine in congestive heart failure. *American Journal of Cardiology* **39:** 442–451.

Cody RJ, Franklin KW, Kluger J et al (1982) Mechanisms governing the postural response and baroreceptor abnormalities in chronic congestive heart failure: effects of acute and long-term converting enzyme inhibition. *Circulation* **66:** 134–142.

Cody RJ, Atlas SA, Laragh JH et al (1986) Atrial natriuretic factor in normal subjects and heart failure patients: plasma levels and renal, hormonal, and hemodynamic responses to peptide infusion. *Journal of Clinical Investigation* **78:** 1362–1374.

Cohen DJ, Loertscher R, Rubin MF et al (1984) Cyclosporine: a new immunosuppressive agent for organ transplantation. *Annals of Internal Medicine* **101:** 667–682.

Cohn JN, Levine TB, Olivari MT et al (1984) Plasma norepinephrine as a guide to prognosis in patients with chronic congestive heart failure. *New England Journal of Medicine* **311:** 819–823.

Cohn JN, Archibald DG, Ziesche S et al (1986) Effect of vasodilator therapy on mortality in chronic congestive heart failure: results of a Veterans Administration Cooperative Study. *New England Journal of Medicine* **314:** 1547–1552.

Creager MA, Faxon DP, Rockwell SM et al (1985) The contribution of the renin–angiotensin system to limb vasoregulation in patients with heart failure: observations during orthostasis and α-adrenergic blockade. *Clinical Science* **68:** 659–667.

Creager MA, Hirsch AT, Dzau VJ et al (1990) Baroreflex regulation of regional blood flow in congestive heart failure. *American Journal of Physiology* **258:** H1409–H1414.

Dargie H (1990) Sympathetic activity and regional blood flow in heart failure. *European Heart Journal* **11(supplement A):** 39–43.

Davis D, Sinoway LI, Robison J et al (1987) Norepinephrine kinetics during orthostatic stress in congestive heart failure. *Circulation Research* **61(supplement I):** I-87–I-90.

Davis D, Baily R & Zelis R (1988) Abnormalities in systemic norepinephrine kinetics in human congestive heart failure. *American Journal of Physiology* **254:** E760–E766.

DiBona GF, Herman PJ & Sawin LL (1988) Neural control of renal function in edema-forming states. *American Journal of Physiology* **254:** R1017–1024.

Eckberg DL, Drabinski M & Braunwald E (1971) Defective cardiac parasympathetic control in patients with heart failure. *New England Journal of Medicine* **285:** 877–883.

Eichhorn EJ, Bedotto JB, Malloy CR et al (1990) Effect of β-adrenergic blockade on myocardial function and energetics in congestive heart failure. *Circulation* **82:** 473–483.

Emori T, Hirata Y, Ohta K et al (1989) Secretory mechanism of immunoreactive endothelin in cultured bovine endothelial cells. *Biochemical and Biophysical Research Communications* **160:** 93–100.

Engelmeier RS, O'Connell JB, Walsh R et al (1985) Improvement in symptoms and exercise tolerance by metoprolol in patients with dilated cardiomyopathy: a double-blind, randomized, placebo-control trial. *Circulation* **72:** 536–546.

Esler MD, Hasking GJ, Willett IR et al (1985) Noradrenaline release and sympathetic nervous system activity. *Journal of Hypertension* **3:** 117–129.

Feng Q, Hedner T, Hedner J et al (1990) Blunted renal response to atrial natriuretic peptide in congestive heart failure rats is reversed by the α_2-adrenergic agonist clonidine. *Journal of Cardiovascular Pharmacology* **16:** 776–782.

Ferguson DW, Abboud FM & Mark AL (1984) Selective impairment of baroreflex-mediated vasoconstrictor responses in patients with ventricular dysfunction. *Circulation* **69:** 451–460.

Ferrari A, Gregorini L, Ferrari MC et al (1981) Digitalis and baroreceptor reflexes in man. *Circulation* **63:** 279–285.

Fowler MB, Laser JA, Hopkins GL et al (1986) Assessment of the β-adrenergic receptor pathway in the intact failing human heart: Progressive receptor down-regulation and subsensitivity to agonist response. *Circulation* **74:** 1290–1302.

Francis GS, Goldsmith SR & Cohn JN (1982) Relationship of exercise capacity to resting left ventricular performance and basal plasma norepinephrine levels in patients with congestive heart failure. *American Heart Journal* **104:** 725–731.

Francis GS, Benedict C, Johnstone DE et al (1990) Comparison of neuroendocrine activation in patients with left ventricular dysfunction with and without congestive heart failure. A substudy of the Studies of Left Ventricular Dysfunction (SOLVD). *Circulation* **82:** 1724–1729.

Ganguly PK & Sherwood GR (1991) Noradrenaline turn over and metabolism in myocardium following aortic constriction in rats. *Cardiovascular Research* **25:** 579–585.

Garty M, Deka-Starosta AG & Chang P (1990) Effects of clonidine on renal sympathetic nerve activity and norepinephrine spillover. *Journal of Pharmacology and Experimental Therapeutics* **254:** 1068–1075.

Genovesi S, Protasoni G, Assi C et al (1990) Interactions between the sympathetic nervous system and atrial natriuretic factor in the control of renal functions. *Journal of Hypertension* **8:** 703–710.

Giles TD, Thomas MG, Quiroz AC et al (1987) Acute and short-term effects of clonidine in heart failure. *Angiology* **38:** 537–548.

Gilson N, Bounani NH, Corsin A et al (1990) Left ventricular function and β-adrenoceptors in rabbit failing heart. *American Journal of Physiology* **258:** H634–H641.

Goldberg LI, McDonald RH Jr & Zimmerman AM (1963) Sodium diuresis produced by dopamine in patients with congestive heart failure. *New England Journal of Medicine* **269:** 1060–1064.

Goldsmith SR, Francis GS, Levine TB et al (1983) Regional blood flow response to orthostasis in patients with congestive heart failure. *Journal of the American College of Cardiology* **1:** 1391–1395.

Goldstein RE, Beiser GD, Stampfer M et al (1975) Impairment of the autonomically mediated heart rate control in patients with cardiac dysfunction. *Circulation Research* **36:** 571–578.

Goldstein DS, McCarty R, Polynsky RJ et al (1983) Relationship between plasma norepinephrine and sympathetic neural activity. *Hypertension* **5:** 552–559.

Greenberg TT, Richmond WH, Stocking RA et al (1973) Impaired atrial receptor responses in dog with heart failure due to tricuspid insufficiency and pulmonary artery stenosis. *Circulation Research* **32:** 424–433.

Guo GB, Sharabi FM, Abboud FM et al (1982) Vasopressin augments baroreflex inhibition of lumbar sympathetic nerve activity in rabbits. *Circulation* **66(supplement II):** 34 (abstract).

Hasking GJ, Esler MD, Jennings GL et al (1986) Norepinephrine spillover to plasma in patients with congestive heart failure: evidence of increased overall and cardiorenal sympathetic nervous activity. *Circulation* **73:** 615–621.

Heilbrunn SM, Shah P, Bristow MR et al (1989) Increased β-receptor density and improved hemodynamic response to catecholamine stimulation during long-term metoprolol therapy in heart failure from dilated cardiomyopathy. *Circulation* **79:** 483–490.

Higgins CB, Vatner SF, Eckberg DL et al (1972) Alterations in the baroreceptor reflex in conscious dogs with heart failure. *Journal of Clinical Investigation* **51:** 715–724.

Hoeldtke RD, Cilmi KM, Reichard GA Jr et al (1983) Assessment of norepinephrine secretion and production. *Journal of Laboratory and Clinical Medicine* **101:** 772–782.

Howes LG, Hodsman GP, Maccarrone C et al (1989) Cardiac 3,4-dihydroxyphenylethylene glycol (DHPG) and catecholamine levels in a rat model of left ventricular failure. *Journal of Cardiovascular Pharmacology* **13:** 348–352.

Imaizumi T, Takeshita A, Higashi H et al (1987) α-ANP alters reflex control of lumbar and renal sympathetic nerve activity and heart rate. *American Journal of Physiology* **253:** H1136–H1140.

Imamura T, Takeshita A, Ashihara T et al (1985) Digitalis-induced augmentation of cardio-pulmonary baroreflex control of forearm vascular resistance. *Circulation* **71:** 11–16.

Ito Y, Ando K, Noda H et al (1988) Evidence for increased sympatho-adrenomedullary activity in young subjects with borderline hypertension. *Japanese Circulation Journal* **52:** 1326–1334.

Kassis E (1989) Baroreflex control of the circulation in patients with congestive heart failure. *Danish Medical Bulletin* **36(3):** 195–211.

Kluger J, Cody RJ & Laragh JH (1982) The contributions of sympathetic tone and the renin–angiotensin system to severe chronic congestive heart failure: response to specific inhibitors (prazosin and captopril). *American Journal of Cardiology* **49:** 1667–1674.

Kubo SH & Cody RJ (1983) Circulatory autoregulation in chronic congestive heart failure: responses to head-up tilt in 41 patients. *American Journal of Cardiology* **52:** 512–518.

Lake CR, Ziegler MG & Kopin IJ (1976) Use of plasma norepinephrine for evaluation of sympathetic neuronal function in man. *Life Sciences* **18:** 1315–1325.

Lake CR, Ziegler MG, Coleman MD et al (1979) Hydrochlorothiazide-induced sympathetic hyperactivity in hypertensive patients. *Clinical Pharmacology and Therapeutics* **26:** 428–432.

Langton D, Jover BF, Trigg L et al (1989) Regional distribution of the cardiac output and renal responses to atrial natriuretic peptide infusion in rabbits with congestive heart failure. *Clinical and Experimental Pharmacology and Physiology* **16:** 939–951.

Langton D, McGrath BP & Ludbrook J (1990a) Cardiovascular responses to graded treadmill exercise during the development of doxorubicin-induced heart failure in rabbits. *Cardiovascular Research* **24:** 959–968.

Langton D, Way D, Trigg L et al (1990b) Vasoconstriction in the renal vascular bed during exercise: studies in control and heart failure rabbits. *Clinical and Experimental Pharmacology and Physiology* **17:** 219–223.

Lehmann M, Hasenfub G, Samek L et al (1990) Catecholamine metabolism in heart failure patients and healthy control subjects. *Arzneimittel-Forschung* **40(II):** 1310–1318.

Leimbach WN, Wallin BG, Victor RG et al (1986) Direct evidence from intraneural recordings for increased central sympathetic outflow in patients with heart failure. *Circulation* **73:** 913–919.

Levine TB, Francis GS, Goldsmith SR et al (1982) Activity of the sympathetic nervous system and renin–angiotensin system assessed by plasma hormone levels and their relation to hemodynamic abnormalities in congestive heart failure. *American Journal of Cardiology* **49:** 1659–1666.

Levine TB, Olivari MT & Cohn JN (1986) Effects of orthotopic heart transplantation on sympathetic control mechanisms in congestive heart failure. *American Journal of Cardiology* **58:** 1035–1040.

Lilly LS, Dzau VJ, Williams GH et al (1984) Hyponatremia in congestive heart failure: implications for neurohumoral activation and responses to orthostasis. *Journal of Clinical Endocrinology and Metabolism* **59:** 924–930.

Ludbrook J (1990) Cardiovascular reflexes from cardiac sensory receptors. *Australian and New Zealand Journal of Medicine* **20:** 597–606.

Mancia G, Parati G, Pomidossi G et al (1982) Modification of arterial baroreflexes by captopril in essential hypertension. *American Journal of Cardiology* **49:** 1415–1419.

McDonald RH Jr, Goldberg LI, McNay JL et al (1964) Effects of dopamine in man: augmentation of sodium excretion, glomerular filtration rate, and renal plasma flow. *Journal of Clinical Investigation* **43:** 1116–1124.

McGrath BP & Arnolda LF (1986) Enalapril reduces the catecholamine response to exercise in patients with heart failure. *European Journal of Clinical Pharmacology* **30:** 485–487.

McGrath BP, Jover BF, Trigg L et al (1987) Adriamycin-induced cardiomyopathic heart failure in the rabbit. In Kawai C & Abelmann WH (eds) *Pathogenesis of Myocarditis and Cardiomyopathy: Cardiomyopathy Update 1*, pp 121–133. Tokyo: University of Tokyo Press.

McGrath BP, Sano N & Way D (1990) Shift in the baroreflex-renal noradrenaline spillover curve during the development of congestive heart failure in the rabbit. *Clinical and Experimental Pharmacology and Physiology* **17:** 303–307.

McMurray JJ, Ray SG, Abdullah I et al (1992) Plasma endothelin in chronic heart failure. *Circulation* **85:** 1374–1379.

Mercuro G, Rossetti Z, Rivaro C et al (1984) Marked increase of plasma 3,4-dihydroxyphenyl-acetic acid in congestive heart failure. *American Heart Journal* **108:** 1588–1589.

Meredith IT, Broughton A, Jennings GL et al (1991) Evidence of a selective increase in cardiac sympathetic activity in patients with sustained ventricular arrhythmias. *New England Journal of Medicine* **325:** 618–624.

Merlet P, Dubois-Rande JL, Adnot S et al (1992) Myocardial β-adrenergic desensitization and neuronal norepinephrine uptake function in idiopathic dilated cardiomyopathy. *Journal of Cardiovascular Pharmacology* **19:** 10–16.

Millard RW, Higgins CB, Franklin D et al (1972) Regulation of the renal circulation during severe exercise in normal dogs and dogs with experimental heart failure. *Circulation* **31:** 881–888.

Minami M, Yasuda H, Yamazaki N et al (1983) Plasma norepinephrine concentration and plasma dopamine-beta-hydroxylase activity in patients with congestive heart failure. *Circulation* **67(6):** 1324–1329.

Mitchell JH & Schmidt RF (1983) Cardiovascular reflex control by afferent fibers from skeletal muscle receptors. In Shepherd JT, Abboud FM & Bethesda SRG (eds) *Handbook of Physiology: The Cardiovascular System III*, pp 623–658. Bethesda, Maryland: The American Physiological Society.

Mohanty PK, Sowers JR, Thames MD et al (1986) Myocardial norepinephrine, epinephrine and dopamine concentration after cardiac autotransplantation in dogs. *Journal of the American College of Cardiology* **7:** 419–424.

Morgan BJ, Lyson T, Scherrer U et al (1991) Cyclosporine causes sympathetically mediated elevations in arterial pressure in rats. *Hypertension* **18:** 458–466.

Noshiro T, Saigusa T, Way D et al (1991a) Norepinephrine spillover faithfully reflects renal sympathetic nerve activity in conscious rabbits. *American Journal of Physiology* **261:** F44–F50.

Noshiro T, Way D & McGrath BP (1991b) Effect of angiotensin-converting enzyme inhibition on renal norepinephrine spillover rate and baroreflex responses in conscious rabbits. *Clinical and Experimental Pharmacology and Physiology* **18:** 375–378.

Olivari MT, Levine TB & Cohn JN (1983) Abnormal neurohumoral response to nitroprusside infusion in congestive heart failure. *Journal of the American College of Cardiology* **2:** 411–417.

Olivari MT, Levine TB, Ring WS et al (1987) Normalization of sympathetic nervous system function after orthotopic cardiac transplant in man. *Circulation* **76(supplement V):** V62–V64.

Osterziel KJ, Roering N, Dietz R et al (1988) Influence of captopril on the arterial baroreceptor reflex in patients with heart failure. *European Heart Journal* **9:** 1137–1145.

Palaic D & Khairallah PA (1967) Inhibition of noradrenaline uptake by angiotensin. *Journal of Pharmacy and Pharmacology* **19:** 396–397.

Pernow J, Lundberg JM & Kaijser L (1988) α-Adrenoceptor influence on plasma levels of neuropeptide Y-like immunoreactivity and catecholamines during rest and sympatho-adrenal activation in humans. *Journal of Cardiovascular Pharmacology* **12:** 593–599.

Petterson A, Hedner J & Hedner T (1989) Renal interaction between sympathetic activity and ANP in rats with chronic ischemic heart failure. *Acta Physiologica Scandinavica* **135**: 487–492.

Pierpont GL, Francis GS, DeMaster EG et al (1987) Heterogeneous myocardial catecholamine concentrations in patients with congestive heart failure. *American Journal of Cardiology* **60**: 316–321.

Pool PE, Covell JW, Levitt M et al (1967) Reduction of cardiac tyrosine hydroxylase activity in experimental congestive heart failure. *Circulation Research* **20**: 349–353.

Rajfer SI, Rossen JD, Douglas FL et al (1986) Effects of long-term therapy with oral ibopamine on resting hemodynamics and exercise capacity in patients with heart failure: Relationship to the generation of *N*-methyldopamine and to plasma norepinephrine levels. *Circulation* **73**: 740–748.

Rajfer SI, Rossen JD, Nemanich JW et al (1987) Sustained hemodynamic improvement during long-term therapy with levodopa in heart failure: Role of plasma catecholamines. *Journal of the American College of Cardiology* **10**: 1286–1293.

Rector TS, Olivari MT, Levine TB et al (1987) Predicting survival for an individual with congestive heart failure using the plasma norepinephrine concentration. *American Heart Journal* **114**: 148–152.

Regitz V, Bossaller C, Strasser R et al (1990) Myocardial catecholamine content after heart transplantation. *Circulation* **82**: 620–623.

Riegger GAJ (1991) Effects of quinapril on exercise tolerance in patients with mild to moderate heart failure. *European Heart Journal* **12**: 705–711.

Riegger GAJ & Liebau G (1982) The renin–angiotensin–aldosterone system, antidiuretic hormone and sympathetic nerve activity in an experimental model of congestive heart failure in dog. *Clinical Science* **62**: 465–469.

Sano N, Way D & McGrath BP (1990) Renal norepinephrine spillover and baroreflex responses in evolving heart failure. *American Journal of Physiology* **258**: F1516–F1522.

Scherrer U, Vissing SF, Morgan BJ et al (1990) Cyclosporine-induced sympathetic activation and hypertension after heart transplantation. *New England Journal of Medicine* **323**: 693–699.

Schwainger M, Hutchins GD, Kalff V et al (1991) Evidence for regional catecholamine uptake and storage sites in the transplanted human heart by positron emission tomography. *Journal of Clinical Investigation* **87**: 1681–1690.

Smith WM (1985) Epidemiology of congestive heart failure. *American Journal of Cardiology* **55**: 3A–8A.

Sole MJ, Kamble AB & Hussain MD (1977) A possible change in the rate-limiting step for cardiac norepinephrine synthesis in the cardiomyopathic Syrian hamster. *Circulation Research* **41**: 814–817.

Sole MJ, Helke CJ & Jacobowitz DM (1982) Increased dopamine in the failing hamster heart: transvesicular transport of dopamine limits the rate of norepinephrine synthesis. *American Journal of Cardiology* **49**: 1682–1690.

Stead SW & Bloor BC (1990) The effects of captopril on the renin–angiotensin system and the sympathetic nervous system during sodium nitroprusside-induced hypotension in the halothane-anaesthetized rabbit. *Journal of Cardiovascular Pharmacology* **15**: 465–471.

Sterns DA, Ettinger SM, Gray KS et al (1991) Skeletal muscle metaboreceptor exercise responses are attenuated in heart failure. *Circulation* **84**: 2034–2039.

Sullivan MJ, Green HJ & Cobb FR (1991) Altered skeletal muscle metabolic response to exercise in chronic heart failure. Relation to skeletal muscle aerobic enzyme activity. *Circulation* **84**: 1597–1607.

Swedberg K, Hjalmarson A, Waagstein F et al (1980) Beneficial effects of long-term beta-blockade in congestive cardiomyopathy. *British Heart Journal* **44**: 117–133.

Szlachcic J, Massie BM, Kramer BL et al (1985) Correlates and prognostic implication of exercise capacity in chronic congestive heart failure. *American Journal of Cardiology* **55**: 1037–1042.

Thomas JA & Marks BH (1978) Plasma norepinephrine in congestive heart failure. *American Journal of Cardiology* **41**: 233–243.

Undesser KP, Hasser EM, Haywood JR et al (1985) Interactions of vasopressin with the area postrema in arterial baroreflex function in conscious rabbits. *Circulation Research* **56**: 410–417.

Viquerat CE, Daly P, Swedberg K et al (1985) Endogenous catecholamine levels in chronic heart failure: Relation to the severity of hemodynamic abnormalities. *American Journal of Medicine* **78**: 455–460.

Waagstein F, Hjalmarson A, Varnauskas E et al (1975) Effect of chronic beta-adrenergic receptor blockade in congestive cardiomyopathy. *British Heart Journal* **37**: 1022–1036.

Weiss RJ, Tobes M, Weritz CE et al (1983) Platelet alpha2 adrenoreceptors in chronic congestive heart failure. *American Journal of Cardiology* **52**: 101–105.

Woodcock EA, Arnolda L & McGrath BP (1988) Ventricular beta-adrenoceptors in adriamycin-induced cardiomyopathy in the rabbit. *Journal of Molecular and Cellular Cardiology* **20**: 771–777.

Yang Z, Richard V, von Segesser L et al (1990) Threshold concentrations of endothelin-1 potentiate contractions to norepinephrine and serotonin in human arteries. *Circulation* **82**: 188–195.

Zelis R & Flaim SF (1982) Alterations in vasomotor tone in congestive heart failure. *Progress in Cardiovascular Disease* **24**: 437–459.

Zimmerman BG, Gomer SK & Liao JC (1972) Action of angiotensin on vascular adrenergic nerve endings: facilitation of norepinephrine release. *Federation Proceedings* **31**: 1344–1350.

Zucker IH, Share L & Gilmore JP (1979) Renal effects of left atrial distension in dogs with chronic congestive heart failure. *American Journal of Physiology* **236**: H554–560.

Zucker IH, Gorman AJ, Cornish KG et al (1985) Impaired atrial receptor modulation or renal nerve activity in dogs with chronic volume overload. *Cardiovascular Research* **19**: 411–418.

Zucker IH, Chen J & Wang W (1991) Renal sympathetic nerve and hemodynamic responses to captopril in conscious dogs: role of prostaglandins. *American Journal of Physiology* **260**: H260–266.

8

Sympathetic nervous system disorders in man

CHRISTOPHER J. MATHIAS

The sympathetic nervous system is a major component of the autonomic nervous system. It is considered mainly as an efferent system, with fibres emerging from the thoracic and upper two or three lumbar spinal segments which synapse in ganglia, from which postganglionic fibres supply virtually every organ in the body. There are, however, a considerable number of nuclei and interconnections within the brain, particularly within the brain stem, which influence the sympathetic outflow. The activity of sympathetic nerves is also regulated by most afferent nerves, a prominent example being the sino-aortic baroreceptor afferents. Disorders of the sympathetic nervous system in humans may result from abnormalities at one or multiple sites.

CLASSIFICATION OF SYMPATHETIC NERVOUS SYSTEM DISORDERS

Disorders can be either localized or generalized (Mathias, 1991). Examples of the former include Horner's syndrome, which affects the sympathetic supply to the face, Hirschsprung's disease, a congenital disorder of the colon, and dysfunction resulting from cardiac transplantation. Some of the generalized disorders are listed in Table 1. They include the primary disorders, where the aetiology is not known. Within these, the chronic syndromes are more common. They may involve the autonomic nervous system alone as part of pure autonomic failure (PAF), previously described as idiopathic orthostatic hypotension (Bradbury and Eggleston, 1925). In such patients there are no additional neurological features, unlike the Shy–Drager syndrome (SDS) (Shy and Drager, 1960), where a variety of neurological signs (parkinsonian, cerebellar and pyramidal) may be present.

The secondary disorders may be associated with certain conditions (as in the elderly) and may be a complication of an established disease process (as in diabetes mellitus), may be due to a specific neurological lesion (as in a high spinal cord transection), or may result from a defect involving specific components of the sympathetic neurotransmitter pathways (as in the dopamine-β-hydroxylase [DBH] deficiency syndrome). Finally, drugs are an important cause of sympathetic dysfunction (Table 2).

Baillière's Clinical Endocrinology and Metabolism—
Vol. 7, No. 2, April 1993
ISBN 0–7020–1698–5

Disorders of sympathetic nerves commonly result in failure. The reverse, however, may occur, as in patients with tetanus (Corbett et al, 1969), high spinal cord lesions (Mathias and Frankel, 1992a), and with drugs such as cyclosporin (Scherrer et al, 1990). In addition, sympathetic impairment may cause or contribute to a relative overactivity of the opposing pathway, resulting in a clinical problem. An example is increased cardiac parasympathetic activity causing severe bradycardia and cardiac arrest during tracheal suction in tetraplegic patients on ventilators (Frankel et al, 1975).

Table 1. Classification of generalized sympathetic nervous system disorders.

PRIMARY AUTONOMIC FAILURE

Chronic:
  Pure autonomic failure
  Shy–Drager syndrome;
    With parkinsonian features
    With cerebellar and pyramidal features
    With multiple system atrophy (combination of above)
Acute or subacute dysautonomias

SECONDARY AUTONOMIC FAILURE OR DYSFUNCTION

Central:
  Brain tumours, especially of the third ventricle or posterior fossa
  Multiple sclerosis
  Syringobulbia
  Elderly
  Tetanus
  Poliomyelitis
Spinal:
  Spinal cord transection—trauma
  Transverse myelitis
  Syringomyelia
  Spinal tumours
Peripheral:
  Afferent:
    Guillain–Barré syndrome
    Holmes–Adie syndrome
    Porphyria
    Carotid sinus hypersensitivity
  Efferent:
    Diabetes mellitus
    Amyloidosis
    Surgery (such as splanchnicectomy)
    Dopamine-β-hydroxylase deficiency
  Afferent/efferent:
    Familial dysautonomia (Riley–Day syndrome)
Miscellaneous:
  Autoimmune and collagen disorders
  Renal failure
  Neoplasia
  Human immunodeficiency virus infection
  Vasovagal syncope

Table 2. Drugs and chemicals with actions executed through the sympathetic nervous system.

Decreasing sympathetic activity
Centrally acting:
  Clonidine
  Methyldopa
  Reserpine
  Barbiturates
  Anaesthetics
Peripherally acting:
  Sympathetic neurone (guanethidine, bethanidine)
  α-Adrenoceptor blockade (phenoxybenzamine)
  β-Adrenoceptor blockade (propranolol)

Increasing sympathetic activity
Amphetamines
Cocaine
Tyramine
Imipramine
Cyclosporin

INVESTIGATION

Overview of investigational strategy

Investigation is directed towards determining if sympathetic function is normal or abnormal. If it is abnormal, additional tests are often needed to assess the functional deficit and determine the underlying aetiological process (Mathias and Bannister, 1992a). An outline of the various investigations which may be needed in the generalized syndromes is provided in Table 3. Investigation of the cardiovascular system is particularly important, and investigational approaches will be described more fully below. It should be noted that the majority of the tests—physiological, biochemical and pharmacological—are designed to assess sympathetic failure rather than overactivity. This is primarily because postural hypotension is a cardinal feature of many sympathetic disorders, and its evaluation is important in determining the site of the lesion and in planning appropriate management.

Physiological tests

These tests are designed to assess sympathetic efferent pathways, although some are dependent on the integrity of the overall baroreceptor reflex. The latter include the cardiovascular response to postural change (using a tilt table with head-up tilt to 45 or 60°, or standing erect) or the Valsalva manoeuvre (when intrathoracic pressure is raised). The responses are dependent upon activation of the afferent arc of the baroreceptor reflex which then increases sympathetic efferent activity. Examples of responses to head-up tilt and to the Valsalva manoeuvre are provided in Figures 1 and 2.

Blood pressure is increasingly being measured using automated devices which provide intermittent readings. More recent advances enable beat-by-beat blood pressure recordings non-invasively, as with the Finapres (Imholz et al, 1991) (see Figure 3). The presence of postural hypotension according to a rigid definition (often a fall of more than 20 mmHg in systolic blood pressure on standing) is not itself of importance, as consideration should also be given to the accompanying symptoms, the basal supine level of blood pressure and associated cardiovascular disease. Furthermore, a range of factors are now recognized as influencing the postural blood pressure response. In primary autonomic failure, postural hypotension is greater in the morning (Mathias et al, 1986) (because of nocturnal diuresis), after food

Table 3. Outline of investigations in sympathetic disorders.

Cardiovascular:	
Physiological:	Head-up tilt (45°); standing; Valsalva manoeuvre
	Pressor stimuli—isometric exercise, cutaneous cold, mental arithmetic
	Heart rate responses—deep breathing, hyperventilation, standing, head-up tilt, 30:15 ratio
	Carotid sinus massage
	Liquid meal ingestion
Biochemical:	Plasma noradrenaline—supine and standing
	Urinary catecholamines
	Plasma renin activity and aldosterone
Pharmacological:	Noradrenaline—α-adrenoceptors (vascular)
	Isoprenaline—β-adrenoceptors (vascular and cardiac)
	Tyramine—pressor and noradrenaline response
	Edrophonium—noradrenaline response
	Atropine—parasympathetic cardiac blockade
Sweating:	Central regulation—increase core temperature by 1°C
	Sweat gland response—intradermal
	Acetylcholine—quantitative sudomotor
	Axon reflex test (Q-SART)—spot test
Gastrointestinal:	Barium studies
	Video cinefluoroscopy
	Endoscopy
	Gastric emptying studies
Renal function and urinary tract:	Day and night urine volumes and sodium/potassium excretion
	Urodynamic studies
	Intravenous urography
	Ultrasound examination
	Sphincter electromyography
Sexual function:	Penile plethysmography
	Intracavernosal papaverine
Respiratory:	Laryngoscopy
	Sleep studies to assess apnoea/oxygen desaturation
Eye:	Schirmer's test
	Pupil function—pharmacological and physiological

Noradrenaline = norepinephrine *USP*; isoprenaline = isoproterenol *USP*.

ingestion (Mathias, 1991) (as a result of vasodilatation in the splanchnic region), when the environmental temperature is elevated in hot weather, after a hot bath or with central heating (because of cutaneous vaso-dilatation), and after exercise (Marshall et al, 1961) (through skeletal

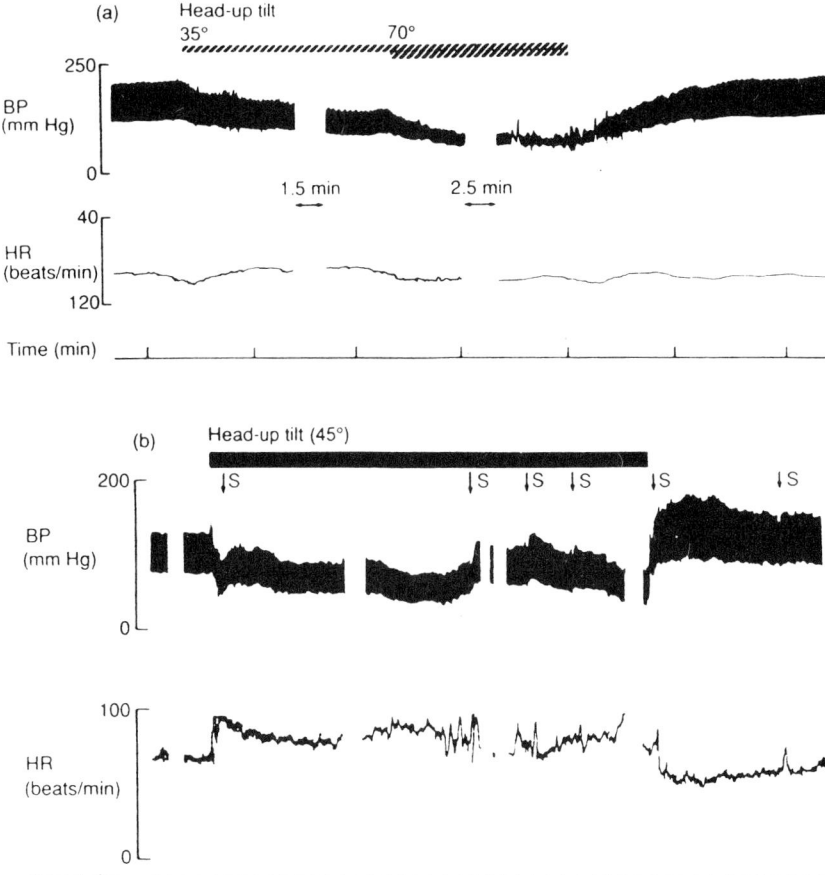

Figure 1. (a) Continuous intra-arterial recording of blood pressure (BP) and heart rate (HR) in a patient with postural hypotension and the Holmes–Adie syndrome. The systolic and diastolic blood pressure falls progressively during tilt, with no recovery. There are minimal changes in heart rate. There is no change in plasma noradrenaline levels following tilt. Other investi-gations indicated that the lesion was likely to be on the afferent side of the baroreflex arc. From Mathias (1987). (b) Blood pressure (BP) and heart rate (HR) in a tetraplegic patient before, during and after head-up tilt to 45°. Blood pressure promptly falls but with partial recovery, which in this case is linked to skeletal muscle spasms (S) inducing spinal sympathetic reflexes. Some of the later oscillations may be due to the rise in plasma renin, which was measured where there are interruptions in the intra-arterial record. In the later phases of tilt, skeletal muscle spasms occur more frequently, and further elevate the blood pressure. On return to the horizontal, blood pressure rises rapidly above the previous level and then slowly levels out. Heart rate usually moves in the opposite direction, except during skeletal muscle spasms, when there is a rise. From Mathias and Frankel (1988).

muscle vasodilatation). In high spinal cord lesions, other factors play a role in modifying the postural response (Figure 1b).

Increased sympathetic efferent activity and an elevation in blood pressure follows activation of afferents in skin (with cutaneous cold), in muscle (with isometric exercise) and following cerebral stimulation (with mental stress). The lack of a pressor response favours a sympathetic efferent defect. It is wise to use a range of these tests, as sympathetic responses can vary even in normal subjects and are influenced by task difficulty and stress perception, among other factors (Callister et al, 1992).

The tests described above form the basis for a range of variables which are being continuously devised, and revised, to assess baroreflex pathways and sympathetic efferent activity (Ewing, 1992; Wieling, 1992). The data obtained are often subjected to analysis, which varies between laboratories

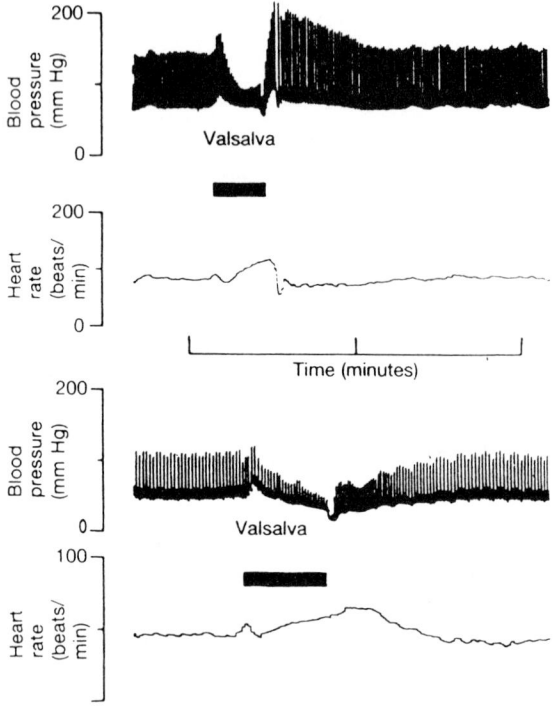

Figure 2. Changes in blood pressure and heart rate measured by an intra-arterial catheter, before, during and after a Valsalva manoeuvre, when intrathoracic pressure was raised to 40 mmHg. In the normal subject (upper trace) in the later phases of the manoeuvre there is recovery of blood pressure; with the release of intrathoracic pressure there is a rapid increase in blood pressure above the basal values, together with reduction in heart rate below basal levels. In a patient with sympathetic failure (lower trace), there is a continuing fall in blood pressure even in the later stages of the Valsalva manoeuvre, with no blood pressure overshoot; blood pressure slowly returns to basal levels. Heart rate rises, suggesting some cardiac para-sympathetic activity in response to the blood pressure fall. From Mathias and Bannister (1992a).

and is often computer assisted. Such variables are valuable for providing quantitative information which may be essential in the study of groups of subjects, especially in longitudinal studies aimed at defining the natural history of sympathetic disorders. Their value in individual cases is questionable, since in the clinical situation many other variables, which cannot be rigidly controlled, are encountered.

Some additional investigations may be performed in specific clinical situations. In subjects with recurrent syncope who have normal sympathetic function based on the above tests, carotid sinus hypersensitivity or vasovagal syncope needs to be considered. The former can be assessed by carotid sinus massage, ideally both while supine and during head-up tilt (Mathias et al, 1991a). The potential risks of carotid massage should be borne in mind and resuscitation facilities should be available. In subjects with vasovagal syncope it is often difficult to reproduce the event in the laboratory, and various modifications, from prolonged head-up tilt to infusion of vasodilators such as nitroprusside and β-adrenoceptor stimulants such as isoprenaline (isoproterenol *USP*) have been utilized to unmask an episode. It is important to exclude cardiac dysrhythmias as a cause of syncope.

The role of 24-h non-invasive ambulatory blood pressure monitoring in the diagnostic work-up of sympathetic dysfunction is not clear (Figure 4). At present this technique is capable of determining whether factors such as time of day, food and exercise can contribute to hypotension, and in assessing the

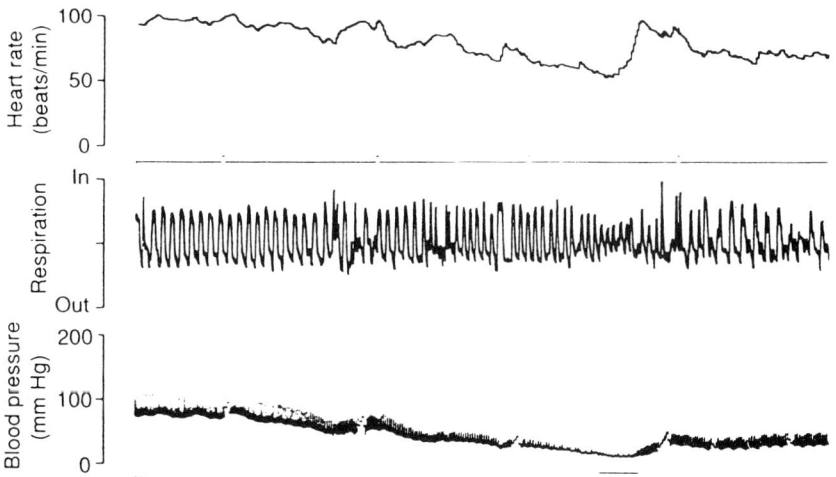

Figure 3. Blood pressure changes towards the end of the period of head-up tilt in a patient with recurrent episodes of vasovagal syncope. Blood pressure, which was previously maintained, begins to fall. There is also a fall in heart rate. Initially there are relatively minor changes in respiratory rate, which can be derived from the time signal above it, each minor dot indicating a second and the bolder mark indicating a minute. The patient was about to faint and was put back to the horizontal, indicated by the elevated time signal below, and then to 5° head-down tilt. Blood pressure and heart rate recover but still remain lower than previously. This patient had no other autonomic abnormalities on detailed testing. Beat-by-beat blood pressure was measured non-invasively using the Finapres. From Mathias and Bannister (1992a).

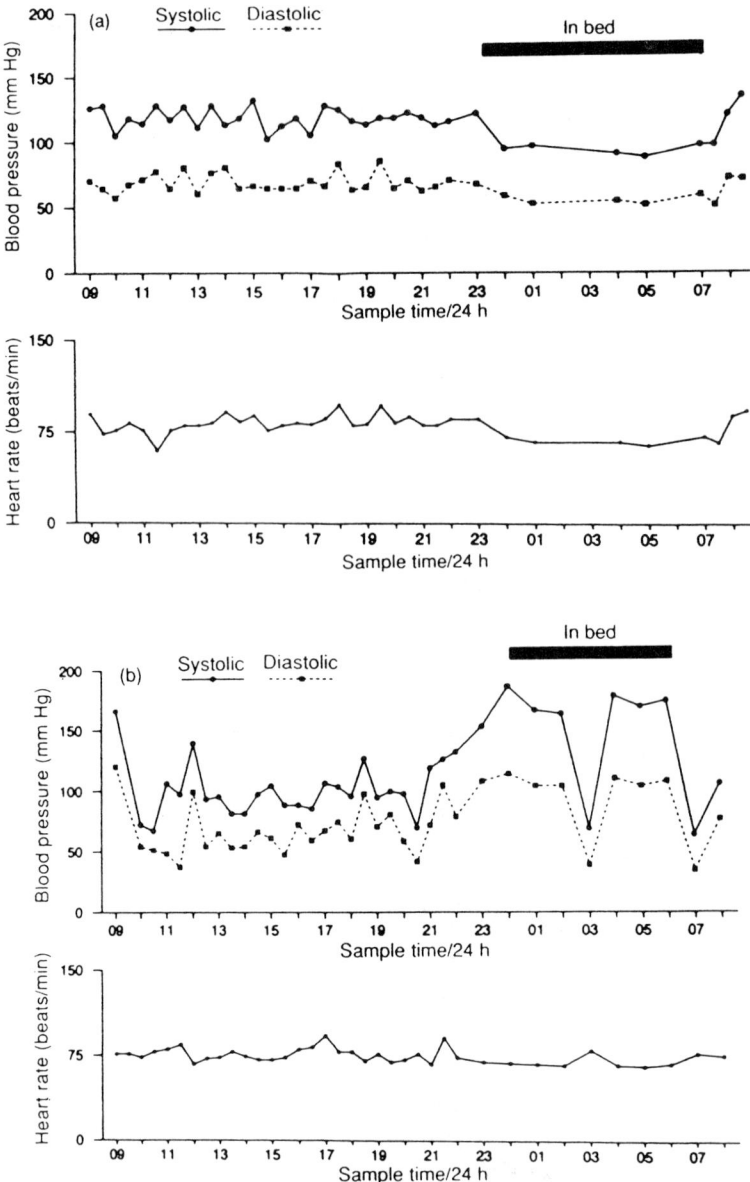

Figure 4. Twenty-four hour non-invasive ambulatory blood pressure profile, showing systolic and diastolic blood pressure and heart rate at intervals throughout the day and night. (a) Changes in a normal subject with no postural fall in blood pressure; there was a fall in blood pressure at night while asleep, with a rise in blood pressure on wakening. (b) Marked fluctuations in blood pressure in a patient with autonomic failure. This is often the result of postural change, either sitting or standing. Supine blood pressure, particularly at night, is elevated. Getting up to micturate causes a marked fall in blood pressure (at 0300 hours). There is a reversal of the diurnal changes in blood pressure, with relatively small changes in heart rate considering the marked changes in blood pressure. From Mathias and Bannister (1992b).

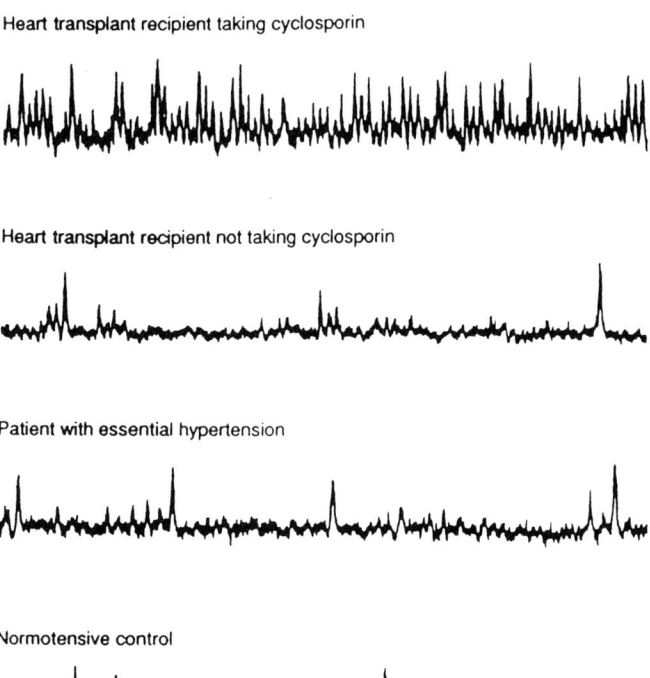

Figure 5. Recordings of muscle sympathetic nerve activity in a heart transplant recipient on cyclosporin showing a greater degree of sympathetic nerve discharge compared with a heart transplant patient not on cyclosporin, a patient with essential hypertension and a normotensive control. From Scherrer et al (1990).

degree of supine hypertension. It may be of value in evaluating therapeutic approaches to reduce postural hypotension.

The specialized technique of microneurography enables continuous recording of skin and muscle sympathetic nerve activity in peripheral nerves in the arm or leg. This technique has been of particular value in understanding various physiological and pathophysiological processes (Wallin, 1992). It is highly dependent upon operator skill, is invasive, and is of greater value in the presence of excessive sympathetic activity (Figure 5) than when there is a chronic reduction, or absence, of sympathetic discharge.

Pharmacological tests

A wide variety of drugs can help to determine aspects of central or peripheral sympathetic function. An example of the former is the use of the predominantly centrally acting α_2-adrenoceptor agonist drug, clonidine. It lowers supine blood pressure in normal subjects and in patients with

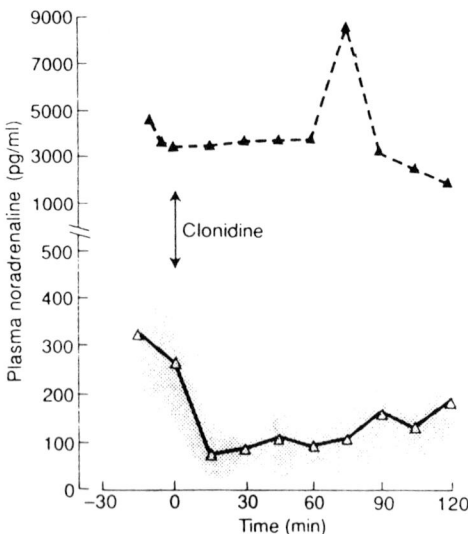

Figure 6. Plasma noradrenaline levels in a patient with phaeochromocytoma (filled triangles) and in a group of patients with essential hypotension (open triangles) before and after intravenous clonidine as indicated by the arrow (2 μg/kg over 10 min). Plasma noradrenaline levels fall rapidly in the essential hypertensive patients after clonidine, and remain low over the period of observation. The stippled area indicates the standard error of the mean. Plasma noradrenaline levels are considerably higher in the phaeochromocytoma patient and are not affected by clonidine. From Mathias and Bannister (1992a).

essential hypertension, but not when there is autonomous secretion of catecholamines, as in phaeochromocytoma (Figure 6). Clonidine does not lower blood pressure in tetraplegics with complete cervical spinal cord lesions because the descending sympathetic pathways have been interrupted (Reid et al, 1977). In peripheral sympathetic failure (as in PAF), clonidine does not lower blood pressure and may even raise it, presumably because of persistence of its initial, transient peripheral α-adrenoceptor agonist effects in the presence of adrenoceptor supersensitivity. The responses in PAF differ from those in patients with central autonomic failure (Shy–Drager syndrome), in whom blood pressure often falls (Thomaides et al, 1992a).

Clonidine stimulates growth hormone release and this effect has been recently used to help separate central from peripheral autonomic failure (Thomaides et al, 1992b) (Figure 7). The lack of a rise in growth hormone may be a useful marker in the early detection of central sympathetic failure, and it may distinguish patients with idiopathic Parkinson's disease from patients with the SDS who may have similar neurological features, especially in the early stages. Other approaches include drugs such as edrophonium, which acts on nicotinic cholinergic receptors in sympathetic ganglia and raises plasma noradrenaline levels in patients with pre- but not postganglionic sympathetic lesions (Gemmill et al, 1988).

Information on peripheral adrenergic receptors can be obtained using adrenoceptor agonists such as noradrenaline (norepinephrine *USP*) or

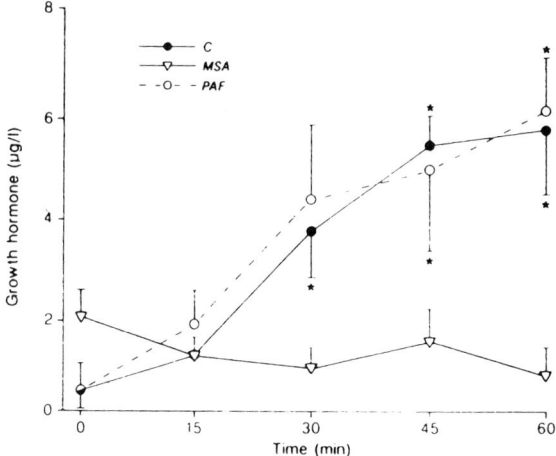

Figure 7. Plasma growth hormone concentrations before (0) and 15, 30, 45 and 60 min after intravenous clonidine (2 μg/kg bodyweight given at time 0) in normal subjects (controls, C) and patients with multiple system atrophy (MSA; Shy–Drager syndrome) or pure autonomic failure (PAF). The bars indicate the standard error of the mean. * = $P < 0.05$. From Thomaides et al (1992b).

isoprenaline to determine if there is pressor or chronotropic supersensitivity. Determination of lymphocyte and platelet adrenoceptor numbers and their characteristics may provide valuable information (Davies et al, 1982; Zoukos et al, 1992). The administration of tyramine may determine if noradrenaline is present within sympathetic nerve terminals. In patients with depleted noradrenaline stores there is no pressor response or elevation in plasma noradrenaline levels. However, in incomplete lesions there may be difficulties in interpretation, as even small amounts of noradrenaline released may result in a marked pressor response in the presence of supersensitivity.

Biochemical tests

The measurement of catecholamines and their metabolites provides an important means of assessing sympathetic neural function (Goldstein et al, 1989; Polinsky, 1992) and enabling diagnosis of specific biochemical defects, as in DBH deficiency. Measurements in plasma are of particular value, and supine basal levels alone may contribute to the diagnosis (Figure 8). In distal sympathetic lesions (as in PAF), levels of noradrenaline are low with no change during head-up tilt or standing. In DBH deficiency, however, levels of both plasma noradrenaline and adrenaline are undetectable, unlike levels of plasma dopamine, which are raised compared with normal subjects and other groups with sympathetic failure. An undetectable level of the enzyme DBH in plasma (Figure 9) and in tissues provides further confirmation of the diagnosis (Mathias et al, 1990).

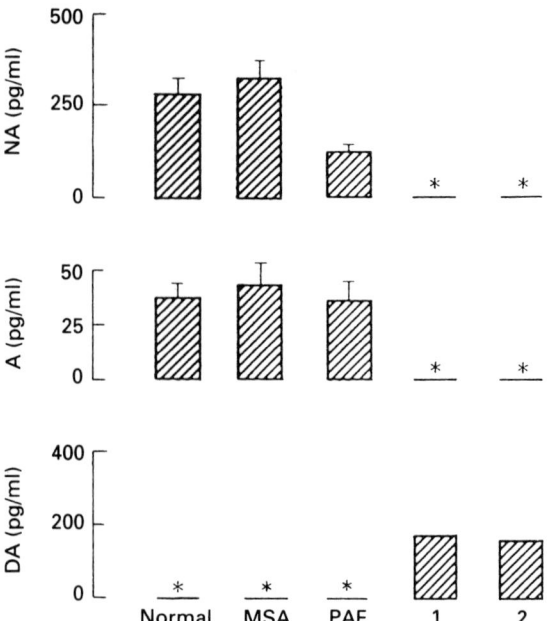

Figure 8. Mean levels (± SEM) of plasma noradrenaline (NA), adrenaline (A) and dopamine (DA) in ten normal subjects, twelve patients with multiple system atrophy (MSA; Shy–Drager syndrome) and eight patients with pure autonomic failure (PAF). Individual values in patients 1 and 2 with DBM deficiency are indicated. The asterisk indicates undetectable levels, which were below 5 pg/ml for NA and A, and below 20 pg/ml for DA. From Mathias et al (1990).

In addition to postural change, insulin-induced hypoglycaemia and exercise may be used to stimulate catecholamine release, and other endocrine and cardiovascular responses; these responses are usually abnormal in sympathetic failure (Polinsky et al, 1980; Mathias et al, 1987). The reverse, using suppression tests as in phaeochromocytoma, are of value when overactivity is suspected.

Measurements of catecholamines and their metabolites in urine may be helpful, especially in DBH deficiency (Figure 10). Measurements in cerebrospinal fluid may provide additional information (Polinsky et al, 1984).

CLINICAL FEATURES AND MANAGEMENT OF MAJOR DISORDERS

Primary chronic autonomic failure

Conditions in which there is primary chronic autonomic failure are currently divided into two major groups, PAF and the SDS. It is likely that, with time, discrete subgroups with distinct entities will be identified. This is important

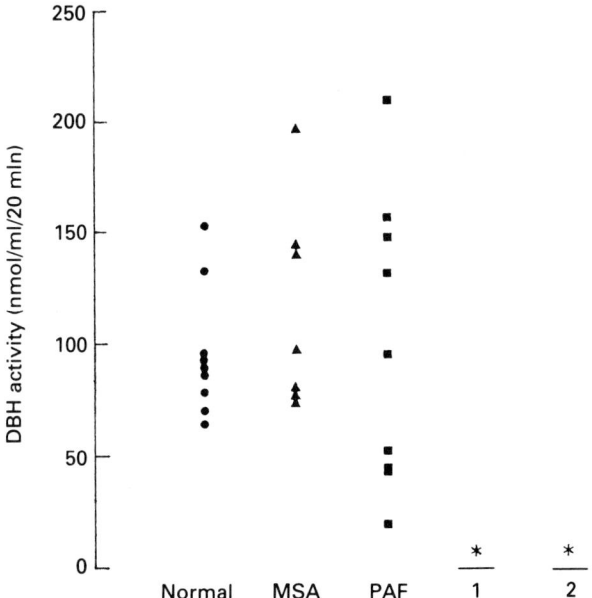

Figure 9. Scattergram showing DBH activity in ten normal subjects, seven patients with multiple system atrophy (MSA; Shy–Drager syndrome) and nine patients with pure autonomic failure (PAF). In patients 1 and 2 with DBH deficiency, activity was undetectable (shown by an asterisk). From Mathias et al (1990).

as the aetiology and management of specific disorders may differ. One example is DBH deficiency, which previously would have been classified under PAF.

The majority of patients with chronic autonomic failure are in their 50s or 60s, although younger patients are being increasingly recognized. There are usually no other affected members in the family. The presenting features may vary. Autonomic involvement in both PAF and the SDS may result in similar symptoms, although these are often, but not necessarily, progressive in the SDS. Features may have been present for many years but may not have prompted a medical consultation. In the male this includes erectile failure and impotence, which may antedate the symptoms of postural hypotension or other neurological features by years. The wide variety of system involvement is outlined in Table 4.

Of the autonomic features, those affecting the cardiovascular system and urinary bladder usually lead patients to seek medical advice. Postural hypotension may be missed if not specifically tested for, especially if the accompanying features are unusual, or if the postural drop is initially small and needs unmasking by stimuli such as food (Mathias et al, 1991b), exercise or vasodilator agents. Urinary bladder symptoms in older male patients may be attributed to prostatic hypertrophy, and this may lead to an unnecessary, often unhelpful, operative procedure.

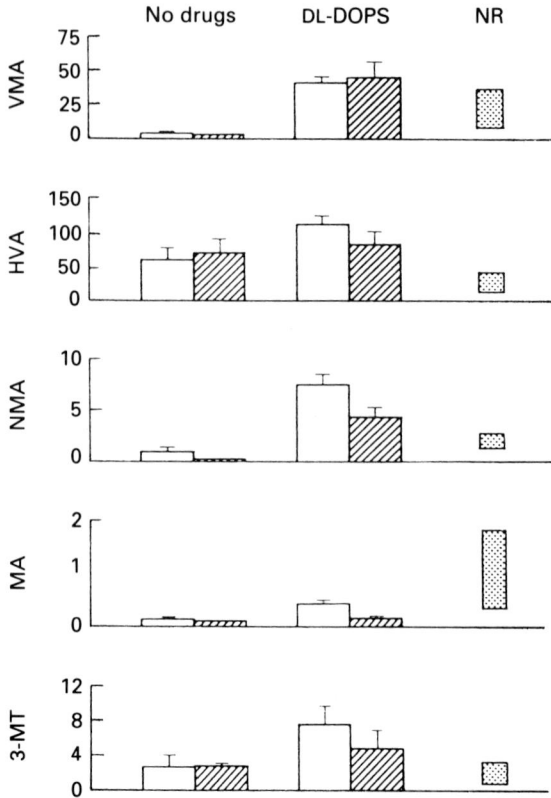

Figure 10. Twenty-four hour urinary secretion of catecholamine metabolites in patient 1 (open histograms) and patient 2 (filled histograms) with the DBH deficiency syndrome, before and after treatment with DL-dihydroxyphenylserine (DL-DOPS). Bars indicate mean ±SEM and relate to collections over three consecutive days. VMA = vanillylmandelic acid, HVA = homovanillic acid, 3-MT = 3-methoxy-tyramine, MA = metadrenaline, NMA = normet-adrenaline. The normal range (NR) is indicated by the stippled histogram on the right. HVA and 3-MT are metabolites of dopamine. From Mathias et al (1990).

Table 4. Some clinical manifestations in patients with primary chronic autonomic failure.

Cardiovascular system:	Postural hypotension
Urinary bladder:	Frequency, urgency, incontinence, retention
Large bowel:	Constipation, occasionally diarrhoea
Genital tract:	Impotence in the male
Sweating:	Anhidrosis
Respiratory system:	Stridor
Pupils:	Anisocoria, Horner's syndrome
Other neurological deficits:	Parkinsonian, cerebellar and pyramidal signs

The symptoms of postural hypotension mainly result from cerebral ischaemia and include lightheadedness, dizziness, weakness, a variety of visual disturbances and, sometimes, loss of consciousness. In addition to the relationship to posture, a number of situations are often recognized as exacerbating symptoms; in the morning, after ingestion of food and alcohol, following exercise, whilst straining during micturition or defecation, and during an elevation in environmental temperature. Lying flat, or a variety of postures such as squatting or stooping, alleviate the symptoms. With time patients often are able to tolerate a considerably lower level of perfusion pressure. Many are able to avoid syncope by anticipating predisposing situations or by responding to presyncopal symptoms with appropriate action, although this may be a problem in those with neurological deficits. Ischaemia to other organs may result in additional symptoms. Neck and shoulder ache in the 'coathanger' distribution is often associated with postural hypotension and is resolved by sitting or lying flat. This may result from ischaemia of tonically contracting muscles. Central chest discomfort or pain akin to angina may occur even in those without electrocardiographic changes indicative of ischaemia. A cauda equina-like ischaemic syndrome affecting the lower limbs may occur when the blood pressure falls.

Impairment of sudomotor function results in hypohidrosis or anhidrosis, although in the initial phases compensatory hyperhidrosis in 'spared' areas may be a distressing symptom. Thermoregulation may be impaired and in hot weather may result in hyperpyrexia, which can increase the tendency to low blood pressure and cause collapse. In incomplete lesions, as in some patients with the SDS, there may be patchy supersensitivity of peripheral hand vessels, with symptoms and signs suggestive of Raynaud's phenomenon. Other features which are related to sympathetic malfunction include ejaculatory failure or retrograde ejaculation. Erectile failure, an early manifestation, is related to parasympathetic involvement, as is involvement of the urinary bladder and large bowel. Nocturnal polyuria is common and may result from a variety of changes, including redistribution of blood from the peripheral into the central compartment, along with the effects of hormones such as renin, aldosterone and atrial natriuretic factor, each of which are known to influence renal handling of salt and water; this may be compounded by the lack of sympathetic control over renal tubular function. An intermittent Horner's syndrome may occur.

In PAF the sympathetic deficit may not be progressive but may appear to be so as the functional deterioration and enhancement of symptoms are often related to environmental (temperature) and other situations (such as fluid loss due to diarrhoea). This is in contradistinction to the SDS, where exacerbation of functional deficits may also occur but where progression is the rule, although this may be more evident in relation to the deterioration of extrapyramidal and cerebellar function. Newer non-invasive neuro-imaging techniques are being increasingly used to evaluate the non-autonomic neurological aspects (Brooks et al, 1990; Fulham et al, 1991). Treatment of the parkinsonian features with levodopa or dopaminergic agonists may precipitate or exacerbate postural hypotension.

The natural history in PAF indicates a more favourable prognosis than in

Table 5a. Approaches to treatment of postural hypotension.

Advice on factors which influence blood pressure:
    Straining during micturition and defecation
    Diurnal changes in blood pressure
    Exposure to a warm environment
    Effects of food
    Effects of drugs with vasoactive properties
Head-up tilt at night
External support
Cardiac pacing
Drugs (see below)

Table 5b. Drugs used in the treatment of postural hypotension.

Site of action	Drugs	Predominant action
Vessels—vasoconstriction		
Resistance vessels	Ephedrine	Indirectly acting sympathomimetic
	Midodrine, phenylephrine, methylphenidate	Directly acting sympathomimetics
	Tyramine	Release of noradrenaline
	Clonidine	Postsynaptic α-adrenoceptor agonist
	Yohimbine	Presynaptic α_2-adrenoceptor antagonist
	DL-DOPS and L-DOPS	Pro-drugs result in formation of noradrenaline
	Triglycyl-lysine-vasopressin (glypressin)	V_1-receptors on blood vessels
Capacitance vessels	Dihydroergotamine	Direct action on α-adrenoceptors
Vessels—prevention of vasodilatation	Propranolol	Blockade of β_2-adreno-receptors
	Indomethacin	Blockade of prostaglandins
	Metoclopramide	Blockade of dopamine receptors
Vessels—prevention of postprandial hypotension	Caffeine	Blockade of adenosine receptors
	Octreotide	Preventing release of vasodilator peptides
Heart—stimulation	Pindolol, Xamoterol	Intrinsic sympathetic action
Plasma volume	Fludrocortisone	Mineralocorticoid effects Increased plasma volume (large dose) Sensitization of α-adrenoreceptors to noradrenaline (small dose)
Kidney—reducing diuresis	Desmopressin	V_2-receptors on renal tubules

DOPS = dihyroxyphenylserine.

the SDS. In PAF, life expectancy is broadly within normal limits, especially if patients avoid the serious injury which may complicate severe postural hypotension. In the SDS, however, the majority are dead within 5 to 7 years of diagnosis; this is often the result of increasing neurological disability. Drug refractory rigidity and bradykinesia may occur in those with parkinsonian features. This may be compounded by dysphagia (with the tendency to aspirate) and involvement of laryngeal muscles, causing obstructive respiratory failure, in addition to central respiratory dysfunction.

Investigations usually indicate that the lesions are peripheral in PAF and central in the SDS. Management often involves multiple treatments, with an emphasis on reducing postural hypotension through a variety of mechanisms (Table 5). In the SDS, attention also needs to be directed to the other autonomic and neurological deficits.

Primary acute and subacute dysautonomias

The sympathetic nervous system may be affected as part of a pure pandysautonomia or in combination with other sensory and motor abnormalities. Severe postural hypotension may occur. There are often associated parasympathetic abnormalities, which may result in gastric and intestinal stasis and urinary retention. The prognosis varies. Complete recovery may occur in some, while in others the deficits persist. Management will depend on the functional deficit and is often similar to that in the chronic syndromes.

DBH

This is a recently described syndrome where there is a deficiency of DBH, resulting in an elevation of the precursor, dopamine, and undetectable levels of noradrenaline and adrenaline (Robertson et al, 1976; Man in't Veld et al, 1987a). DBH cannot be detected in plasma or in tissues.

The patients have many of the features of PAF, but with certain exceptions and characteristics. Although the diagnosis is often made later in life (after 20 years in the reported cases), the history indicates abnormalities from birth; hypoglycaemia and epilepsy are often considered as an explanation. A brother and sister with the disorder have been reported, favouring a genetic basis to the abnormality (Mathias et al, 1990). The DBH gene has been located at chromosome 9q34 (Craig et al, 1988), but no major genetic abnormality has as yet been detected in the two siblings with DBH deficiency (Craig et al, 1992). The features of postural hypotension, with exacerbating and relieving factors, are similar to those described in the chronic syndromes. Sweating, and therefore sympathetic cholinergic function, is preserved. Parasympathetic function of the heart, along with urinary bladder and large bowel function, is intact. In studies in a male patient, penile erection was normal but ejaculation was difficult to achieve (Mathias et al, 1990). There are no associated neurological deficits. The features therefore are consistent with selective noradrenergic involvement, with sparing of sympathetic cholinergic and parasympathetic function.

Biochemical investigations are used to confirm the diagnosis. Noradrenaline and adrenaline are undetectable in plasma. Plasma dopamine levels, however, are elevated (Figure 8). Further evidence can be provided from urinary measurements of catecholamines and their metabolites (Figure 10). Activity of DBH in plasma cannot be measured. In the cerebrospinal fluid noradrenaline and adrenaline are not detectable while dopamine and its metabolites are elevated. A range of physiological and pharmacological tests are consistent with preservation of parasympathetic function. Specialized investigations include skin biopsies which indicate lack of DBH immunoreactivity. Microneurographic studies of sympathetic function in the periphery in a single patient indicated preservation of sympathetic electrical discharge (Rea et al, 1990). This is consistent with the electron microscopy studies confirming morphologically normal sympathetic terminals, thus suggesting a localized, specific, biochemical defect. Patients with DBH deficiency have nocturnal and recumbency-induced polyuria but, unlike patients with chronic and primary autonomic failure, do not have food-induced hypotension.

There are a number of other genetically acquired autonomic disorders (Thomas, 1992), including familial amyloid polyneuropathy. However, a number of other neurological or endocrine features usually distinguish these

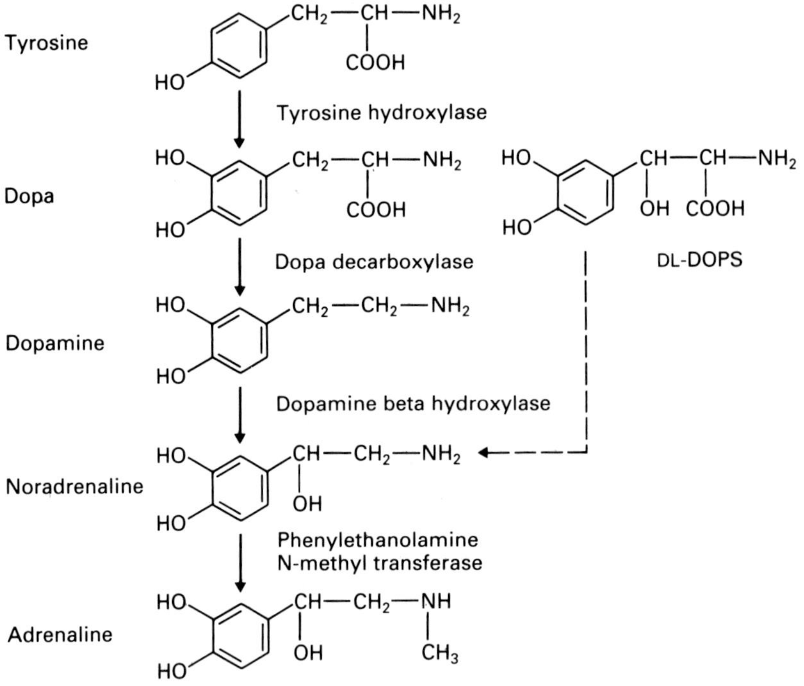

Figure 11. Biosynthetic pathway for the formation of noradrenaline and adrenaline. The structure of DL-DOPS is indicated on the right. This is converted directly to noradrenaline by dopa decarboxylase, thus bypassing the necessity for DBH. From Mathias et al (1990).

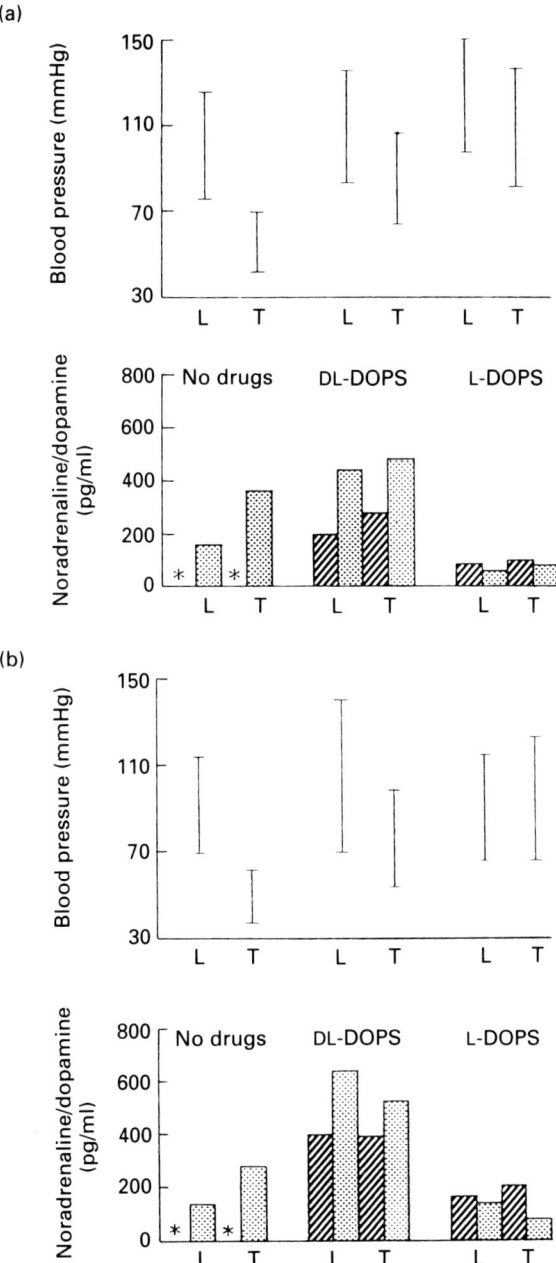

Figure 12. Blood pressure (systolic and diastolic) while lying (L) and during 45° head-up tilt (T) in patient 1 (a) and patient 2 (b) with DBH deficiency, before and during treatment with DL-DOPS and L-DOPS. Plasma noradrenaline (hatched histogram) and dopamine (stippled histogram) levels are indicated before and during tilt. Plasma noradrenaline was undetectable (indicated by asterisk) in both patients while off drugs. From Mathias et al (1990).

patients from those with DBH deficiency (Mathias and Bannister, 1992b). Variants have been, and are likely to be, described (Cortelli et al, 1992). Recently, a patient has been reported with clinical features of DBH deficiency, but with deficiency of tyrosine hydroxylase and the sensory neuropeptides, substance P and calcitonin gene-related peptide (Anand et al, 1991). There were low levels of nerve growth factor in skin, suggesting a trophic basis for this particular syndrome, as distinct from isolated DBH deficiency.

The diagnosis is of importance, as such patients (unlike most others with chronic autonomic failure) can be satisfactorily treated with the precursor drug, DL- or L-dihydroxyphenylserine (DL- or L-DOPS) (Biaggioni and Robertson, 1987; Man in't Veld et al, 1987b; Mathias et al, 1990) (see Figure 11). This is converted to noradrenaline by dopa carboxylase, thus bypassing the enzymatic block. The drug elevates noradrenaline levels in plasma and reduces postural hypotension (Figure 12). In a male subject it improved ejaculatory function. It has been successfully used in our patients for over 5 years without the need for other drugs except for desmopressin.

High spinal cord lesions

In cervical and high thoracic spinal cord lesions either a substantial part of, or the entire, sympathetic outflow may be separated from cerebral control.

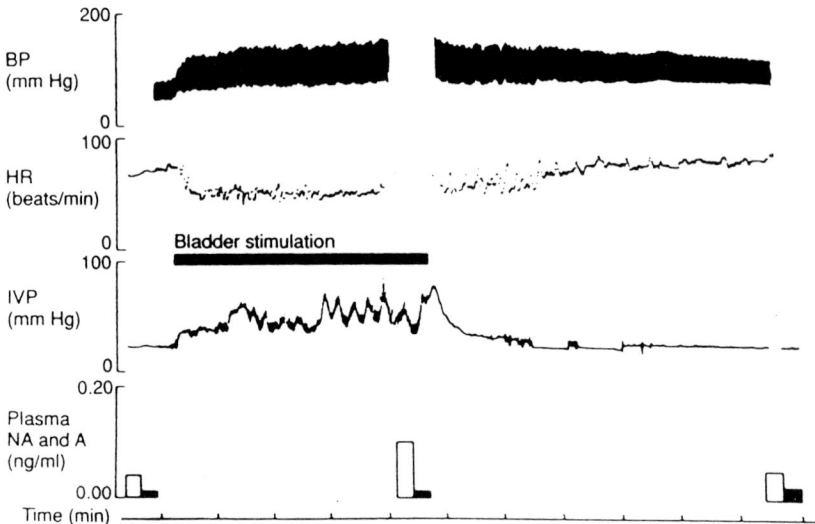

Figure 13. Blood pressure (BP), heart rate (HR), intravascular pressure (IVP) and plasma noradrenaline (NA; open histogram) and adrenaline (A; filled histogram) levels in a tetraplegic patient before, during and after bladder stimulation induced by suprapubic percussion of the anterior abdominal wall. The rise in blood pressure is accompanied by a fall in heart rate as a result of increased vagal activity and in response to the rise in blood pressure. Noradrenaline but not adrenaline levels rise, suggesting an increase in sympathoneural activity independent of adrenomedullary activation. From Mathias and Frankel (1986).

This results in a number of abnormalities, many of which are directly related to impaired sympathetic control.

The inability to activate peripheral sympathetic nerves during head-up postural change causes postural hypotension, which can be severe, especially in the early stages of rehabilitation. This tends to improve later (Figure 1b) for a variety of reasons, which could include improved cerebrovascular autoregulation, activation of spinal sympathetic reflexes, and the compensatory effects of hormones such as renin, aldosterone and vasopressin (Mathias et al, 1975, 1980; Poole et al, 1987). There is usually no need for the range of drugs used to improve postural hypotension in chronic autonomic failure. Head-up tilt at night, together with repeated head-up tilt during the day, is often sufficient. In some, ephedrine (15 mg) given half an hour before postural change is of value.

The reverse, a paroxysmal rise in blood pressure, may occur as a result of stimuli applied below the level of the lesion, such as cutaneous stimulation, activation of viscera such as the urinary bladder or bowel, and during skeletal muscle spasms (Guttmann and Whitteridge, 1947) (Figure 13). This does not usually occur in the early stages, when patients are in spinal shock,

Table 6. Causes of autonomic dysreflexia.

Abdominal or pelvic visceral stimulation
Ureter:
    Calculus
Urinary bladder:
    Distension by blocked catheter or discoordinated bladder infection
    Irritation by calculus, catheter, or bladder washout
Rectum and anus:
    Enemata
    Faecal retention
    Anal fissure
Gastrointestinal organs:
    Gastric dilatation
    Gastric ulceration
    Cholecystitis or cholelithiasis
Uterus:
    Contraction during pregnancy
    Menstruation, occasionally

Cutaneous stimulation
Pressure sores
Infected ingrowing toenails
Burns

Skeletal muscle spasms
Especially in limbs with contractures

Miscellaneous
Intrathecal neostigmine
Electroejaculatory procedures
Ejaculation
Vaginal dilatation
Urethra—insertion of catheter or abscess
Fractures of bones

(Mathias et al, 1979a), but invariably occurs in the chronic phase, with return of the spinal reflexes. The paroxysmal hypertension and subsequent bradycardia is part of the syndrome of autonomic dysreflexia. There is a rise in levels of plasma noradrenaline but not adrenaline, indicative of an increase in sympathoneural but not adrenomedullary activity (Mathias et al, 1976b). Basal levels of plasma noradrenaline in high lesions are usually a third of the resting levels in normal humans. However, during the hypertension, plasma noradrenaline levels do not rise above normal levels despite the exaggerated pressor response. This is consistent with microneurographic studies which indicate only a modest sympathetic discharge during the rise in blood pressure (Stjernberg et al, 1986), when there is usually marked and prolonged vasoconstriction in the periphery. There is thus both biochemical and physiological data indicating that a marked increase in sympathetic reflexes (hyperreflexia) does not occur, but that other mechanisms, including supersensitivity of blood vessels, may account for the abnormalities. The enhanced pressor response to agents such as noradrenaline and angiotensin II favours non-specific vascular supersensitivity. There is also marked hypotension in response to vasodilator agents, including isoprenaline and glyceryl trinitrate. It may be that disruption of descending pathways in the cervical spinal cord, accounting for both constrictor and dilator effects which contribute to blood pressure homeostasis, may be a key factor.

The management of autonomic dysreflexia is of importance, as the hypertension may result in complications, ranging from a throbbing headache, epileptic seizures and visual deficits to myocardial failure and even death from cerebral haemorrhage. It is important to determine the cause of the problem (Table 6) and rectify it. Drugs, however, are often needed, as detection of the underlying cause might be difficult. The approaches used are outlined in Table 7.

Table 7. Some of the drugs used in the management of autonomic dysreflexia classified according to their major site of action on the reflex arc or on target organs.

Afferent:	Topical lignocaine
Spinal cord:	Clonidine*
	Reserpine*
	Spinal anaesthetics
Efferent	
Sympathetic ganglia	Hexamethonium
Sympathetic nerve terminals	Guanethidine
α-Adrenoceptors	Phenoxybenzamine
Target organs:	
Blood vessels	Glyceryl trinitrate
	Nifedipine
Sweat glands	Propantheline

*Clonidine and reserpine have multiple effects, some of which are peripheral.
Lignocaine = lidocaine *USP*.

SUMMARY

The sympathetic nervous system innervates most organs in the body and controls their function. A variety of disease processes, surgery or drugs can result in disordered sympathetic nerve function, which can be either localized or more generalized. Malfunction can result in either sympathetic underactivity (causing postural hypotension, impotence or anhidrosis) or overactivity (causing paroxysmal hypertension or hyperhidrosis). The investigation of sympathetic disorders depends upon the system and organs involved and should include, where relevant, investigation of the possible aetiological processes. The clinical features and management of some of the major disorders affecting the sympathetic nervous system, including the recently described syndrome of DBH deficiency, are described.

Acknowledgements

We thank Miss Tina Holmes for secretarial assistance. The author thanks the Wellcome Trust for their sustained support.

REFERENCES

Anand P, Rudge P, Mathias CJ et al (1991) New autonomic and sensory neuropathy with loss of adrenergic sympathetic function and sensory neuropeptides. *Lancet* **33:** 1253–1254.

Bannister R & Mathias CJ (1992) The management of postural hypotension. In Bannister R & Mathias CJ (eds) *Autonomic Failure: A Textbook of Clinical Disorders of the Autonomic Nervous System* 3rd edn, pp 622–645. Oxford: Oxford Medical Publications.

Biaggioni I & Robertson D (1987) Endogenous restoration of noradrenaline by precursor therapy in dopamine beta-hydroxylase deficiency. *Lancet* **ii:** 1170–1172.

Bradbury S & Eggleston C (1925) Postural hypotension: a report of three cases. *American Heart Journal* **1:** 73–86.

Brooks DJ, Salmon EP, Mathias CJ et al (1990) The relationship between locomotor disability, autonomic dysfunction, and the integrity of the striatal dopaminergic system in patients with multiple system atrophy, pure autonomic failure, and Parkinson's disease, studied with PET. *Brain* **113:** 1539–1552.

Callister R, Suwarno NO & Seals DR (1992) Sympathetic activity is influenced by task difficulty and stress perception during mental challenge in humans. *Journal of Physiology* **454:** 373–387.

Corbett JL, Kerr JH, Prys-Roberts C, Smith AC & Spalding JMK (1969) Cardiovascular disturbances in severe tetanus due to over-activity of the sympathetic nervous system. *Anaesthesia* **24:** 198–212.

Cortelli P, Parchi P, Contin M et al (1992) Isolated failure of noradrenergic transmission in a case with orthostatic hypotension and hyperactivity of gastric-colic reflex. *Clinical Autonomic Research* **2:** 177–182.

Craig SP, Buckle VJ, Lamouroux A et al (1988) Localization of the human dopamine beta hydroxylase (DBH) gene to chromosome 9q34. *Cytogenetics and Cell Genetics* **48:** 48–50.

Craig I, Porter C & Craig SB (1992) The molecular genetics of dopamine β-hydroxylase. In Bannister R & Mathias CJ (eds) *Autonomic Failure: A Textbook of Clinical Disorders of the Autonomic Nervous System* 3rd edn, pp 749–758. Oxford: Oxford Medical Publications.

Davies IB, Mathias CJ, Sudera D & Sever PS (1982) Agonist regulation of alpha-adrenergic receptor responses in man. *Journal of Cardiovascular Pharmacology* **4:** s139–144.

Ewing DJ (1992) Analysis of heart rate variability and other non-invasive tests with special reference to diabetes mellitus. In Bannister R & Mathias CJ (eds) *Autonomic Failure: A*

Textbook of Clinical Disorders of the Autonomic Nervous System 3rd edn, pp 312–333. Oxford: Oxford Medical Publications.

Frankel HL, Mathias CJ & Spalding JMK (1975) Mechanisms of reflex cardiac arrest in tetraplegic patients. *Lancet* ii: 1183–1185.

Fulham MJ, Dubinsky RM, Polinsky RJ et al (1991) Computerized tomography, magnetic resonance imaging and positron emission tomography with [18F] fluorodeoxyglucose in the assessment of multiple system atrophy and pure autonomic failure. *Clinical Autonomic Research* 1: 27–36.

Gemmill JD, Venables GS & Ewing DJ (1988) Noradrenaline response to edrophonium in primary autonomic failure: distinction between central and peripheral damage. *Lancet* i: 1018–1021.

Goldstein DS, Polinsky RJ, Garty M et al (1989) Patterns of plasma levels of catechols in neurogenic orthostatic hypotension. *Annals of Neurology* 26: 558–563.

Guttmann L & Whitteridge D (1947) Effects of bladder distension on autonomic mechanisms after spinal cord injury. *Brain* 70: 361–404.

Imholz BPM, Wieling W, Langewouters GJ & van Montfrans GA (1991) Continuous finger arterial pressure: utility in the cardiovascular laboratory. *Clinical Autonomic Research* 1: 43–53.

Man in't Veld AJ, Boomsma F, Moleman P & Schalekamp MADH (1987a) Congenital dopamine beta-hydroxylase deficiency. A novel orthostatic syndrome. *Lancet* i: 183–187.

Man in't Veld AJ, Van den Meiracker AH, Boomsma F & Schalekamp MADH (1987b) Effect of unnatural noradrenaline precursor on sympathetic control and orthostatic hypotension in dopamine beta-hydroxylase deficiency. *Lancet* ii: 1172–1175.

Marshall RJ, Schirger A & Shepherd JT (1961) Blood pressure during supine exercise in idiopathic autostatic hypotension. *Circulation Research* 24: 76–81.

Mathias CJ (1987) Autonomic dysfunction. *British Journal of Hospital Medicine* 38: 238–243.

Mathias CJ (1991) Disorders of the autonomic nervous system. In Bradley WG, Daroff RB, Fenichel GM & Marsden CD (eds) *Neurology in Clinical Practice*, pp 1661–1685. Massachusetts: Butterworth–Heinemann.

Mathias CJ & Bannister R (1992a) Investigation of autonomic disorders. In Bannister R & Mathias CJ (eds) *Autonomic Failure: A Textbook of Clinical Disorders of the Autonomic Nervous System* 3rd edn, pp 255–290. Oxford: Oxford Medical Publications.

Mathias CJ & Bannister R (1992b) Postcibal hypotension in autonomic disorders. In Bannister R & Mathias CJ (eds) *Autonomic Failure: A Textbook of Clinical Disorders of the Autonomic Nervous System* 3rd edn, pp 489–509. Oxford: Oxford Medical Publications.

Mathias CJ & Bannister R (1992c) Dopamine β-hydroxylase deficiency and other genetically determined causes of autonomic disorders. A. Clinical features, investigation, and management. In Bannister R & Mathias CJ (eds) *Autonomic Failure: A Textbook of Clinical Disorders of the Autonomic Nervous System* 3rd edn, pp 721–748. Oxford: Oxford Medical Publications.

Mathias CJ & Frankel HL (1986) The neurological and hormonal control of blood vessels and heart in spinal man. *Journal of the Autonomic Nervous System* supplement: 457–464.

Mathias CJ & Frankel HL (1988) Cardiovascular control in spinal man. *Annual Review of Physiology* 50: 577–592.

Mathias CJ & Frankel HL (1992a) Autonomic disturbances in spinal cord lesions. In Bannister R & Mathias CJ (eds) *Autonomic Failure: A Textbook of Clinical Disorders of the Autonomic Nervous System* 3rd edn, pp 839–881. Oxford: Oxford Medical Publications.

Mathias CJ & Frankel HL (1992b) The cardiovascular system in tetraplegia and paraplegia. In Vinken PJ, Bruyn GW & Klawans HL (eds) *Handbook of Clinical Neurology*, Vol. 61 spinal cord trauma. Series editor HL Frankel. Chap. 25 (in press). pp 435–456. Amsterdam: Elsevier Science Publishers.

Mathias CJ, Christensen NJ, Corbett JL et al (1975) Plasma catecholamines, plasma renin activity and plasma aldosterone in tetraplegic man, horizontal and tilted. *Clinical Science and Molecular Medicine* 49: 291–299.

Mathias CJ, Frankel HL, Christensen NJ & Spalding JMK (1976a) Enhanced pressor response to noradrenaline in patients with cervical spinal cord transection. *Brain* 99: 757–770.

Mathias CJ, Christensen NJ, Corbett JL, Frankel HL & Spalding JMK (1976b) Plasma catecholamines during paroxysmal neurogenic hypertension in quadriplegic man. *Circulation Research* 39: 204–208.

Mathias CJ, Christensen NJ, Frankel HL & Spalding JMK (1979a) Cardiovascular control in recently injured tetraplegics in spinal shock. *Quarterly Journal of Medicine* 48: 273–287.

Mathias CJ, Frankel HL, Turner RC & Christensen JN (1979b) Physiological responses to insulin hypoglycaemia in spinal man. *Paraplegia* 17: 319–326.

Mathias CJ, Christensen JN, Frankel HL & Peart WS (1980) Renin release during head-up tilt occurs independently of sympathetic nervous activity in tetraplegic man. *Clinical Science* 59: 251–256.

Mathias CJ, Frankel HL, Davies IB, James VHY & Peart WS (1981) Renin and aldosterone release during sympathetic stimulation in tetraplegia. *Clinical Science* 60: 399–604.

Mathias CJ, Fosbraey P, da Costa DF, Thornley A & Bannister R (1986) Desmopressin reduces nocturnal polyuria, reverses overnight weight loss and improves morning postural hypotension in autonomic failure. *British Medical Journal* 293: 353–354.

Mathias CJ, da Costa DF, Fosbraey P, Christensen JN & Bannister R (1987) Hypotensive and sedative effects of insulin in autonomic failure. *British Medical Journal* 295: 161–163.

Mathias CJ, Bannister R, Cortelli P et al (1990) Clinical, autonomic and therapeutic observations in two siblings with postural hypotension and sympathetic failure due to an inability to synthesize noradrenaline from dopamine because of a deficiency of dopamine beta-hydroxylase. *Quarterly Journal of Medicine* 75: 617–633.

Mathias CJ, Armstrong E, Browse N et al (1991a) Value of non-invasive continuous blood pressure monitoring in the detection of carotid sinus hypersensitivity. *Clinical Autonomic Research* 1: 157–159.

Mathias CJ, Holly ER, Armstrong E, Shareef M & Bannister R (1991b) The influence of food and postural hypotension in three groups of chronic autonomic failure; clinical and therapeutic implications. *Journal of Neurology, Neurosurgery and Psychiatry* 54: 726–730.

Polinsky RJ (1992) Neuropharmacological investigation of autonomic failure. In Bannister R & Mathias CJ (eds) *Autonomic Failure: A Textbook of Clinical Disorders of the Autonomic Nervous System* 3rd edn, pp 334–358. Oxford: Oxford Medical Publications.

Polinsky RJ, Kopin IJ, Ebert MH & Weise V (1980) The adrenal medullary response to hypoglycaemia in patients with orthostatic hypotension. *Journal of Clinical Endocrinology and Metabolism* 51: 1401–1406.

Polinsky RJ, Jimerson DC & Kopin IJ (1984) Chronic autonomic failure: CSF and plasma 3-methoxy-4-hydroxyphenylglycol. *Neurology* 34: 979–983.

Poole CJM, Williams TDM, Lightman SL & Frankel HL (1987) Neuroendocrine control of vasopressin secretion and its effect on blood pressure in subjects with spinal cord transection. *Brain* 110: 727–735.

Rea R, Biaggioni I, Robertson RM, Haile V & Robertson D (1990) Reflex control of sympathetic nerve activity in dopamine beta-hydroxylase deficiency. *Hypertension* 1: 107–112.

Reid JL, Wing LMH, Mathias CJ, Frankel HL & Neill E (1977) The central hypotensive effect of clonidine: studies in tetraplegic subjects. *Clinical Pharmacology and Therapeutics* 21: 375–381.

Robertson D, Goldberg MR, Onrot J et al (1986) Isolated failure of autonomic noradrenergic neurotransmission. Evidence for impaired beta-hydroxylation of dopamine. *New England Journal of Medicine* 314: 1494–1497.

Scherrer U, Vissing SF, Morgan BJ et al (1990) Cyclosporine-induced sympathetic activation and hypertension after heart transplantation. *New England Journal of Medicine* 323: 693–699.

Shy GM & Drager GA (1960) A neurological syndrome associated with orthostatic hypotension. *Archives of Neurology* 3: 511–527.

Stjernberg L, Blumberg H & Wallin BG (1986) Sympathetic activity in man after spinal cord injury: outflow to muscle below the lesion. *Brain* 109: 695–715.

Thomaides TN, Chaudhuri KR, Maule S & Mathias CJ (1992a) Differential responses in superior mesenteric artery blood flow may explain the varying pressor responses to clonidine in two groups with sympathetic denervation. *Clinical Science* 83: 59–64.

Thomaides TN, Chaudhuri KR, Maule S, Watson L, Marsden CD & Mathias CJ (1992b) Growth hormone response to clonidine in central and peripheral primary autonomic failure. *Lancet* 340: 263–266.

Thomas PK (1992) Autonomic involvement in inherited neuropathies. *Clinical Autonomic Research* 2: 51–56.

Wallin BG (1992) Intraneural recordings of normal and abnormal sympathetic activity in man. In Bannister R & Mathias CJ (eds) *Autonomic Failure: A Textbook of Clinical Disorders of the Autonomic Nervous System* 3rd edn, pp 359–377. Oxford: Oxford Medical Publications.

Wieling W (1992) Non-invasive continuous recording of heart rate and blood pressure in the evaluation of neurocardiovascular control. In Bannister R & Mathias CJ (eds) *Autonomic Failure: A Textbook of Clinical Disorders of the Autonomic Nervous System* 3rd edn, pp 291–311. Oxford: Oxford Medical Publications.

Williams TDM, Lightman SL & Bannister R (1985) Vasopressin secretion in progressive autonomic failure: evidence for defective afferent cardiovascular pathways. *Journal of Neurology, Neurosurgery and Psychiatry* **48:** 225–228.

Zerbe RL, Henry DP & Robertson GL (1983) Vasopressin response to orthostatic hypotension: etiologic and clinical implications. *American Journal of Medicine* **74:** 265–271.

Zoukos Y, Thomaides T, Pavitt DV et al (1992) Up-regulation of β-adrenoceptors on circulating mononuclear cells after reduction of central sympathetic outflow by clonidine in normal subjects. *Clinical Autonomic Research* **2:** 165–170.

9

Imaging of catecholamine-secreting tumours: uses of MIBG in diagnosis and treatment

BRAHM SHAPIRO

Metaiodobenzylguanidine (MIBG), which was introduced into clinical practice over 10 years ago (Sisson et al, 1981), is now widely employed for the routine diagnostic localization of phaeochromocytomas and neuroblastomas (McEwan et al, 1985; Shapiro and Sisson, 1988). When administered in large doses, it has shown some promise as a therapeutic radiopharmaceutical (Sisson et al, 1984b; Hoefnagel, 1991; Shapiro, 1992). MIBG is a good example of a rational radiopharmaceutical design which exploits a physiological mechanism present primarily in the tissues from which the tumours in question derive, and a tracer which undergoes limited metabolism or loss of the radiolabel.

HISTORICAL BACKGROUND

The development of MIBG represents the culmination of a prolonged search at the University of Michigan for a sympathomedullary-avid radiopharmaceutical which began with studies of carbon-14 (^{14}C) labelled catecholamines and catecholamine precursors in animals in 1967 and subsequently in human neuroblastoma and phaeochromocytoma (Morales et al, 1967, McEwan et al, 1985). This led to the investigation of γ-ray emitting labels on compounds including iododopamine, bretylium and a large number of aralkylguanidines (Korn et al, 1977). Of the latter, iodobenzylguanidine had the best adrenal medulla to blood and liver ratios and was able to depict the canine and primate adrenal medulla and cardiac sympathetic innervation in vivo (Wieland et al, 1979; McEwan et al, 1985). Of the three isomers of iodobenzylguanidine, the meta-isomer is least susceptible to in vivo deiodination and iodine-131 (^{131}I) labelled MIBG was successfully used by Sisson et al (1981) to locate human phaeochromocytomas.

PHARMACOLOGICAL PRINCIPLES

Knowledge of the pharmacology of MIBG is derived from a number of sources, including in vitro studies using isolated cells and cultures of bovine adrenal medulla, human and animal phaeochromocytoma and neuro-blastoma cell lines, biodistribution and pharmacological intervention studies in animals, and pharmacological interventions in humans. The current model of MIBG action is one of so-called 'type I', specific, high affinity, energy- and sodium-dependent uptake by the peripheral sympathetic autonomic nerves and the adrenal medulla and tumours derived from these structures (Jacques et al, 1984; Tobes et al, 1985). In the adrenal medulla and phaeochromo-cytomas (but probably not neuroblastomas), a significant fraction of the

Table 1. Drugs which may potentially reduce MIBG uptake. Modified from Khafagi et al (1989).

Drugs	Mechanism
KNOWN	
Tricyclic antidepressants Amitriptyline and derivatives Imipramine and derivatives Others	Uptake 1 inhibition

Sympathomimetics
Phenylephrine, phenylpropanolamine,
    pseudoephedrine, ephedrine
	Depletion of storage vesicle contents
	(These drugs occur in numerous non-prescription
	    decongestants and 'diet aids'—their use should
	    be ruled out)

Cocaine	Uptake 1 inhibition
Antihypertensive/cardiovascular Labetalol Reserpine	 Uptake 1 inhibition Depletion of storage vesicle contents Inhibition of vesicle active transport

Calcium-channel blockers	Uncertain
	(May also enhance retention of previously stored
	    MIBG by blocking calcium-mediated release
	    from vesicles)

EXPECTED	
Antihypertensive/cardiovascular Adrenergic neurone blockers Bethanidine, debrisoquine, bretylium, guanethidine	 Depletion of storage vesicle contents Competition for transport into vesicles
'Atypical' antidepressants Maprotiline Trazodone	Uptake 1 inhibition
Antipsychotics ('major tranquillizers') Phenothiazines* Thioxanthines Butyrophenones	Uptake 1 inhibition
Sympathomimetics Amphetamine and related compounds β-Sympathomimetics† Dobutamine Dopamine Metaraminol	Depletion of storage vesicle contents

* Frequently also used as antiemetic/antipruritic agents.
† Systemic use. Effect unlikely with aerosol administration in conventional doses.

MIBG appears to enter the intravesicular storage compartment (Guilloteau et al, 1984; Gasnier et al, 1986). In all tissues, including those lacking the specific type I uptake, there is some non-specific uptake which is diffusional and non-energy-dependent; this contributes to the general background activity, but tissue retention is transient and diminishes over time more rapidly than that in tissues with specific uptake and storage. This permits the visualization of phaeochromocytomas, neuroblastomas, cardiac and salivary gland sympathetic innervation and, in some cases, the normal adrenal medulla (Nakajo et al, 1983, 1984b; Sisson et al, 1987). Because of the mechanisms on which MIBG imaging is dependent, a number of drugs may interfere with the procedure and must be avoided (Khafagi et al, 1989; Petry and Shapiro, 1989) (see Tables 1 and 2).

Table 2. Commonly used drugs without obvious effect on MIBG uptake. Modified from Khafagi et al (1989).

Antihypertensive/cardiovascular
α-Adrenergic blockers (clonidine, phenoxybenzamine, phentolamine, prazosin)
α-Methyldopa†
Angiotensin converting enzyme inhibitors (captopril, enalapril)
β-Adrenergic blockers (except labetalol)
Digitalis glycosides
Diuretics

Analgesics
Major (morphine and other opioids)
Minor (aspirin, paracetamol [acetaminophen *USP*])*

Hypnotics, minor tranquillizers

α-Methylparatyrosine†

* Often combined with sympathomimetic agents in non-prescription 'cold remedies', use of which should be specifically ruled out.
† Will falsely elevate catecholamine and metabolite levels in fluorimetric assays.

Within 24 h, 55% of the injected radioactivity is excreted in the urine, rising to 90% by 4 days; in renal failure, clearance is markedly reduced (Mangner et al, 1986; Tobes et al, 1989). Most radioactivity is excreted as unchanged MIBG, with 2–16% in the form of free iodide, metaiodobenzoic acid and 4-hydroxy-3-iodobenzylguanidine (Mangner et al, 1986). A small fraction of activity (<5%) appears in the faeces (Geatti et al, 1988). The prominent hepatic uptake appears to be due to metabolism and not type I uptake.

Radiolabels

The most widely used radioisotope of iodine used to label MIBG is ^{131}I, which has suboptimal imaging characteristics and high radiation dosimetry that limits the dose to 0.5–1.0 mCi in adults (Swanson et al, 1981; Petry and Shapiro, 1989). The 8-day half-life permits a shelf life of up to 2 weeks. A more expensive but superior alternative is ^{123}I with a high γ-ray flux well suited to modern instrumentation and with few particulate emissions;

10 mCi can be administered with similar radiation dosimetry to 0.5 mCi
^{131}I-MIBG, and thus ^{123}I-MIBG is enjoying increasingly wide usage (Lynn
et al, 1984). Preparations should use ^{123}I which is free of ^{125}I or [124]I contamination, which increase dosimetry and degrade image quality (Swanson et al,
1981). For the experimental radiotherapy of the bone marrow micro-
metastases of neuroblastoma, the non-penetrating low energy Auger
electrons of ^{125}I may offer advantages (Sisson et al, 1990). The various
characteristics of different radiolabels for MIBG are presented in Table 3.

Table 3. Characteristics of various radiolabels for MIBG.

	^{131}I-MIBG	^{123}I-MIBG*	^{125}I-MIBG
Main photon energy (utility for imaging)	364 KeV (suboptimal)	159 KeV (optimal)	25–30 KeV (unsuitable)
Particulate emissions	Many moderate energy β	Few particles	Low energy Auger electrons
Half-life	8 days	13 h	60 days
Relative costs	Low	High	High
Uses (usual doses)	Diagnosis (0.5–1.0 mCi) Radiotherapy (100–300 mCi)	Diagnosis (3–10 mCi)	Radiotherapy (300–800 mCi)
Adult dosimetry (rad/mCi)			
Adrenals	4.80	0.14	8.4
Bladder	2.80	0.24	0.54
Liver	0.44	0.04	0.09
Ovaries	1.18	0.07	0.22
Red marrow	0.74	0.06	0.24
Spleen	1.60	0.11	0.28
Testis	0.70	0.04	0.13
Thyroid†	34.00	2.1	3.7
Whole body	0.70	0.04	0.16

* Pure ^{123}I with no [124]I or ^{125}I contamination.
† Radiation dose may be decreased to 1–3% by iodide administration.

Imaging protocols

No medical imaging procedure should be performed until the history,
physical examination and biochemical evaluation support the diagnosis of
phaeochromocytoma or neuroblastoma with a reasonable level of certainty
(a pretest probability of at least 5–10%) (Bravo and Gifford, 1984; Shapiro
and Fig, 1989; Young et al, 1989; Stein and Black, 1990).

The thyroidal uptake of free radioiodine liberated by in vivo deiodination
may be minimized by the administration of iodides (Lugol's solution three
drops t.i.d. or saturated solution of potassium iodide one drop t.i.d.—begun
1 day before and continued for 1 week after ^{131}I-MIBG) or thyroxine and
perchlorate (Petry and Shapiro, 1989). The administration of potentially
interfering drugs must be excluded, and, if present, they must be withdrawn
(Khafagi et al, 1989).

MIBG is administered by slow intravenous injection of 0.5–1.0 mCi ^{131}I-MIBG or 3–10 mCi ^{123}I-MIBG in adults and with proportional adjustment to weight or body surface area in children. Multiple overlapping images are obtained from the skull to the upper femurs in adults and extended to the feet in children. Imaging is performed at 1 and 2 days with ^{123}I-MIBG and 1, 2 and 3 days with ^{131}I-MIBG (Shapiro and Sisson, 1988). Both digital computer-stored and analogue images are obtained; ^{123}I-MIBG also permits single photon emission computed tomography (SPECT) in trans-axial, coronal and parasagittal planes (Lynn et al, 1984). For potential MIBG therapy candidates, additional dosimetric studies of whole body and blood tracer clearance and quantification of tumour uptake using conjugate imaging are performed over 5–7 days (Shulkin et al, 1988). The abnormal foci of MIBG uptake may be better located by using radioactive surface markers and the simultaneous scintigraphic depiction of other structures, including: the kidneys and bladder, using technetium-99m (^{99m}Tc) labelled diethylenetriaminepentaacetic acid (DTPA); the skeleton, using ^{99m}Tc-methylenediphosphonate; the blood pool, using ^{99m}Tc-labelled red blood cells; the liver and spleen, using ^{99m}Tc-sulphur colloid; or the myocardium, using thallium-201 (Shapiro et al, 1984a,b; Shapiro and Sisson, 1988). Anatomical imaging modalities (e.g. computed tomography, magnetic resonance imaging or angiography) can also be directed to sites of abnormal

Table 4. Scintigraphic biodistribution of MIBG.

(a) Normal distribution

Usually present	Commonly present	Unusually present
Salivary glands	Adrenal medulla*	Lacrimal glands*
Nasopharynx	Colon	Lungs
Heart	Thyroid (if blockade inadequate)	Brain
Liver		Menstruating uterus
Bladder		Kidney (if obstructed or dilated)

(b) Decreased tracer in normal structures

Common	Uncommon
Interfering drugs	Autonomic neuropathy
High circulating catecholamine levels	Denervation (e.g. heart transplant or Horner's
Intense uptake by neoplasm	syndrome)
Widespread neoplasm	

(c) Focal abnormal increased tracer uptake

Common	Uncommon	Rare
Phaeochromocytoma	Carcinoid	Retinoblastoma
Neuroblastoma	Medullary thyroid carcinoma	Merkel tumour
Paraganglioma	Ganglioneuroma	Islet cell tumour
		Parathyroid adenoma

* Rarely depicted by ^{131}I-MIBG, more often depicted by ^{123}I-MIBG.
Data from Nakajo et al (1983), Nakajo et al (1984a,b), Parisi et al (1992) and Von Moll et al (1987).

MIBG uptake to demonstrate the detailed anatomical relationship and vascular anatomy for the planning of curative resection (Francis et al, 1983; Shapiro et al, 1984a).

Normal biodistribution of MIBG

MIBG is taken up by the adrenergic sympathetic innervation of some organs (e.g. heart, salivary glands, adrenal medulla), sites of metabolism (e.g. liver or thyroid) or excretion (e.g. kidney, bladder, gut) (Nakajo et al, 1983; Shulkin et al, 1987; Parisi et al, 1992) (see Table 4).

THE IMAGING OF PHAEOCHROMOCYTOMAS

The management of phaeochromocytoma requires that all tumour deposits be extirpated and recognition of those patients in whom this is not possible (Bravo and Gifford, 1984; Shapiro and Fig, 1989). The majority of medical imaging procedures used for these purposes depict the non-specific anatomical features of the lesion and will not distinguish between phaeo-chromocytomas and other tumours.

Relatively insensitive techniques such as plane radiography, intravenous urography and retroperitoneal air insufflation must be considered obsolete. The chest X-ray often depicts lung metastases and posterior mediastinal tumours. Bone radiography and bone scintigraphy may reveal skeletal metastases (Shapiro et al, 1984b). Ultrasound may reveal intra-adrenal lesions in thin patients and the more obvious liver metastases (Bowerman et al, 1981).

Angiography is invasive and the radiographic contrast may provoke phaeochromocytoma crisis. This technique now has limited utility in tumour location. In specific cases it may be useful to aid in the planning of resection of some extra-adrenal lesions (Rossi et al, 1968; Smith et al, 1987).

Venography with venous sampling of catecholamine levels permits the functional location of phaeochromocytomas but is invasive, technically demanding, particularly in previously operated patients, and not without risk of contrast-induced crises or tumour infarction or rupture (Harrison et al, 1967; Jones et al, 1979).

X-ray computed tomography (CT) using modern instrumentation and techniques will depict almost all intra-adrenal lesions, but is less accurate for smaller extra-adrenal and metastatic tumours. It is not well suited to screen-ing the entire body for occult tumours, and it may fail in very thin patients or children without adequate retroperitoneal fat and in postoperative patients, particularly those with metallic surgical clips (Laursen and Damgaard-Pederson, 1984; Moulton and Moulton, 1988).

Magnetic resonance imaging (MRI) may have some advantages over CT, including the absence of ionizing radiation or the need for iodinated contrast, reconstruction of images in any plane, and the depiction of vascular structures due to the absence of signal from flowing blood (Fink et al, 1985; Quint et al, 1987). Phaeochromocytomas are intensely bright on

T2-weighted images but this is not a totally specific characteristic. MRI is especially well suited to lesions of the spine and mediastinum, but offers limited advantages in the abdomen (Quint et al, 1987; Schmedtje et al, 1987).

Diagnostic results of MIBG scintigraphy in phaeochromocytoma and paraganglioma

Multiple investigators have shown that MIBG scintigraphy can safely and accurately depict the location of the vast majority of phaeochromocytomas and paragangliomas in a single, non-invasive procedure (McEwan et al, 1985; Shapiro and Sisson, 1988; Gross and Shapiro, 1989) (Table 5). This

Table 5. Summary of results of ^{131}I-MIBG scintigraphy for suspected phaeochromocytoma.

Reference	No. of patients	Sensitivity (%)	Specificity (%)	Prevalence (%)
Shapiro and Sisson, 1988	927	88	99	20
Hanson et al, 1991	64	88	88	47
Anonymous, 1983 (combined German series)	191	88	99	34
Baulieu et al, 1984	99	91	96	46
Ackery et al, 1986	46	88	95	52
Swenson et al, 1985	42	79	96	45
Chatal and Charbonnel, 1985	27	89	94	33

includes: benign, sporadic, intra-adrenal (Ackery et al, 1984; Shapiro et al, 1984b, 1985) (see Figure 1) and extra-adrenal lesions (Chatal and Charbonnel, 1985; Shapiro et al, 1985; Hanson et al, 1992) (cervical, thoracic, abdominal and pelvic); malignant metastases (Shapiro et al, 1984b) (see Figure 2); and familial lesions (Valk et al, 1981; Kalff et al, 1982; Sisson et al, 1984a; Glowniak et al, 1985) (multiple endocrine neoplasia syndromes types IIA and IIB, neurofibromatosis, Von Hippel–Lindau

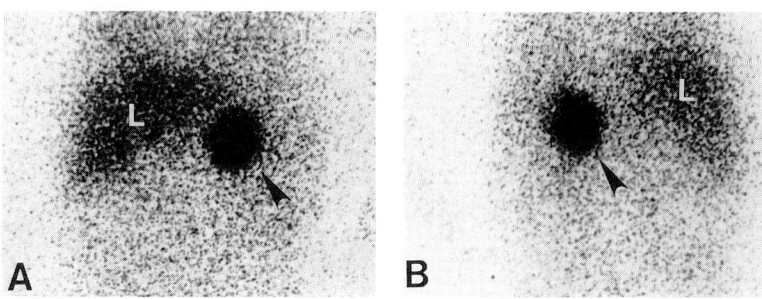

Figure 1. Anterior (A) and posterior (B) abdominal scintigrams performed 24 h after injection of 0.5 mCi ^{131}I-MIBG, demonstrating intense left adrenal tracer uptake in a phaeochromocytoma (arrow). L = normal liver uptake. The patient was a 57-year-old man with neurofibromatosis who presented with a hypertensive crisis and right-sided cerebral infarct during an elective hernia repair operation.

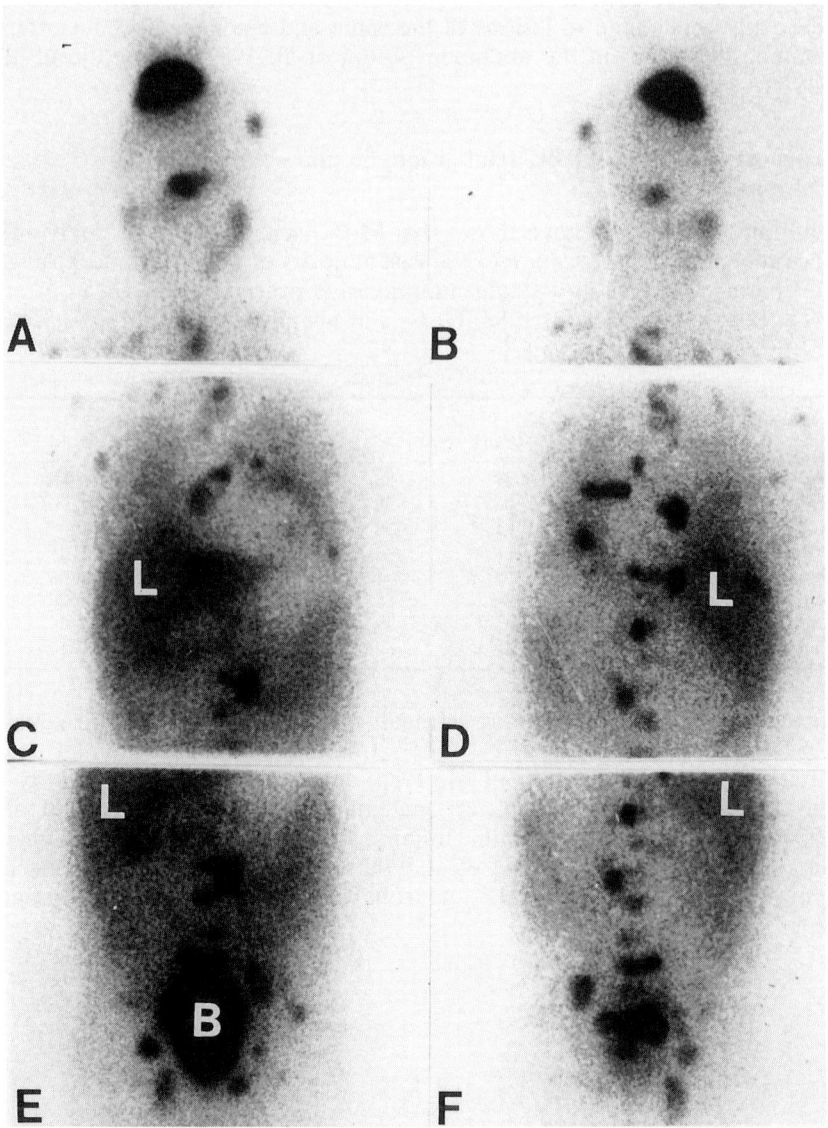

Figure 2. Anterior and posterior scintigrams performed 24 h after injection of 10 mCi ^{123}I-MIBG demonstrating multiple intense abnormal tracer uptake in phaeochromocytoma metastases in bone, lung and lymph nodes. A and B = head and neck; C and D = chest and abdomen; E and F = abdomen and pelvis. L = normal liver uptake; B = normal bladder excretion. The patient was a 36-year-old man who initially presented at age 10 with a malignant abdominal lesion. The patient currently has diabetes mellitus and polycythaemia in addition to labile hypertension and headaches. He has failed to respond to attempts at surgical resection, chemotherapy and ^{131}I-MIBG therapy (cumulative dose 606 mCi).

disease, and isolated familial phaeochromocytoma). The technique is also efficacious for childhood phaeochromocytomas (Khafagi et al, 1991). It is especially useful in patients with suspected recurrent, residual or metastatic disease in whom previous surgery renders anatomical imaging techniques inaccurate due to metallic clips, artefacts and disruption of normal tissue planes (Shapiro et al, 1984b; Swenson et al, 1985). MIBG scintigraphy can distinguish phaeochromocytoma (positive) from neurofibroma (negative) in neurofibromatosis, phaeochromocytoma (positive) from other tumours such as hypernephroma (negative) in Von Hippel–Lindau disease, and phaeochromocytoma (positive) from gastric leiomyosarcoma or pulmonary hamartoma (negative) in Carney's syndrome.

The overall sensitivity of ^{131}I-MIBG scintigraphy is in the range 80–90% (see Table 5). Experience with ^{123}I-MIBG is as yet smaller, but the higher photon flux and better image quality probably makes it somewhat more sensitive (Lynn et al, 1984; Gross and Shapiro, 1989).

Suggested approaches to the imaging of phaeochromocytomas

Where available, MIBG scintigraphy permits the screening of the entire body in a single, safe, sensitive and specific procedure, and we advise this as the initial medical imaging procedure of choice (Shapiro and Sisson, 1988; Shapiro and Fig, 1989). If positive, MIBG-directed anatomical studies may be obtained to establish anatomical relationships and vascular anatomy. If MIBG scintigraphy is suspected of being falsely negative, CT, MRI and venous sampling may then be used for tumour location (Francis et al, 1983).

An alternative approach is CT of the adrenal region, which should reveal 80% of lesions, including almost all intra-adrenal lesions. However, even if CT locates a tumour, the mass lesion may not be due to a phaeochromocytoma and in up to 10% of patients there may be occult metastatic or second primary tumours. Thus, MIBG scintigraphy may still be useful when an anatomical imaging modality has located a tumour (Chatal and Charbonnel, 1985; Shapiro and Fig, 1989).

THE IMAGING OF NEUROBLASTOMAS

Neuroblastoma is a relatively common and highly lethal childhood tumour, the prognosis and management of which are highly dependent on tumour staging (Shapiro and Sisson, 1988). Primary tumours and liver or lymph node metastases are usually well depicted by CT, MRI or ultrasound, but these techniques do not distinguish neuroblastoma from other childhood tumours. The presence of metastases results in a very poor prognosis. The most common sites for metastases are bone and bone marrow. Radiographic skeletal survey is insensitive and has been replaced by the ^{99m}Tc-methylene-diphosphonate bone scan, but even this is imperfect for detecting early marrow involvement. MRI is expensive and bone marrow biopsy is invasive and may also give a false-negative result unless performed at multiple sites.

Diagnostic results of MIBG scintigraphy in neuroblastoma

MIBG scintigraphy has been shown to have a high sensitivity and specificity for neuroblastoma (Hoefnagel et al, 1985; Lumbroso et al, 1985; Heyman and Evans, 1986; Feine et al, 1987) (Table 6). Scintigraphy may occasionally

Table 6. Summary of results of MIBG scintigraphy in neuroblastoma.

Reference	No. of patients	Sensitivity (%)	Specificity (%)	Prevalence (%)
Hoefnagel et al, 1992*	138	96	100	88
Shapiro and Sisson, 1988	36	85	100	92
Lumbroso et al, 1985	24	70	100	83
Munkner, 1985	16	75	—	100
Heyman and Evans, 1986	19	57	60	74
Feine et al, 1984	5	100	100	80

* C. Hoefnagel, May 1992, personal communication.

aid in the diagnosis of the disease prior to histological confirmation or in cases where histology is non-diagnostic (MIBG is only taken up by neuroblastoma and not by other small, round cell tumours of childhood). The main uses of MIBG are in the staging of neuroblastoma at presentation and for monitoring the extent of the disease during and following therapy (see Figure 3). MIBG scintigraphy may often provide data on disease extent in a single non-invasive procedure which is otherwise available only from combinations of other modalities (e.g. CT, ultrasound, bone scan) (Shapiro and Sisson, 1988). In a small number of cases, MIBG may depict disease not demonstrable by any other procedure, with important consequences for staging and prognosis.

Neuroendocrine tumours other than neuroblastoma and phaeochromocytoma may also be depicted by MIBG scintigraphy (Hoefnagel et al, 1985; Von Moll et al, 1987).

MIBG SCINTIGRAPHY AS AN IN VIVO PROBE OF AUTONOMIC INNERVATION

The uptake of MIBG by the salivary glands and heart is dependent on the integrity of the adrenergic sympathetic innervation of these organs (Nakajo et al, 1984b; Sisson et al, 1987; Dae et al, 1989). Thus, decreased MIBG uptake has been demonstrated in the surgical denervation of Horner's syndrome (Nakajo et al, 1984b) (Figure 4) and cardiac transplantation, experimental epicardial phenol patch, ischaemic interruption due to myocardial infarction (Dae et al, 1989; Stanton et al, 1989), and autonomic neuropathy due to diabetes mellitus, the Shy–Drager syndrome or idiopathic aetiologies (Sisson et al, 1987).

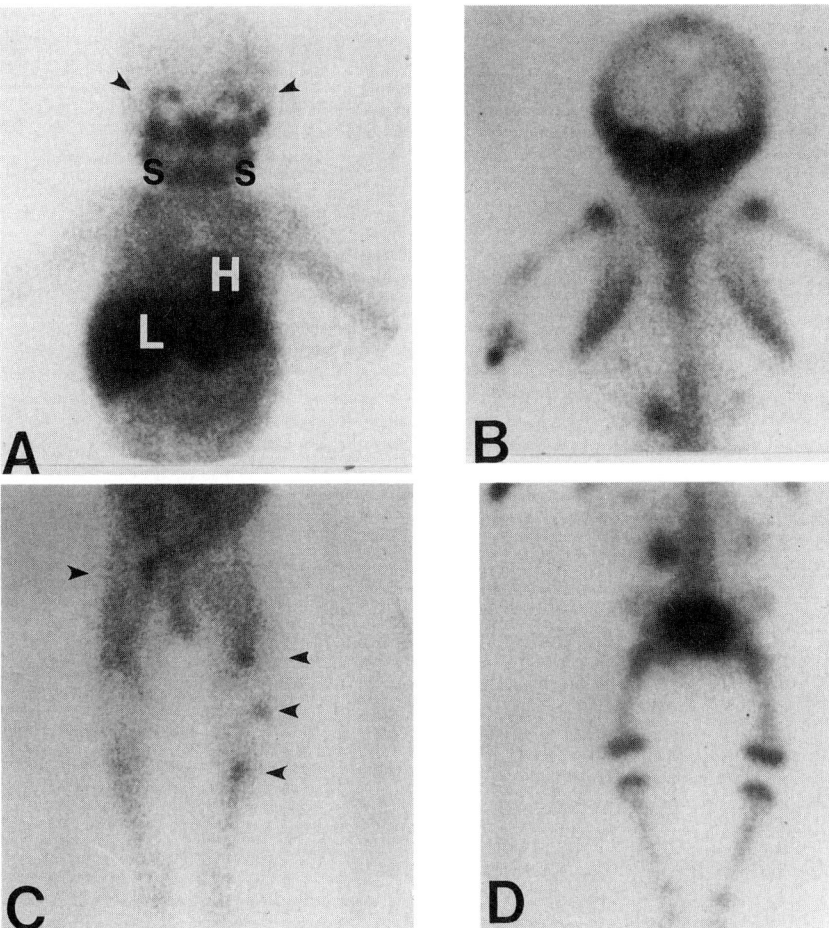

Figure 3. Anterior ^{123}I-MIBG (A and C) and ^{99m}Tc-methylenediphosphonate (B and D) scintigrams demonstrating intense abnormal MIBG uptake in periorbital, femoral and tibial deposits of neuroblastoma (arrows). Note the bone scan of the legs is only subtly abnormal. L = normal liver uptake; H = normal heart uptake; S = normal salivary gland uptake. The patient was a 3½-year-old boy with stage IV neuroblastoma arising from a paraspinous thoracic primary tumour which has been resected.

The intensity of cardiac MIBG uptake is reduced in the presence of the hypercatecholaminaemia of phaeochromocytoma, probably due to dilution of the tracer and downregulation of cellular uptake processes (Nakajo et al, 1984a). MIBG scintigraphy, particularly with ^{123}I-MIBG, provides an attractive experimental in vivo probe for the study of catecholamine uptake and storage within peripheral, presynaptic adrenergic neurones (Sisson et al, 1987).

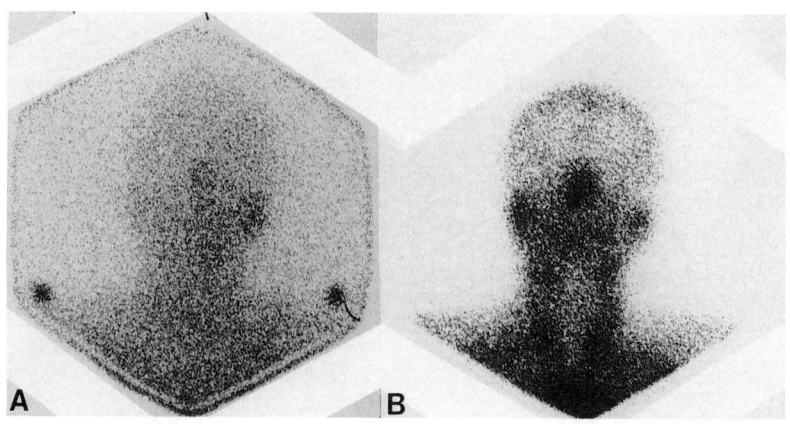

Figure 4. Anterior head and neck images 24 h after 0.5 mCi ^{131}I-MIBG (A) and 20 min after 5.0 mCi ^{99m}Tc-O$_4$ (B) in a patient with right-sided Horner's syndrome showing decreased ^{131}I-MIBG uptake into the sympathetic innervation of the parotid gland which retains normal glandular uptake of ^{99m}Tc-O$_4$. From Nakajo et al (1984b), with permission.

RADIOPHARMACEUTICAL THERAPY OF PHAEOCHROMOCYTOMA AND NEUROBLASTOMA USING ^{131}I- OR ^{125}I-MIBG

The intense and prolonged uptake and retention of tracer doses of MIBG by many malignant or otherwise unresectable phaeochromocytomas and advanced neuroblastomas which have resisted conventional therapies provided the rationale for the therapeutic use of large doses of MIBG (Sisson et al, 1984b; Hoefnagel et al, 1985). This general approach is well established for the use of ^{131}I-iodide in thyroid cancer. The criteria for phaeochromocytoma and neuroblastoma patient selection are listed in Table 7. After whole-body, blood and tumour radiation dosimetric determinations performed over 5–7 days using a tracer dose of ^{131}I-MIBG (Shulkin et al, 1988; Sisson et al, 1988), a therapeutic dose of high specific activity (33–50 Ci/mg) ^{131}I-MIBG is infused over 90 min; blood pressure and ECG

Table 7. University of Michigan selection criteria for ^{131}I-MIBG therapy.

	Phaeochromocytoma	Neuroblastoma
Histological diagnosis	Yes	Yes
Tumour location	Metastatic	Recurrent or residual despite
	Primary but locally invasive or otherwise unresectable	standard therapy
Anticipated survival	12 months	3 months
MIBG uptake	All known tumour sites	All known tumour sites
Dosimetric studies	Whole body	Whole body
	Tumour (where possible)	Tumour (where possible)
Informed consent	Yes	Parent or guardian if < 18 years

are monitored continuously for the 90 min infusion, then measured at frequent intervals for 24 hours (Hutchinson et al, 1992; Shapiro et al, 1992). The patient remains in a restricted, specially prepared ward until the body burden of ^{131}I is below 30 mCi, at which time the distribution of the therapy dose is confirmed by scintigraphy and the patient is discharged to a follow-up protocol which examines bone marrow, liver, kidney, thyroid, adreno-cortical and autonomic neuronal function and tumour response. Thyroidal blockade is continued for a total of at least 4 weeks.

Doses were initially limited to approximately 100 mCi due to difficulties with synthesis (Sisson et al, 1984b). Currently large quantities are readily prepared, and doses of 200–300 mCi are administered to adults and doses calculated to deliver 100–200 cGY whole-body radiation to children (Hutchinson et al, 1992; Shapiro et al, 1992). Calculated tumour doses have ranged from 2550–34 000 cGy per dose (19–162 cGy/mCi). Therapy has been repeated at various intervals and cumulative doses of up to 900 mCi (Shapiro, 1992; Shapiro et al, 1992) or even 2300 mCi (Krempf et al, 1991) have been administered.

Therapy with ^{131}I-MIBG results in no significant pharmacological toxicity, but mild to moderate acute radiation sickness results in anorexia, nausea and vomiting in some patients (Sisson et al, 1988; Shapiro et al, 1992). In adults, myelosuppression is not significant, but in children with neuroblastoma it may be severe and in a few patients has been permanent (Sisson et al, 1988; Shapiro et al, 1992). Prior bone marrow transplantation appears to sensitize patients to this complication (Sisson et al, 1988). A few patients have developed hypothyroidism despite iodide administration to block thyroid uptake of free [131]I. No significant injury to liver, kidney, adrenal cortex or autonomic nerves has been observed (Sisson et al, 1988).

Multiple investigators have demonstrated significant responses to ^{131}I-MIBG (Shapiro, 1992) (Table 8). In phaeochromocytoma this may be in the form of tumour shrinkage and/or reduced catecholamine secretion; results are similar to those of chemotherapy (Averbuch et al, 1988). Complete responses are rare. Significant partial responses are more frequent, but many are not durable and may last from weeks to many months or even years (Shapiro, 1992; Hutchinson et al, 1992; Shapiro et al, 1992).

Table 8. Summary of pooled data on therapeutic responses to ^{131}I-MIBG reported at the 1991 Rome Symposium. From Shapiro (1992)*, with permission.

	Phaeochromocytoma	Neuroblastoma	Carcinoid	Medullary thyroid cancer
Complete response	3	13	0	1
Partial response	34	60	10	—
Stable disease (including mixed and minimal responses)	33	74	28	—
Progressive disease	27	75	11	—
Non-evaluable	10	33	2	—
Total	107	255	51	18

* Data provided by L. Troncone.

MIBG therapy remains a promising but still experimental modality and much needs to be learned about patient selection, radiation dosimetry, the size and frequency of therapeutic doses, and optimal integration with other therapies (e.g. chemotherapy, teleradiotherapy and surgery) (Shapiro, 1992). The relatively high energy β-particles of ^{131}I can penetrate several millimetres of tissue and thus are not well suited to treating micro-metastases, which in neuroblastoma are frequently present in the bone marrow and which may be responsible for relapse (Sisson et al, 1990). The low energy, non-penetrating Auger electrons of ^{125}I may be better suited to these lesions (Sisson et al, 1990). Preliminary therapies have been conducted with ^{125}I-MIBG in doses in excess of 800 mCi (Sisson et al, 1990). The problems related to radiochemical synthesis and radiation protection have been solved, but it is too early to determine if ^{125}I-MIBG is superior to ^{131}I-MIBG. In the future, both of these radiopharmaceuticals may be used in combination.

SUMMARY

MIBG radiolabelled with ^{131}I or ^{123}I is a radiopharmaceutical which is concentrated in neuroendocrine tumours, particularly phaeochromocytomas and neuroblastomas. This permits non-invasive whole-body scintigraphic screening for benign and malignant, familial and sporadic, intra-adrenal and extra-adrenal phaeochromocytomas and primary and metastatic neuroblastomas, with high sensitivity (85–90%) and specificity (> 95%). MIBG is also concentrated in presynaptic terminals of adrenergic, autonomically innervated organs such as the heart, and may be used as a non-invasive in vivo probe to study this system. Large doses of ^{131}I-MIBG and ^{125}I-MIBG have been used experimentally to selectively deliver therapeutic doses of radiotherapy to malignant phaeochromocytomas and refractory advanced neuroblastomas.

Acknowledgements

The author owes much to Barbara Burton for typing and editing the manuscript and Shirley Zempel for data management. This work was supported by the following grants: FDA 1RO1 FD01257, NCI15-PO1 CA42768, NCI5T32 CA 09015 and MO1 RR00042. Synthesis of diagnostic and therapeutic MIBG was performed at the Phoenix Memorial Laboratory at the University of Michigan.

REFERENCES

Ackery DM, Tippett PA, Condon BR et al (1986) New approach to the localization of phaeochromocytoma: Imaging with iodine-131-meta-iodobenzylguanidine. *British Medical Journal* **288**: 1587–1591.
Anonymous (1983) Clinical value of adrenomedullary scintigraphy with ^{131}I-MIBG. *Nuclear Compact* **14**: 318–320.
Averbuch SD, Steakley CS, Young RC et al (1988) Malignant phaeochromocytoma: Effective treatment with a combination of cyclophosphamide, vincristine, and dacarbazine. *Annals of Internal Medicine* **109**: 267–273.

Baulieu JL, Guilloteau D, Chambon C et al (1984) Meta-iodobenzylguanidine (MIBG) scintigraphy: A one year experience. *Journal of Nuclear Medicine* **25**: 111(abstract).

Bowerman RA, Silver TM, Jaffe MJ et al (1981) Sonography of adrenal phaeochromocytoma. *American Journal of Roentgenology* **137**: 1227–1231.

Bravo EL & Gifford RW (1984) Phaeochromocytoma: Diagnosis, localisation and management. *New England Journal of Medicine* **311**: 1298–1303.

Chatal JF & Charbonnel B (1985) Comparison of iodobenzylguanidine imaging with computed tomography in locating phaeochromocytoma. *Journal of Clinical Endocrinology and Metabolism* **61**: 769–772.

Dae MW, O'Connell JW, Botvinick EH et al (1989) Scintigraphic assessment of regional cardiac adrenergic innervation. *Circulation* **79**: 634–644.

Feine U, Muler-Schauenburg W, Treuner J & Klingebiel TH (1984) Meta-iodobenzylguanidine (MIBG) labeled with I-123/I-131 in neuroblastoma. *Medical and Pediatric Oncology* **15**: 181–187.

Fink IJ, Reining JW, Dwyer AJ et al (1985) MR imaging of phaeochromocytomas. *Journal of Computer Assisted Tomography* **9**: 454–458.

Francis IR, Glazer G, Shapiro B et al (1983) Complementary roles of CT scanning and ^{131}I-MIBG scintigraphy in the diagnosis of phaeochromocytoma. *American Journal of Roentgenology* **141**: 719–725.

Gasnier B, Rosin MP, Scherman D et al (1986) Uptake of meta-iodobenzylguanidine by bovine chromaffin granule membranes. *Molecular Pharmacology* **29**: 275–280.

Geatti O, Shapiro B, Shulkin B, Hutchinson R & Sisson JC (1988) Gastrointestinal iodine-131-meta-iodobenzylguanidine activity. *American Journal of Physiologic Imaging* **3**: 189–191.

Glowniak JV, Shapiro B, Sisson JC et al (1985) Familial extra-adrenal phaeochromocytoma: A new syndrome. *Archives of Internal Medicine* **145**: 257–261.

Gross MD & Shapiro B (1989) Adrenal hypertension. *Seminars in Nuclear Medicine* **19**: 122–143.

Guilloteau D, Baulieu J-L, Huguet F et al (1984) Meta-iodobenzylguanidine adrenal medulla localization: Autoradiographic and pharmaceutical studies. *European Journal of Nuclear Medicine* **9**: 278–281.

Hanson MW, Feldman JM, Beam CA et al (1991) Iodine 131-labeled meta-iodobenzylguanidine scintigraphy and biochemical analyses in suspected phaeochromocytoma. *Archives of Internal Medicine* **151**: 1397–1402.

Harrison TS, Seaton RF & Cerney JC (1967) Localization of phaeochromocytoma by caval catheterization. *Archives of Surgery* **95**: 339–343.

Heyman S & Evans AE (1986) I-131-meta-iodobenzylguanidine (I-131-MIBG) in the diagnosis of neuroblastoma. *Journal of Nuclear Medicine* **27**: 931(abstract).

Hoefnagel CA (1991) Radionuclide therapy revisited. *European Journal of Nuclear Medicine* **18**: 408–431.

Hoefnagel CA, Dekraker J, Marcuse HR & Voute PA (1985) Detection and treatment of neural crest tumours using ^{131}I-MIBG. *European Journal of Nuclear Medicine* **11**: A73.

Hutchinson RJ, Sisson JC, Miser JS et al (1992) Long-term results of ^{131}I-metaiodobenzyl-guanidine treatment of refractory advanced neuroblastoma. *Journal of Nuclear Medicine* **36** (in press).

Jacques S Jr, Tobes MC, Sisson JC et al (1984) Comparison of the sodium dependence of uptake of meta-iodobenzylguanidine and norepinephrine into cultured bovine adreno-medullary cells. *Molecular Pharmacology* **26**: 539–546.

Jones DH, Allison DJ, Hamilton CA et al (1979) Selective venous sampling in the diagnosis and localization of phaeochromocytoma. *Clinical Endocrinology* **10**: 179–183.

Kalff V, Shapiro B, Lloyd R et al (1982) The spectrum of phaeochromocytoma in hypertensive patients with neurofibromatosis. *Archives of Internal Medicine* **142**: 2092–2098.

Khafagi FA, Shapiro B, Fig LM et al (1989) Labetalol reduces iodine-131-MIBG uptake by phaeochromocytoma and normal tissues. *Journal of Nuclear Medicine* **30**: 481–489.

Khafagi FA, Shapiro B, Fischer M et al (1991) Phaeochromocytoma and functioning para-ganglioma in childhood and adolescence: Role of iodine-131-metaiodobenzylguanidine. *European Journal of Nuclear Medicine* **18**: 191–198.

Korn N, Buswink A, Yu T et al (1977) A radioiodinated bretylium analog as a potential agent for scanning the adrenal medulla. *Journal of Nuclear Medicine* **18**: 87–89.

Krempf M, Lumbroso J, Mornex R et al (1991) Use of m-[131I]iodobenzylguanidine in the treatment of malignant phaeochromocytoma. *Journal of Clinical Endocrinology and Metabolism* **72:** 455–461.

Laursen K & Damgaard-Pederson K (1984) CT for phaeochromocytoma diagnosis. *Journal of Computer Assisted Tomography* **8:** 895–899.

Lumbroso J, Hartmann O, Lemerle J et al (1985) Scintigraphic detection of neuroblastoma using ^{131}I and ^{123}I labelled metaiodobenzylguanidine. *European Journal of Nuclear Medicine* **11:** A16(abstract 71).

Lynn MD, Shapiro B, Sisson JC et al (1984) Portrayal of phaeochromocytoma and normal human adrenal medulla by *m*-[I-123]-iodomethylguanidine: concise communication. *Journal of Nuclear Medicine* **25:** 436–440.

Mangner TJ, Tobes MC, Wieland DM et al (1986) Metabolism of meta-I-131-iodobenzylguanidine in patients with metastatic phaeochromocytoma: Concise communication. *Journal of Nuclear Medicine* **27:** 37–44.

McEwan AJ, Shapiro B, Sisson JC et al (1985) Radio-iodobenzylguanidine for the scintigraphic location and therapy of adrenergic tumours. *Seminars in Nuclear Medicine* **15:** 132–153.

Morales JO, Beierwaltes WH, Counsell RE & Meier DE (1967) The concentration of radioactivity from labeled epinephrine and its precursors in the dog adrenal medulla. *Journal of Nuclear Medicine* **8:** 800–809.

Moulton JS & Moulton JS (1988) CT of the adrenal glands. *Seminars in Roentgenology* **23:** 288–303.

Munkner T (1985) I-131 meta-iodobenzylguanidine scintigraphy of neuroblastomas. *Seminars in Nuclear Medicine* **15:** 154–160.

Nakajo M, Shapiro B, Copp J et al (1983) The normal and abnormal distribution of the adrenomedullary imaging agent *m*-[I-131]-iodobenzylguanidine (I-131-MIBG) in man: Evaluation by scintigraphy. *Journal of Nuclear Medicine* **24:** 672–682.

Nakajo M, Shapiro B, Glowniak J et al (1984a) Inverse relationship between cardiac accumulation of ^{131}I-MIBG and circulating catecholamines in suspected phaeochromocytoma. *Journal of Nuclear Medicine* **24:** 1127–1134.

Nakajo M, Shapiro B, Sisson JC et al (1984b) Salivary gland accumulation of meta-131-iodobenzylguanidine. *Journal of Nuclear Medicine* **25:** 2–6.

Parisi MT, Sandler EP & Hattner RS (1992) The biodistribution of meta-iodobenzylguanidine. *Seminars in ¡Nuclear Medicine* **22:** 46–48.

Petry NA & Shapiro B (1989) Radiopharmaceuticals for the endocrine system: Adrenomedullary imaging. In Swanson D, Chilton H & Thrall JH (eds) *Pharmaceuticals in Medical Imaging*, pp 368–393. New York: Macmillan.

Quint LE, Glazer GM, Francis IR et al (1987) MR imaging and in vitro relaxation time measurements in phaeochromocytoma and paraganglioma: A comparison with MIBG scintigraphy and CT. *Radiology* **165:** 89–93.

Rossi P, Young IS & Panke WF (1968) Techniques, usefulness, and hazards of arteriography of phaeochromocytoma: Review of 99 cases. *Journal of the American Medical Association* **205:** 547–553.

Schmedtje JF Jr, Sax S, Pool JE et al (1987) Localization of ectopic phaeochromocytomas by magnetic resonance imaging. *American Journal of Medicine* **83:** 770–772.

Shapiro B (1992) Summary, conclusions and future directions of ^{131}I-metaiodobenzylguanidine therapy in the treatment of neural crest tumours. *Journal of Nuclear Biology and Medicine* **36** (in press).

Shapiro B & Fig LM (1989) Management of phaeochromocytoma. *Endocrinology and Metabolism Clinics of North America* **18(2):** 443–481.

Shapiro B & Sisson JC (1988) Sympatho-adrenal imaging with radioiodinated meta-iodobenzylguanidine. In VanNostrand B & Baum S (eds) *Atlas of Nuclear Medicine*, pp 72–114. Philadelphia: Lippincott.

Shapiro B, Sisson JC, Kalff V et al (1984a) The location of middle mediastinal phaeochromocytoma. *Journal of Thoracic and Cardiovascular Surgery* **87:** 814–820.

Shapiro B, Sisson JC, Lloyd R et al (1984b) Malignant phaeochromocytoma: Clinical, biochemical and scintigraphic characterization. *Clinical Endocrinology* **20:** 189–203.

Shapiro B, Copp JE, Sisson JC et al (1985) Iodine-131-meta-iodobenzylguanidine for location of suspected phaeochromocytoma: Experience in 400 cases. *Journal of Nuclear Medicine* **26:** 576–585.

Shapiro B, Sisson JC, Beierwaltes WH et al (1992) Long term results of ^{131}I-MIBG therapy for malignant phaeochromocytoma. *Journal of Nuclear Biology and Medicine* **36** (in press).

Shulkin B, Shen S-W, Sisson JC et al (1987) Normal and abnormal ^{131}I-meta-iodobenzylguanidine scintigraphy of the extremities. *Journal of Nuclear Medicine* **28**: 315–318.

Shulkin B, Sisson JC, Koral KF et al (1988) Conjugate view gamma camera method for estimating tumour uptake of iodine-131 metaiodobenzylguanidine. *Journal of Nuclear Medicine* **29**: 542–548.

Sisson JC, Frager MS, Valk TW et al (1981) Scintigraphic localization of phaeochromocytoma. *New England Journal of Medicine* **305**: 12–17.

Sisson JC, Shapiro B & Beierwaltes WH (1984a) Scintigraphy with I-131-MIBG as an aid to the treatment of phaeochromocytomas in patients with the MEN-2 syndromes. *Henry Ford Hospital Medical Journal* **32**: 254–261.

Sisson JC, Shapiro B & Beierwaltes WH (1984b) Radiopharmaceutical treatment of malignant phaeochromocytoma. *Journal of Nuclear Medicine* **25**: 197–206.

Sisson JC, Shapiro B, Meyers L et al (1987) Metaiodobenzylguanidine to map scintigraphically the adrenergic nervous system in man. *Journal of Nuclear Medicine* **28**: 1625–1636.

Sisson JC, Hutchinson RJ, Carey JE et al (1988) Toxicity from treatment of neuroblastoma with ^{131}I meta-iodobenzylguanidine. *European Journal of Nuclear Medicine* **14**: 337–340.

Sisson JC, Hutchinson RJ, Shapiro B et al (1990) Iodine-125-MIBG to treat neuroblastoma: preliminary report. *Journal of Nuclear Medicine* **31**: 1479–1485.

Smith EJ, McPherson GAD & Lynn J (1987) Inferior vena cava involvement by a phaeochromocytoma. *British Journal of Surgery* **74**: 597.

Stanton MS, Tuli MM, Radtke NL et al (1989) Regional sympathetic denervation after myocardial infarction in humans detected noninvasively using I-123 metaiodobenzylguanidine. *Journal of the American College of Cardiology* **14**: 1519–1529.

Stein PP & Black HP (1990) A simplified diagnostic approach to phaeochromocytoma: A review of the literature and report of one institution's experience. *Medicine* **70**: 46–66.

Swanson DP, Carey JE, Brown LE et al (1981) Human absorbed dose calculations for iodine-131 and iodine-123 labeled MIBG: A potential myocardial and adrenal medulla imaging agent. In *Proceeding of the Third International Radiopharmaceutical Dosimetry Symposium Health and Human Services Publications*, pp 213–224. Rockville: FDA 81-8166.

Swenson SJ, Brown MI, Sheps SG et al (1985) Use of ^{131}I-MIBG scintigraphy in the evolution of suspected phaeochromocytoma. *Mayo Clinic Proceedings* **60**: 299–304.

Tobes MC, Jacques S, Wieland DM et al (1985) Effect of uptake-one-inhibitors on the uptake of norepinephrine and meta-iodobenzylguanidine. *Journal of Nuclear Medicine* **26**: 897–907.

Tobes MC, Fig LM, Carey L et al (1989) Alterations of iodine-131-MIBG biodistribution in an anephric patient: Comparisons to normal and impaired renal function. *Journal of Nuclear Medicine* **30**: 1476–1482.

Valk TW, Frager MS, Gross MD et al (1981) Spectrum of phaeochromocytoma in multiple endocrine neoplasia. *Annals of Internal Medicine* **94**: 762–767.

Von Moll L, McEwan AJ, Shapiro B et al (1987) ^{131}I-MIBG scintigraphy of neuroendocrine tumours other than phaeochromocytoma and neuroblastoma. *Journal of Nuclear Medicine* **28(6)**: 979–988.

Wieland DM, Swanson DP, Brown LE & Beierwaltes WM (1979) Imaging the adrenal medulla with an I-131-labeled anti-adrenergic agent. *Journal of Nuclear Medicine* **20**: 155–158.

Young MJ, Dmuchowski C, Wallis J et al (1989) Biochemical tests for phaeochromocytoma: Strategies in hypertensive patients. *Journal of General Internal Medicine* **4**: 273–276.

10

Phaeochromocytoma and paraganglioma

VIVIAN FONSECA
PIERRE-MARC BOULOUX

Phaeochromocytoma has been called the great mimic because of its protean manifestations and the variety of clinical conditions for which it has been mistaken. It is a potentially lethal condition and was first described by Frankel (1886) in the adrenal glands of an 18-year-old girl who had died suddenly in collapse. Manasse (1896) demonstrated that a similar adrenal tumour could be stained brownish when exposed to chromium salts, a reduction phenomenon responsible for the name given to the tumour (*phaeo* = dusky, *chroma* = colour). In 1908 Alezais and Peyron introduced the term paraganglioma to designate extra-adrenal chromaffin tumours arising in paraganglia. The first documented case of bilateral phaeochromocytoma was reported by Hyman and Mencher in 1943.

ORIGIN OF CHROMAFFIN CELLS

The embryonic origin of adrenergic cells and tumours is shown in Figure 1. The sympathetic ganglia are formed in the embryo by cells that migrate from the thoracic region of the neural crest about the fifth week and settle

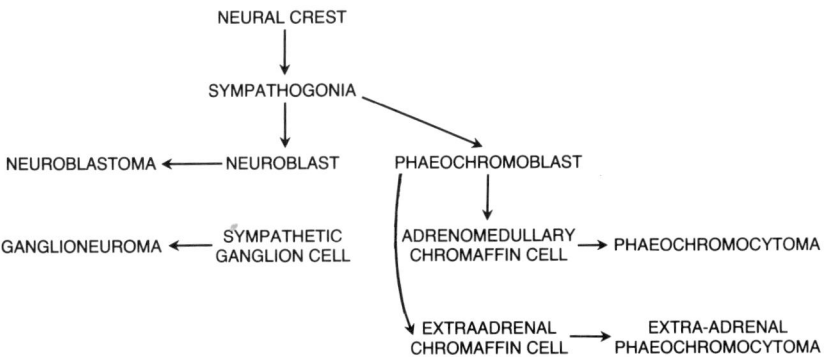

Figure 1. Cells of origin of the adrenal medulla and the sympathetic ganglia and their tumours.

Baillière's Clinical Endocrinology and Metabolism—
Vol. 7, No. 2, April 1993
ISBN 0–7020–1698–5

dorsolaterally to the aorta to form the sympathetic chains (Langman, 1969). Some sympathetic neuroblasts migrate anteriorly to the aorta to form other ganglia. A second migration occurs during the seventh week to form phaeochromoblasts. These invade the mesenchymal cells that make up the adrenal cortex to form the adrenal medulla (Hervonen, 1971). Certain neural crest cells form the primitive cells, the sympathogonia, which differentiate into sympathoblasts and also phaeochromoblasts. Sympathoblasts differentiate into sympathetic ganglia, whereas the phaeochromoblasts differentiate into phaeochromocytes. However, since both differentiation and dedifferentiation can occur, this can cause doubt as to the precise cell of origin of the resultant tumours. Small clusters of extra-adrenal chromaffin cells may be found in and about the sympathetic ganglia. While these are numerous during fetal life and infancy, they tend to regress during childhood. Remnants of chromaffin cells may, however, remain along the vagus, in the paravertebral sympathetic ganglia, and along the paraganglia associated with the great vessels such as the carotid arteries, arch of the aorta and the abdominal aorta (especially at the inferior mesenteric artery origin as the 'organ of Zuckerkandl', a bilateral structure frequently fused by an isthmus). These nests can give rise to paragangliomas. Rarer sites of chromaffin tissue deposition include the wall of the urinary bladder, the prostate, behind the liver, in the hilus of the liver or kidney, and in the region of the rectum, testicles, spermatic cord (Eusebi and Massarelli, 1971) or ovary. Certain specialized structures can give rise to paraganglioma-like lesions that occasionally hypersecrete catecholamines. These include carotid and aortic body tumours (chemodectomas) and glomus jugulare tumours. A full classification of paragangliomas is given in Table 1.

Table 1. Classification of paragangliomas.

Branchiomeric:
Intercarotid
Jugulotympanic
Orbital
Laryngeal
Subclavian
Aorticopulmonary
Coronary
Pulmonary

Intravagal

Aorticosympathetic:
Neck
Thoracic
Abdominal

Visceral autonomic
Atria of heart
Urinary bladder
Liver hilum
Mesenteric vessels

ANATOMY OF THE ADRENAL MEDULLA

The adrenal glands weigh about 4–6 g in adult life, of which about 10% is friable reddish adrenal medulla. Arterial inflow arises from the superior adrenal artery (a branch of the inferior phrenic artery), the middle adrenal artery (from the aorta) and the inferior adrenal artery (a branch of the renal artery or the aorta). The medulla receives a dual blood supply. The cortico-medullary veins draining the cortex deliver cortisol-rich blood into the substance of the medulla, while the medullary arteries largely bypass the cortex. The adrenaline-secreting cells of the medulla are found predominantly at the corticomedullary junction; this arrangement can be rationalized in terms of the high concentrations of cortisol required for the induction of the enzyme phenylethanolamine-N-methyltransferase (PNMT) required for the synthesis of adrenaline.

INCIDENCE AND ASSOCIATIONS OF PHAEOCHROMOCYTOMA AND PARAGANGLIOMA

The incidence of catecholamine-secreting tumours has been estimated to be about 0.1–1.0% of hypertensive patients (van Heerden et al, 1982; Manger et al, 1985). However, from post-mortem studies it is evident that many such tumours are not diagnosed in life (Bittar, 1982). The tumour affects both sexes equally, except in childhood. The peak incidence is between the third and fourth decade (Modlin et al, 1979). Although most tumours are sporadic (90%) and solitary, they may also occur in association with a number of familial neurocristopathic syndromes, including multiple endocrine neoplasia type II (medullary carcinoma of the thyroid, hyperparathyroidism and phaeochromocytoma) or type IIb (medullary carcinoma of the thyroid with ganglioneuromatosis, hypertrophic corneal nerves and phaeochromocytomas), Von Hippel–Lindau disease (retinal haemangiomatosis, cerebellar haemangiomatosis, phaeochromocytoma and hypernephromas; Horton et al, 1976; Hubschmann et al, 1981), and the phakomatoses such as neurofibromatosis (Humble, 1967), ataxia telangiectasia, tuberous sclerosis and the Sturge–Weber syndrome. More rarely, phaeochromocytomas have been associated with the multiple neoplasia triad (Margulies, 1988; extra-adrenal paragangliomas, gastric epithelioid leiomyosarcomas and pulmonary chondromas). Phaeochromocytomas can also occur as an isolated inherited trait with an autosomal dominant mode of inheritance (Smits and Huizinga, 1961; Samaan and Hickley, 1987).

PATHOLOGICAL FEATURES OF PHAEOCHROMOCYTOMA

Solitary phaeochromocytomas are more frequent on the right; about 5–10% are bilateral, and about 10% are extra-adrenal and solitary. Paragangliomas can be located anywhere from the base of the brain to the testicle, including the heart and pericardium. Most of the extra-adrenal tumours are located within the peritoneal cavity. Among children, bilateral and multiple tumours of the adrenal are more common, whereas in familial cases bilaterality, multicentricity and multiplicity are commoner. The tumours are variable in size, ranging from a few grams to lesions in excess of 1 kg. However, symptoms appear to bear little relationship to size and the smaller tumours can be associated with significant symptoms. Since tumours can be multicentric in origin, the diagnosis of malignancy may be difficult to establish (Shapiro et al, 1984; Medeiros et al, 1985). Malignancy may be diagnosed with certainty only by the demonstration of tumour cells in sites where chromaffin tissue would not normally occur (e.g. lymph nodes, liver, bone, muscle, lung). The incidence of malignancy is almost certainly underestimated, ranging from 3 to 14%. The study of chromosomal ploidy from tumour material may assist in predicting malignant potential: normal DNA histograms predict a benign course, whereas aneuploid peaks (e.g. tetraploidy/polyploidy) have a 30–40% incidence of malignancy (Hosaka et al, 1986). Macroscopically, tumours are usually encapsulated, the cut surface being dark, with haemorrhagic areas and areas of necrosis. The normal adrenal tissue is usually displaced and compressed. The microscopic features are similar to those of the normal adrenal, although tumour cells are bigger; ultrastructurally the secretory chromaffin granules are larger.

SECRETORY PRODUCTS OF PHAEOCHROMOCYTOMA

The dominant products, and those largely responsible for the clinical symptomatology, are noradrenaline, adrenaline and, to a lesser extent,

Table 2. Secretory peptides from phaeochromocytomas and their biological actions.

Peptide	Symptoms
Vasoactive intestinal peptide	Flushing, diarrhoea
Substance P	Flushing
Somatostatin	Constipation
Enkephalins	Constipation
Motilin	Diarrhoea
Neuropeptide Y	Vasoconstriction
Renin	Vasoconstriction
Corticotrophin-releasing factor, adrenocorticotrophin	Hypercortisolism
Parathormone	Hypercalcaemia
Parathormone-related peptide	Hypercalcaemia
Endothelin	Vasoconstriction
Erythropoietin-like factor	Polycythaemia
Angiotensin-converting enzyme	Hypertension
Human growth hormone releasing hormone	Acromegaly
Interleukin 6	Pyrexia
Neurone-specific enolase	
Atrial natriuretic factor	Polyuria, hypotension?
Insulin-like growth factor II	Related to tumour growth?
S100 protein	
Chromogranin A	
Calcitonin	
CGRP (Calcitonin gene-related peptide)	Vasodilatation
Pituitary adenylate cyclase activating polypeptide	Vasodilatation, interleukin 6 release

dopamine. Some tumours secrete L-dopa. Chromaffin cells belong to the APUD series of cells (amine precursor uptake decarboxylase; Pearse and Polak, 1974); these cells can also elaborate and secrete other peptide hormones (Table 2), some of which may cause symptoms not blockable by pharmacological α-and β-blockade (Landsberg and Young, 1985; Stewart et al, 1987; Helman et al, 1989). Such peptides may also permit differentiation between benign and malignant lesions. In one study, neurone-specific enolase (NSE) (an isoform of enolase, a glycolytic enzyme found in the neuroendocrine system) was raised in 50% of malignant phaeochromocytomas but normal in all benign lesions (Grouzmann et al, 1990).

TUMOUR BIOLOGY OF PHAEOCHROMOCYTOMA

Receptors for both IgFI and IgFII have been documented in phaeochromocytomas. These tumours also have increased levels of IgFII without increased peripheral levels, suggesting an autocrine growth-promoting action (Gelato and Vassaloti, 1990). Tumours also express high affinity somatostatin receptors (Reubi et al, 1991), and the use of γ-camera scanning techniques after injection of radiolabelled octreotide analogues has enabled in vivo labelling of tumours in about 33% of cases. The biological function of these receptors is uncertain; somatostatin binding appears to be guanosine triphosphate dependent, which is in agreement with a G protein coupled receptor. Somatostatin causes mild suppression of potassium-induced catecholamine release from tumour cells.

MOLECULAR GENETICS OF PHAEOCHROMOCYTOMA

Most of the currently available information is derived from the study of families with the multiple endocrine neoplasia syndromes (MEN 2a and 2b). The use of an 'exclusion map' and subsequent linkage analysis indicated that the MEN 2a gene was located on chromosome 10, linkage being established between the MEN 2a gene and the retinol-binding protein (RBP3) locus and the D10S5 locus, thereby mapping the responsible gene to the 10cen–10q11.2 (Mathew et al, 1987a,b; Simpson et al, 1987). More recently the locus has been narrowed down to between D10S34 and RPB3 (Mathew et al, 1991). Loss of heterozygosity in the region of the predisposing locus is rarely found in phaeochromocytomas, and it seems probable that malignant transformation in the MEN 2 syndromes is caused by mechanisms other than those occurring in MEN 1 syndromes; these may involve oncogene activation or the inactivation of a tumour suppressor gene at a different chromosomal locus. Using RFLP (restriction fragment length polymorphism) analysis identification of loss of all or a portion of 1p in 12 out of 18 phaeochromocytomas has been documented, and further studies have indicated that the region bounded by D1S15 (1pter–p22) and D122 (1p36.3) may harbour tumour suppressor genes whose inactivation may be important in the development of these tumours (Moley et al, 1991).

CLINICAL FEATURES OF PHAEOCHROMOCYTOMA

Cardiovascular sequelae of catecholamine-secreting tumours

Paroxysmal hypertension is the clinical hallmark of catecholamine-secreting tumours. In 50% of cases, the episodic surges of hypertension with associated symptomatology lead to 'crises' (Bravo and Gifford, 1984). These can be superimposed on a background of constant blood pressure elevation or normotension, or more rarely the pressor episodes can alternate with episodes of hypotension. 'Crises' tend to have a characteristic and reproducible pattern for each individual, although the duration and severity is usually variable, often increasing with time (Ross and Griffith, 1989). Typically, two or more symptoms occur synchronously with sudden onset and a peak severity occurring within a few minutes, with a slower offset. In most patients, the duration of the crisis is between 15 and 60 min (Thomas et al, 1966). An associated feeling of intense malaise and impending doom is characteristic, as is headache (often throbbing), pallor (often followed by flushing), perspiration and palpitations. Crises may be spontaneous, or provoked by exercise, bending over, urination or defecation. Induction of anaesthesia, tumour palpation and the administration of a large number of drugs (Table 3) can precipitate hypertensive episodes. Severe paroxysms

Table 3. Drugs whose administration has been associated with pressor crises in phaeochromocytoma.

Glucagon
Histamine
Metoclopramide
Droperidol
Tyramine
Adrenocorticotrophin
Saralasin
Tricyclic antidepressants
Phenothiazines
Naloxone
Imipramine

may be associated with severe peripheral vasospasm, with falsely low blood pressure measurements but severe central hypertension (Hull, 1986). Raynaud's phenomenon and acral gangrene have been reported in some cases (Manger and Gifford, 1977).

The most common symptoms associated with phaeochromocytoma are summarized in Table 4. While the inappropriately elevated levels of circulating catecholamines acting on α-receptors account for the blood pressure elevation, the circulation continues to be under sympathetic regulation. Thus administration of the α_2-agonist clonidine is associated with a lowering of blood pressure in patients with phaeochromocytomas (Bravo and Gifford, 1984). Since the effects of clonidine are mediated via postsynaptic brain stem α_2-receptors and peripheral presynaptic α_2-adrenergic receptors (inhibiting noradrenaline release), this suggests that tonic sympathetic

Table 4. Symptoms associated with phaeochromocytoma/ paraganglioma and their frequency. From Thomas et al (1966) and Landsberg and Young (1985).

Clinical feature	Frequency (%)
Headache (throbbing)	80
Diaphoresis	71
Palpitations	64
Pallor	42
Nausea, vomiting	42
Tremor	31
Weakness/exhaustion	28
Nervousness/anxiety	22
Abdominal/epigastric pain	22
Chest pain	19
Dyspnoea	19
Flushing	18
Weight loss	
Postural hypotension	
Micturition headache	

regulation of arteriolar tone operates even in the presence of elevated circulating catecholamines. This phenomenon is more easily understood if it is appreciated that intrasynaptic noradrenaline concentrations are in the 10^{-6} mol/litre range, whereas plasma noradrenaline levels are usually in the 8–80 nmol range in phaeochromocytoma patients (P. M. Bouloux, personal observations). It seems likely that extrasynaptic vascular α_2-receptors may be a major target of action of tumour catecholamines. Continuous blood pressure measurement in patients with phaeochromocytomas suggests that the expected nocturnal fall in blood pressure is absent in some though not all patients (Padfield and Stewart, 1991). There have been no attempts to correlate tumour size and secretory behaviour (i.e. episodic versus continuous catecholamine secretion) with 24-h continuous blood pressure recordings, and it is unclear why some patients experience the normal falls in blood pressure at night.

Chronic blood pressure elevation leads to left ventricular hypertrophy, while sudden massive catecholamine release can in addition cause severe venoconstriction, increasing preload at a time when afterload has been acutely increased. This may lead to sudden pulmonary oedema, and dysrhythmias which may be life threatening (Sode et al, 1967). Hypokalaemia caused by adrenaline release can compound the problem. A specific catecholamine cardiomyopathy has been clearly documented in patients with phaeochromocytoma; this can be dilated or hypertrophic.

Histologically focal myocardial necrosis may be seen. This usually resolves with removal of the tumour (Scott et al, 1988; Sardesai et al, 1990; Hicks et al, 1991).

Effects of phaeochromocytoma on muscles

Catecholamine-induced vasoconstriction and skeletal muscle ischaemia has been suggested as the cause of acute rhabdomyolysis and myoglobinuric renal failure in one case (Shermin et al, 1990).

Phaeochromocytoma and cytokine production

Phaeochromocytomas can cause several paraneoplastic syndromes. There have been reports of adrenal and extra-adrenal tumours presenting with fever, hypertension, anaemia, thrombocytosis, megakaryocytosis, hyperfibrinogenaemia and hypouricaemia. All symptoms resolved after tumour resection, and immunohistochemical analysis of the supernatant of the tumour culture showed high levels of interleukin 6 (Fukumoto et al, 1991; Suzuki et al, 1991). Interleukin 6 stimulates the synthesis of acute phase proteins and inhibits synthesis of albumin. Polycythaemia and venous thrombosis have also been reported and may have a humoral origin (Shulkin et al, 1987).

Phaeochromocytoma and the gastrointestinal system

Chronic constipation has been noted as a symptom in 13% of patients with phaeochromocytoma, and is occasionally so severe as to result in marked ileus and pseudo-obstruction of the large bowel (Turner, 1983). Gastrointestinal bleeding, intestinal ischaemia and enterocolitis have been documented in extreme cases. The combination of a distended adynamic intestine from α_2- and β_2-receptor stimulation and a compromised blood flow from α_1- and α_2-receptor stimulation causing vascular smooth muscle contraction are considered contributory factors. However, tumour production of enkephalins may also account for some of these symptoms. Phaeochromocytomas are rich in messenger RNA (mRNA) for all three classes of endogenous opioids, and elevated opioid peptides have been documented in plasma during phaeochromocytoma crisis.

There have been seven reports of vasoactive intestinal peptide (VIP) secreting phaeochromocytomas (Sackel et al, 1985), but with concurrent hypertension noted in only two. Watery diarrhoea (six cases) and hypokalaemia (five cases) were present, and the authors speculate that the mechanism of the normotension was the vasodilating actions of VIP.

Phaeochromocytoma and psychiatric symptoms

Cognitive impairment may be present in long-standing phaeochromocytoma, and reversible dementia has been associated with this diagnosis. In one case report, improvement of cognitive function occurred after surgical removal of bilateral phaeochromocytomas (White et al, 1986). Tremor has been reported in phaeochromocytoma, presumably the result of β_2-stimulation of muscle spindles. During paroxysmal attacks, patients may appear anxious and frightened because of the fear of impending death.

Phaeochromocytoma and the thyroid

Acute thyroid swelling has been noted in association with phaeochromocytoma crises (Bauer and Belt, 1947; Buckels et al, 1983). Since acute thyroid swelling has been observed during L-noradrenaline (norepinephrine *USP*) infusion in humans, but not with adrenaline (epinephrine *USP*), it seems that this symptom may be associated with noradrenaline-secreting phaeochromocytomas.

Phaeochromocytoma, weight loss and fever

Weight loss has been reported in patients in whom the hypertension is sustained (Kvale et al, 1956; Gifford et al, 1964). This seems to be associated with increased appetite, and the mechanism is thought to be increased catabolism. Cytokine production by the tumour could also play a role in this symptom, as well as the fever ('pyrexia of unknown origin') with which patients occasionally present.

Phaeochromocytoma and endogenous opioids

The administration of high but not of low doses of intravenous naloxone may precipitate a pressor crisis (Bouloux et al, 1986) (Figure 2). It has been proposed that enkephalins derived from the tumour may act on tumour cell opioid autoreceptors (?kappa subtype) to suppress catecholamine release.

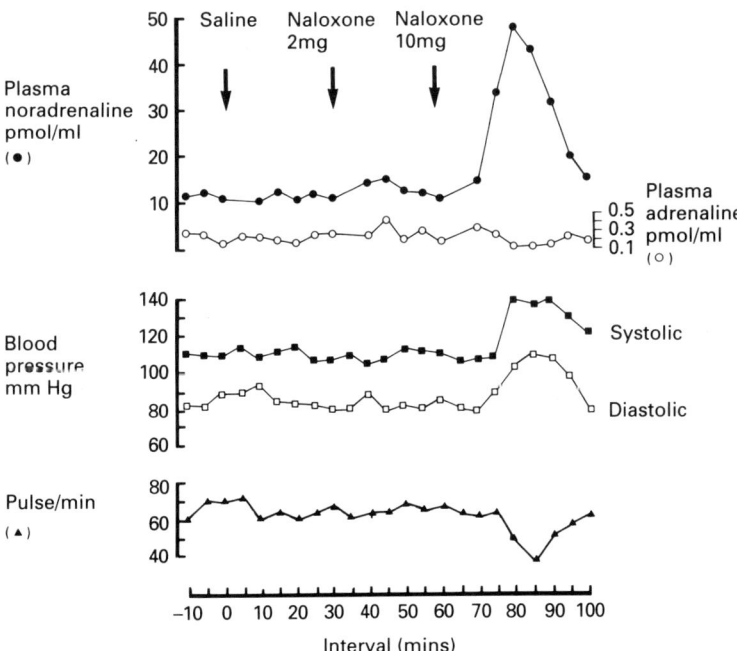

Figure 2. Effect of placebo and increasing doses of intravenous boluses of naloxone on plasma noradrenaline, adrenaline, blood pressure and pulse in a 32-year-old man with disseminated paraganglioma.

However, the latency of 10 min or so before catecholamine release suggests that other mechanisms may be operating.

Who should be screened for phaeochromocytoma?

Patients with progressive or malignant hypertension, hypertension with an early age of onset, resistance to conventional therapy, a paradoxical (i.e. pressor) response to β-blockade (caused by unopposed α-adrenoceptor activity), and a history of pressor responses to induction of anaesthesia, labour and delivery or to invasive investigative procedures where intravenous contrast media are used (e.g. angiographic procedures, intravenous urography), should prompt a search for an underlying catecholamine-secreting tumour. Similarly, patients with episodic symptomatology and hypertension, glucose intolerance/diabetes mellitus or features of hypermetabolism may be harbouring phaeochromocytomas. Patients with neurocutaneous syndromes (see above) or a family history of MEN 2 or familial phaeochromocytoma should also be screened, probably on an annual basis, with urinary free catecholamine estimations. Many of the symptoms of phaeochromocytoma are, however, non-specific, and may be mimicked by a number of conditions (Table 5), many of which are associated with episodic cardiovascular symptomatology (e.g. acute intermittent porphyria; Bravenboer and Erkelens, 1989).

Table 5. Differential diagnosis of phaeochromocytoma.

Hyperadrenergic hypertension ('pseudophaeochromocytoma')
Withdrawal of clonidine/methyldopa therapy
Hyperventilation
Withdrawal from alcohol
Migraine/cluster headaches
Primary cardiac rhythm disturbance
Excess caffeine intake
Anxiety neurosis
Basilar artery aneurysm
Menopausal flushing
Diencephalic epilepsy
Acute intermittent porphyria
Tabetic crisis
Cocaine
Thyrotoxicosis
Toxaemia of pregnancy
Tetanus
Guillain–Barré syndrome
Lead poisoning

Effects of excess catecholamine secretion in phaeochromocytoma

Tumours differ in the proportion of vasoactive biogenic amines they elaborate and secrete. Small adrenal tumours may be predominantly adrenaline secreting, and are associated with β-adrenoceptor stimulation related symptoms such as tachycardia, glucose intolerance and cardiac arrhythmias (Page et al, 1969). The systolic blood pressure is increased, but there is also a rise in pulse pressure. Larger adrenal as well as paragangliomas secrete predominantly noradrenaline. This is because the tumour outstrips its usual blood supply from the adrenal cortex, and thus becomes devoid of the high cortisol concentrations necessary for PNMT induction and hence adrenaline biosynthesis. Similar mechanisms explain the noradrenaline secretion of paragangliomas. Noradrenaline secretion is associated with systolic and diastolic hypertension and reflex bradycardia. The latter is a valuable pointer to the presence of autonomous noradrenaline secretion. It is perceived by the patient as a slow forceful palpitation. Excess noradrenaline secretion may also lead to shrinkage of the plasma volume with a rise in the haematocrit (Brunjes et al, 1960; Pinaud et al, 1985) and the occurrence of postural hypotension. It is rare for only one catecholamine to be secreted by the tumour, so that the symptom complex tends to reflect the actions of both noradrenaline and adrenaline. Dopamine secretion, particularly characteristic of the more aggressive tumours (Tippett et al, 1986), may lead to hypotension (Proye et al, 1986). L-Dopa secretion exerts a similar effect. The pressor episode can be extremely severe, precipitating acute heart failure, stroke and acute renal failure (Northfield, 1967; Radtke et al, 1975).

Childhood phaeochromocytoma

Clinical manifestations of childhood tumours differ in a number of ways from those in adults (Farquhar, 1958; Hume, 1960; Stackpole et al, 1963). Firstly only about 8% of children have paroxysmal hypertension, and two-thirds are male. Sweating and visual complaints (due to hypertensive retinopathy) are also more common than in adults, as are symptoms of nausea, vomiting (occasionally projectile) and weight loss. Polydipsia and polyuria (Tevetoglu and Lee, 1956) occur in 25% of childhood phaeochromocytomas. This may be related to increased renal blood flow secondary to raised cardiac output, causing polyuria. Thirst may be secondary to increased urine output as well as excessive sweating. Increased secretion of L-dopa or dopamine from childhood tumours may also cause polyuria. Polyphagia (Hume, 1960), convulsions and reddish blue mottling of the skin are seen more frequently in childhood tumours.

COURSE AND PROGNOSIS OF PHAEOCHROMOCYTOMA

Tumours may go unrecognized in life and up to 50% may be found incidentally at post mortem (Bittar, 1982). Untreated, tumours are associated with morbidity and mortality due to sustained hypertension, diabetes, left ventricular hypertrophy and catecholamine cardiomyopathy. Sudden death is also well recognized as an initial and final manifestation of phaeochromocytoma. This occurs as part of a sudden massive crisis.

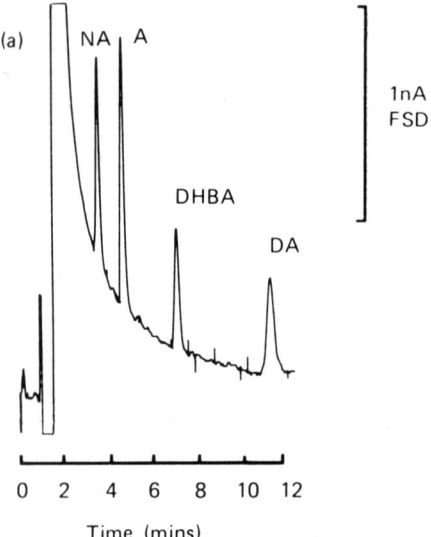

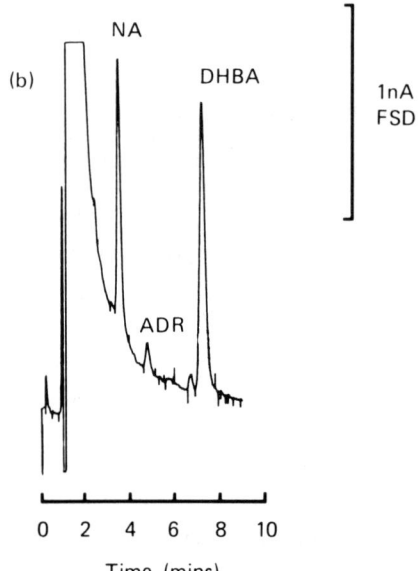

Figure 3. (a) High performance liquid chromatography coupled to electrochemical detection (HPLC-ECD) of a 2 pmol standard catecholamine solution. (b) HPLC-ECD of a 2 ml plasma extract showing physiological catecholamine levels. NA = noradrenaline; A and ADR = adrenaline; DHBA = dihydroxybenzylamine, the internal standard; DA = dopamine. 1 nA FSD = 1 nanoamp per full-scale deflection.

THE DIAGNOSIS OF PHAEOCHROMOCYTOMA

Once the condition is suspected on clinical grounds, it is customary to proceed to biochemical screening and confirmatory tests. This is followed by investigations to localize the tumour. Over the past 20 years microanalytical techniques using reversed phase high performance liquid chromatography coupled to electrochemical detection (HPLC-ECD) (Figure 3) and single or double isotope radioenzymatic assays have enabled the quantification of both plasma and urinary catecholamines with a high degree of sensitivity and specificity. These have or are in the process of displacing the older assays for urinary metabolites (vanillylmandelic acid (VMA)/HMMA, 4-hydroxy 3-methoxy mandelic acid, and metanephrines), which are more susceptible to inaccuracies by virtue of interference by dietary constituents (Quinn, 1988). A 24-h urinary collection into a container with 30 ml 6N (normal) HCl is the screening method of choice, although 12-h samples or timed 2–3 h collections to coincide with 'crises' are also useful. The sample must be acidified and the patient must be told the container contains concentrated acid! The completeness of the collection must be verified by urinary creatinine measurement. Upper limits of the normal ranges for 24 h urinary free catecholamines in our laboratory are 290 nmol for noradrenaline, 90 nmol for adrenaline and 2500 nmol for dopamine. The upper limit for VMA is 35 µmol/24 h, and for metanephrines 5 µmol/24 h. If only metabolite estimations are available, urinary metanephrines are to be preferred (normetanephrine and metanephrine) (Manu and Runge, 1984; Sheps et al, 1988, 1990). Depending on which cut-off point is used the specificity of the latter is about 93% (7% false positive), with a sensitivity of about 79%. The corresponding figures for VMA are 42% sensitivity and 100% specificity (see Table 6).

Table 6. Performance of biochemical tests in the diagnosis of phaeochromocytoma and paraganglioma: sensitivity and specificity at various cut-off points.

	Cut-off point (Normal range)	Sensitivity %	Specificity %
Urinary Metanephrines	>9 µmol/24 h (<5 µmol/24 h)	79	93
Urinary VMA (vanillylmandelic acid)	>55 µmol/24 h (<35 µmol/24 h)	42	100
Urinary free Noradrenaline	>720 nmol/24 h (<290 nmol/24 h)	95	95
Adrenaline*	>200 nmol/24 h (<90 nmol/24 h)	95	95
Plasma Noradrenaline	>5 nmol/l (0.3–2.8 nmol/l)	94	97
Adrenaline*	>1.5 nmol/l (0.1–0.52 nmol/l)	90	90

* Interference by labetalol (adrenaline).

Plasma catecholamines

The advent of methodologies for accurate quantification of plasma noradrenaline, adrenaline and dopamine has been a powerful adjunct to the diagnosis of phaeochromocytomas. Plasma catecholamine estimation can be useful in a number of ways. First, if a plasma sample taken during a hypertensive episode is found to be normal, the presence of a phaeochromocytoma is effectively excluded. Conversely, in the presence of normal blood pressure and urinary indices (VMA, metanephrines, urinary free catecholamines), a raised plasma catecholamine measurement taken during a 'crisis' may be diagnostic of a phaeochromocytoma. A recent patient under our care illustrates this principle:

> A 54-year-old woman was referred for investigation of a right adrenal mass, found incidentally during an ultrasound of the liver for right hypochondrial pain. She was not hypertensive, but gave a history of 'panic/anxiety' attacks occurring every 2–3 months lasting about 30 min. Urinary free cortisols were normal, and she had normal plasma cortisol suppressibility to a low dose dexamethasone suppression test. Two urinary free catecholamines estimations and three VMA and metanephrine estimations were within normal limits. An iodine-123 meta-iodobenzylguanidine (^{123}I-MIBG) scan showed no uptake of radionuclide within the right adrenal. Resting plasma catecholamines were normal. While on the ward, she experienced one of her infrequent attacks. A blood sample was immediately taken for plasma catecholamine estimation. The results showed a plasma noradrenaline of 8.6 nmol/litre and a plasma adrenaline of 23.7 nmol/litre. A right adrenal phaeochromocytoma was subsequently excised.

There are a number of important principles which govern the diagnostic uses of plasma catecholamines. First, the collection technique must be standardized. It is our practice to cannulate the patient 30 min before collecting a supine sample into a lithium heparin tube. This is cold spun immediately and the plasma flash frozen and stored at $-80°C$ prior to analysis. Situations such as noise, stress, discomfort and anticipation of venepuncture may spuriously elevate plasma catecholamines. Other factors and drugs which may cause spurious changes in plasma noradrenaline and adrenaline are listed in

Table 7. Average changes in plasma catecholamine with various physiological and pathological stimuli (adapted from Cryer, 1980).

	Plasma Noradrenaline	Plasma Adrenaline
Physiological		
Pain	↑ ×2–3	↑ ×2–3
Hypoglycaemia	↑ ×2–3	↑ ×10–40
Age	↑ ×2	→
Luteal phase of menstrual cycle	↑ ×1.5	→
Standing (*vs* supine)	↑ ×2–3	↑ ×1.5
Time of day	↓ 30–40% (at night)	↓ 30–40% (at night)
Pathological		
Cigarette smoking	↑ ×2	↑ ×2–3
Congestive heart failure	↑ ×2–6	→
Myocardial infarction	↑ ×3–5	↑ ×5–20
Cerebrovascular accident	↑ ×2–6	↑ ×2–3

→ = No significant change from basal.

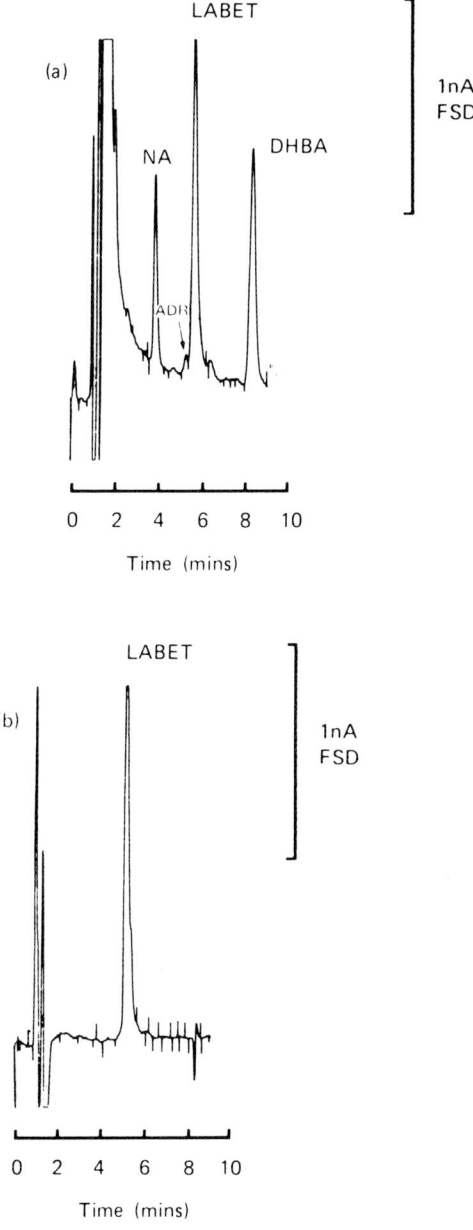

Figure 4. Labetalol interference–HPLC-ECD of 2 ml of plasma extract from a patient on labetalol 200 mg 8-hourly. LABET = the interfering peak, which obscures the adrenaline peak (ADR). (b) Direct injection of 30 pmol of labetalol onto the HPLC-ECD column. NA = noradrenaline; DHBA = dihydroxybenzylamine, the internal standard; 1 nA FSD = 1 nanoamp per full-scale deflection.

Table 7. We draw specific attention to the interference of labetalol in the measurement of adrenaline by HPLC-ECD, which in our experience has resulted in an unnecessary laparotomy in a patient (Figure 4). Plasma catecholamines remain stable for about 3–4 weeks at −20°C but they are stable indefinitely at −80°C (Bouloux et al, 1985). Under most circumstances, the levels of catecholamines fall into an unequivocally abnormal range in phaeochromocytomas. Levels of noradrenaline usually exceed 6 nmol/litre, and adrenaline levels are usually greater than 1 nmol/litre (Figure 6). In our experience, difficulty in establishing the significance of raised plasma catecholamines emanate from the indiscriminate use of this measurement in poorly selected patients; the use of plasma catecholamines for screening of patients with vague and non-specific symptoms has a very low positive yield. Under such circumstances a number of patients will give catecholamine levels in a 'grey' or equivocal range. In this situation, suppressive tests may be particularly useful (see below) in order to rule out a phaeochromocytoma in these patients. While the diagnostic specificity of mildly raised plasma catecholamines can be called into question, it has been shown that diagnostic sensitivity and specificity are superior to the traditional use of VMA and metanephrines (Figure 5).

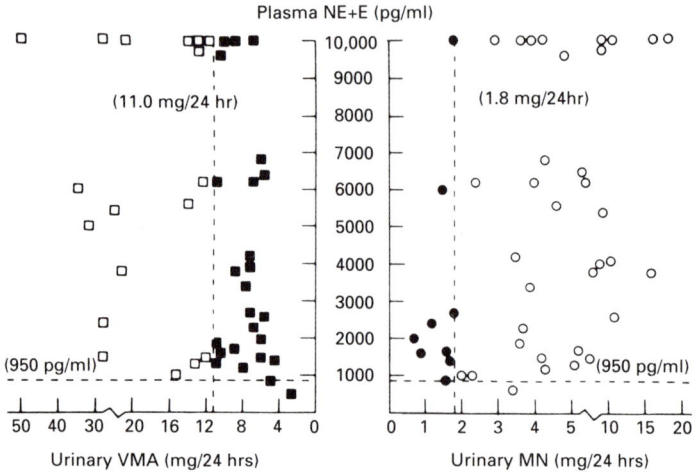

Figure 5. Comparison of the plasma catecholamines Noradrenaline (NE) and adrenaline (E) with simultaneous 24-h urinary vanillylmandelic acid (VMA) and metanephrines (MN) in patients with phaeochromocytoma. The interrupted lines indicate the normal ranges for the plasma and urinary indices; solid symbols denote false negative results; open symbols denote true positive results (Bravo and Gifford, 1984).

Suppressive tests

When studies of catecholamines in the blood give equivocal results (Figure 6), provocative or suppressive tests may be used. The latter are generally considered safer, and two are in clinical use. Clonidine, a centrally post-synaptically acting α_2-agonist, reduces sympathetic tone and plasma noradrenaline levels in normal subjects (Figure 7a,b). After a 300 μg dose, blood is sampled at 30-min intervals for a 2-h period. Suppression of plasma noradrenaline into the normal range effectively rules out phaeochromocytoma, whereas lack of suppression suggests the presence of autonomous

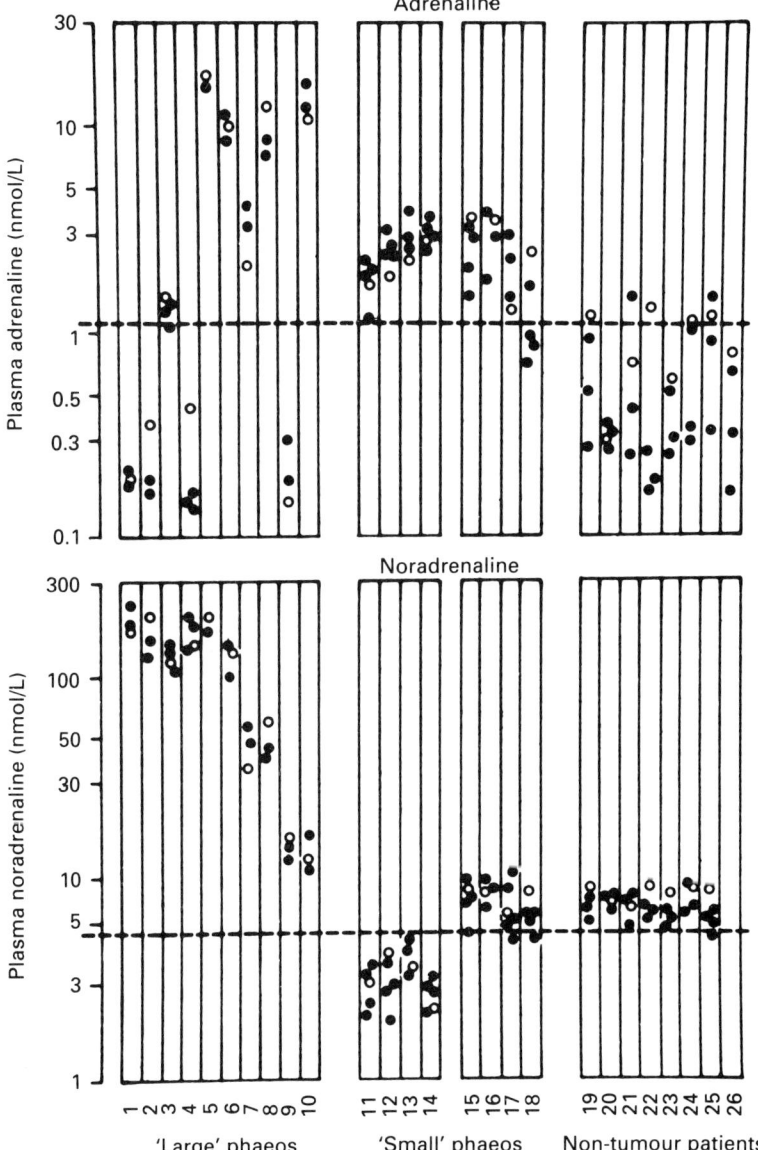

Figure 6. Distribution of adrenaline and noradrenaline in plasma from patients with large phaeochromocytomas, small phaeochromocytomas and non-tumour patients. From Brown et al (1981).

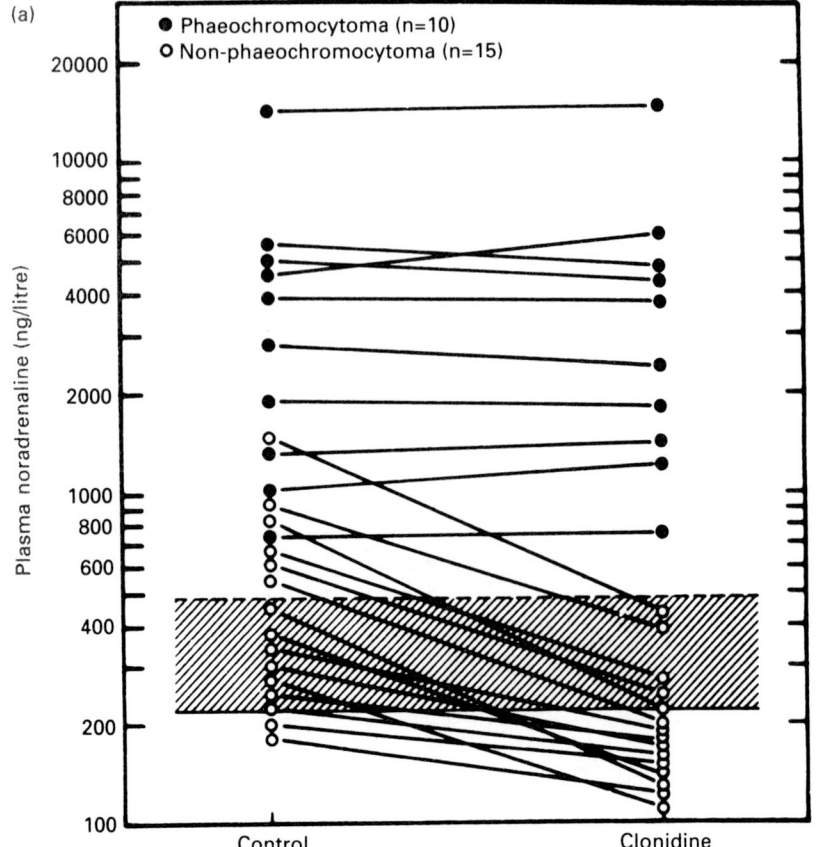

Figure 7. Effect of 300 µg of oral clonidine on (a) plasma noradrenaline and (b) adrenaline in patients with essential hypertension (open circles) or phaeochromocytoma (closed circles). From Bravo and Gifford (1984).

catecholamine secretion (Bravo et al, 1984). The dose of clonidine used causes drowsiness and a dry mouth, and the hypotension that ensues makes the test difficult to perform as a rapid outpatient procedure.

Pentolinium is a short-acting ganglion blocker which, when administered in a 2.5 mg or 5 mg dose, acutely suppresses both plasma noradrenaline and adrenaline. Tumorous catecholamine secretion is once again unaffected by ganglion blockade, and the test has proved useful in the diagnosis of small adrenal tumours (Brown et al, 1981). Postural hypotension and accommodation defects are associated with the 5 mg dosage. The test can be conducted as an outpatient procedure. The main drawback to suppressive tests is the loss of specificity when the basal catecholamines are within the normal range (Elliott and Murphy, 1988).

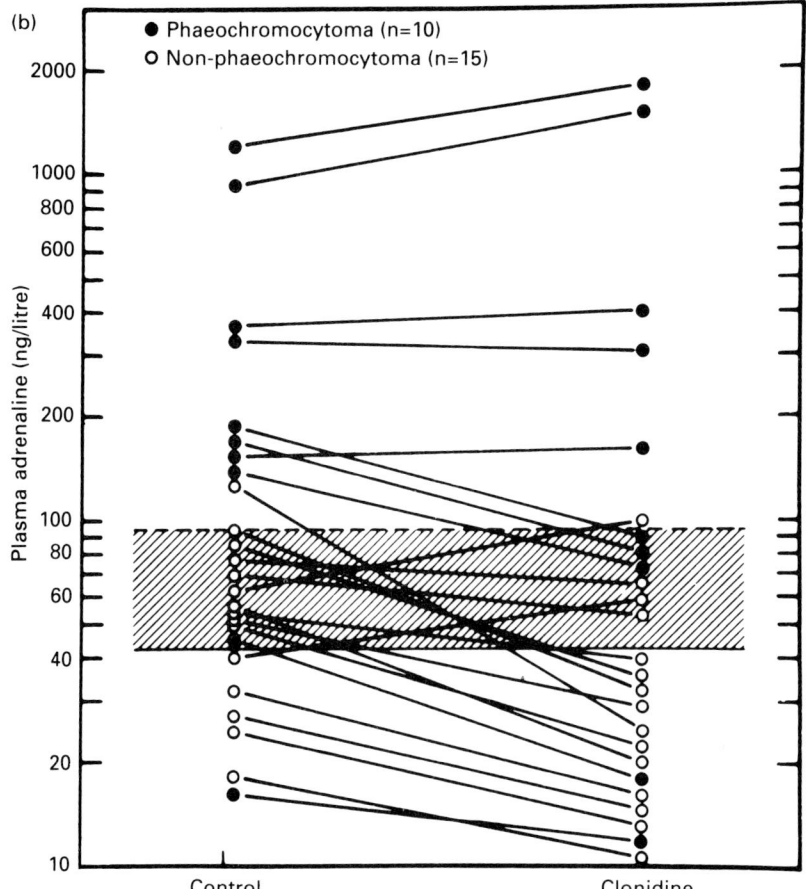

Provocative tests

Provocative tests are rarely indicated and are associated with a high incidence of false positive and false negative results. The exception is in patients with familial phaeochromocytomas or MEN 2 syndromes, where adrenomedullary hyperplasia may be present. In these instances, intravenous glucagon 1 mg may be administered and the ensuing plasma catecholamine response followed over a 10-min period. A significant rise in plasma catecholamines, usually within the first 2–4 min, suggests the presence of underlying tumorous catecholamine-secreting tissue. A further indication for a provocative test is where an adrenal mass is found incidentally, with normal plasma and urinary catecholamines and a negative MIBG scan. Under these circumstances it may be appropriate to administer intravenous glucagon 1 mg and monitor the plasma catecholamine response. The patient should be α- and β-blockaded prior to such a provocative test to mitigate the possible deleterious effects of an uncontrolled pressor response (Elliott et al, 1989).

Nocturnal clonidine suppression test

There is a circadian variation to both plasma and urinary catecholamine levels, with the nadir for both plasma and urinary catecholamines occurring at night. Patients with phaeochromocytomas on the whole continue secreting catecholamines in a constant fashion, and the daytime/night-time difference in urinary catecholamines is small compared with normal and essential hypertensive patients. The difference between urinary catecholamine excretion in essential hypertension and phaeochromocytoma patients may be accentuated by the nocturnal administration of clonidine 0.3 mg, based on observations in 12 patients with proven phaeochromocytoma and 40 non-phaeochromocytoma hypertensive patients (MacDougall et al, 1988). This α_2-agonist reduced plasma and urinary catecholamines in essential hypertension, but failed to do so in cases of phaeochromocytoma. This test has not found widespread use as yet, and there is insufficient experience of it to assess its sensitivity and specificity.

Chromogranin A (CgA) measurement

This is a soluble protein found within chromaffin granules stored with catecholamines. It is released into the circulation along with catecholamines. It can be measured in plasma, with an upper limit of normal (99th centile) of 70 ng/ml, and has been found to be significantly elevated in patients with phaeochromocytoma (O'Connor and Bernstein, 1984) with a sensitivity of 90% (Canale and Bravo, 1992). However, it may also be secreted by other endocrine tumours, e.g. medullary carcinoma of the thyroid, and other tumours of endocrine origin, i.e. polypeptide-secreting tumours. Specificity of CgA measurement in the diagnosis of phaeochromocytoma falls off significantly with renal impairment, with 50% patients with a creatinine clearance of less than 80 ml/min giving false positive results (Canale and Bravo, 1992).

Platelet catecholamine measurement

Platelets actively accumulate catecholamines from the plasma, and platelet catecholamine levels, which do not fluctuate rapidly, have been used in diagnosis (Zweifler and Julius, 1982). In this study of ten patients with proven phaeochromocytoma, six with hypertension and no tumour and 22 controls, platelet noradrenaline levels were 448 + 274 pg/ml, 49.0 + 27 pg/ml and 37.7 + 15.7 pg/ml in the respective groups (mean + SD), and 65.2 + 62.5 pg/ml, 4.1 + 2.2 pg/ml and 2.8 + 1.4 pg/ml for adrenaline, respectively. In this study, all patients with phaeochromocytomas had elevated plasma noradrenaline, and eight of the ten had elevated plasma adrenaline levels. However, five out of six patients without tumours had elevated plasma noradrenaline levels, yet their platelet noradrenaline and adrenaline levels did not differ significantly from levels in the control groups. It is thus evident that the predictive value of the platelet catecholamine assay is hampered by its lack of specificity.

Venous sampling for the diagnosis of phaeochromocytoma

Selective venous sampling is a safe and reliable method of confirming or refuting the diagnosis of phaeochromocytoma (Allison et al, 1983). In the case of a positive result, the sampling method accurately identifies the presence of the tumour, which is particularly useful in the case of ectopic or multiple tumours and bilateral lesions. The method complements computed tomography (CT) and magnetic resonance imaging (MRI), and is useful in situations where ^{123}I-MIBG scanning is negative yet clinical suspicion is high. A recent patient we treated illustrates the principle.

> A 24-year-old hypertensive man known to suffer from Von Hippel–Lindau disease was referred for treatment of a suspected right adrenal phaeochromocytoma. Investigations revealed elevated basal plasma catecholamines (plasma noradrenaline 14.5 nmol/litre and adrenaline 3.7 nmol/litre) and CT scanning showed a 3 × 2 cm right adrenal mass and a slightly enlarged left adrenal. MIBG scanning showed increased uptake only in the right adrenal. Venous catheterization confirmed the presence of a right adrenal tumour, and a sample of left adrenal venous effluent gave a noradrenaline value of 89 nmol/litre and an adrenaline value of 21.4 nmol/litre. At operation bilateral adrenal tumours were resected.

In this case the value of venous sampling was to investigate whether the slightly bulky left adrenal contained a second phaeochromocytoma. Usually adrenal venous blood contains more adrenaline than noradrenaline in a ratio of approximately 4 to 1. Here the reversal of that ratio suggested the presence of a tumour, which was confirmed at surgery. Thus venous catheterization may be used both for diagnostic purposes and localization procedures.

Ratio of 3,4-dihydroxyphenylethylene glycol to noradrenaline

Brown (1984) and Duncan et al (1988) have shown that the ratio of 3,4-dihydroxyphenylethylene glycol (DHPG) to noradrenaline in plasma will distinguish phaeochromocytoma (<0.5) from essential hypertension (>2.0), based on a study of 17 patients with proven phaeochromocytoma (Figures 8a,b,c,d). DHPG reflects mainly nervous release of noradrenaline, whereas noradrenaline released directly into the bloodstream (as in phaeochromocytoma) is not converted into DHPG.

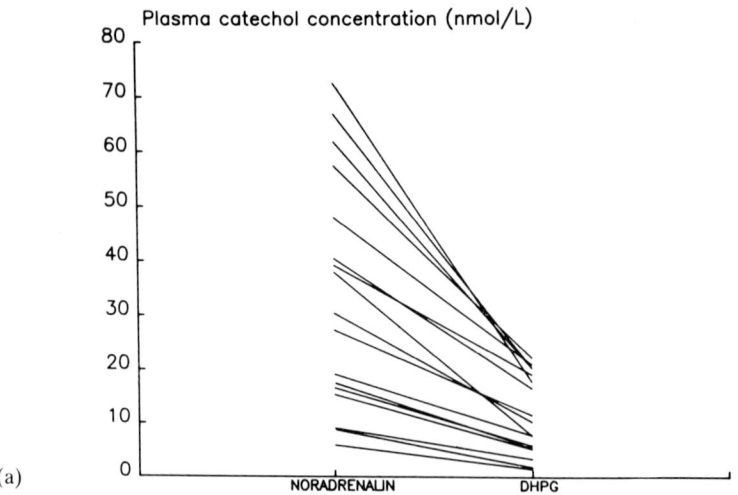

(a)

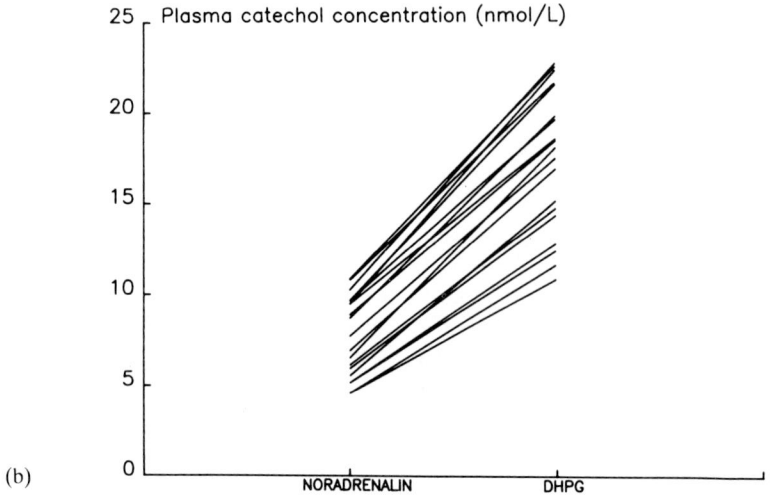

(b)

Figure 8. (a) Distribution of plasma noradrenaline and dihydroxyphenylglycol (DHPG) in plasma in 17 patients with proven phaeochromocytomas. (b) Distribution of plasma noradrenaline and DHPG in 18 patients with essential hypertension. (c) Pre- and postoperative ratio of plasma noradrenaline:DHPG ratio in patients with proven phaeochromocytoma. In patient 10, a disseminated lesion was present. (d) Metabolic pathways for noradrenaline (MAO = monoamine oxidase; COMT = catechol-O-methyltransferase; MHPG = 3 methoxy-4 hydroxyphenyl ethylglycol).

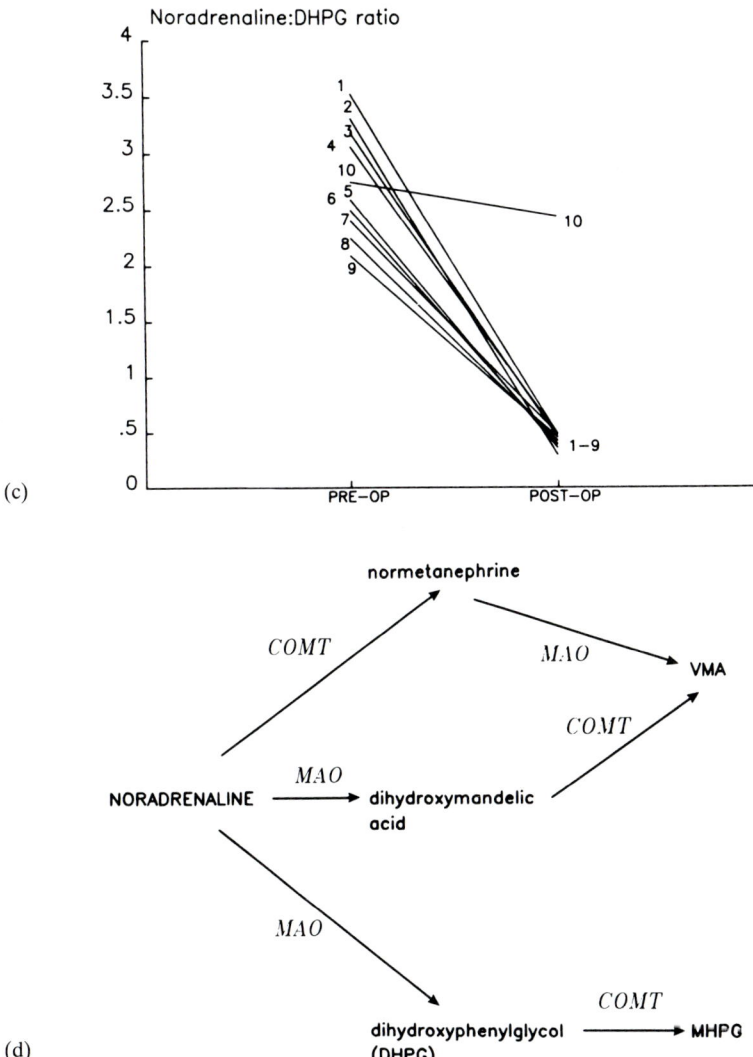

(c)

(d)

TUMOUR LOCALIZATION

Accurate tumour localization is an essential part of phaeochromocytoma management. The three imaging techniques of choice are CT, MRI and ^{123}I-MIBG.

CT scanning

Most tumours can be visualized using CT scanning (Figure 9). This should be

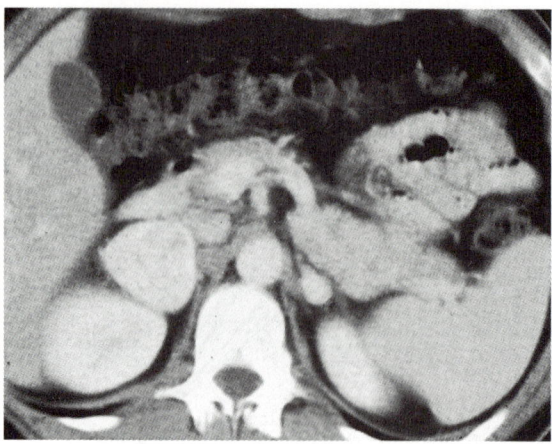

Figure 9. CT scan of adrenal showing a right adrenal phaeochromocytoma.

targeted at the adrenals in the first instance, and if the examination is negative, directed at the thorax and pelvis. Thin sections should be used, with adequate opacification of the bowel with contrast. The patient should have been α- and β-blockaded prior to the administration of intravenous contrast to assist in the diagnosis. CT scanning is less useful in the diagnosis of extra-adrenal tumours and may fail in children and very thin patients where there may be a lack of retroperitoneal fat. Ultrasonic examination is more useful in children.

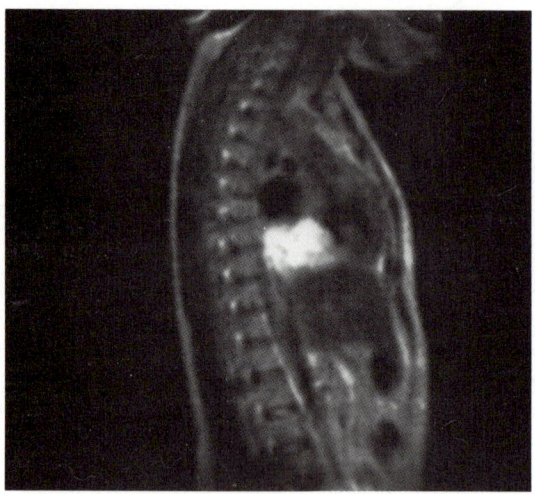

Figure 10. T2 weighted image of intracardiac phaeochromocytoma. By kind permission of Professor G. M. Besser.

MRI scanning

Sectional imaging in multiple planes using MRI allows some degree of in vivo characterization as well as being free of ionizing radiation. Lesions characteristically give out a high T2 weighted signal intensity, appearing bright white, while the normal adrenal has the same intensity as liver (Schmedtje et al, 1987). The technique may be useful in differentiating cortical adenomas from phaeochromocytomas, though not secondary adrenal deposits which may be hyperintense. A further advantage of MRI over CT scanning is that imaging is better in the proximity of large vessels, since flowing blood gives a signal void. We have found it particularly useful in the imaging of tumour deposits within vertebrae and spinal foramina, as well as visualizing intracardiac lesions (Figure 10).

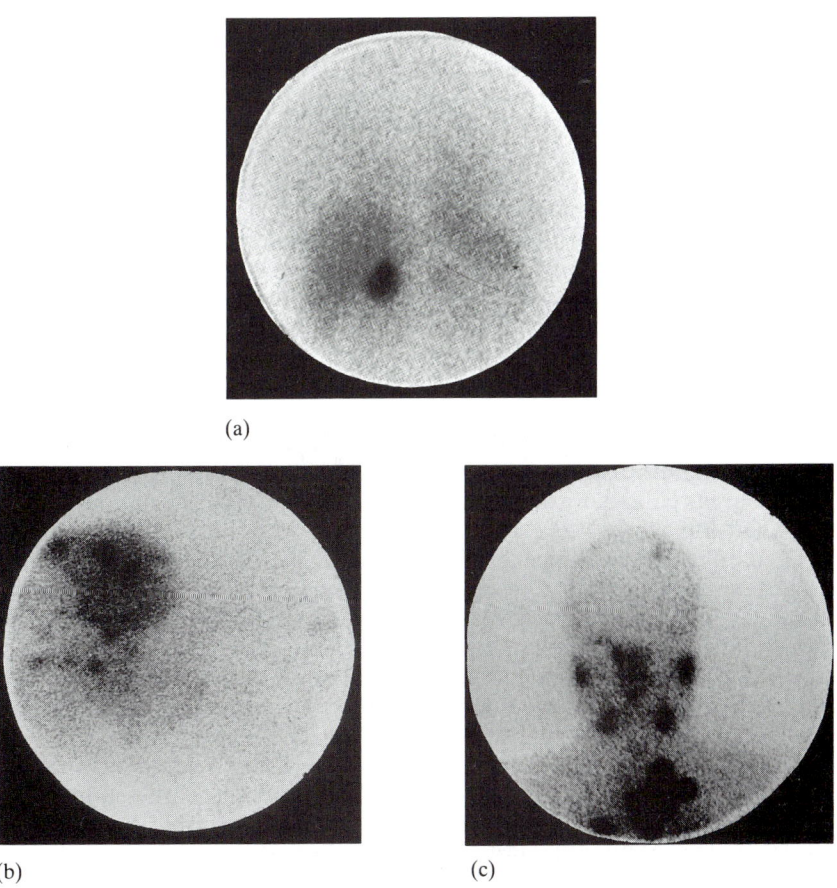

(a)

(b) (c)

Figure 11. (a) ^{123}I-MIBG scan showing right adrenal phaeochromocytoma. (b) ^{123}I-MIBG scan showing disseminated metastatic intrahepatic lesions. (c) ^{123}I-MIBG scan showing intra-thoracic paragangliomas. The salivary glands are visualized, and a small metastatic lesion is seen in the calvarium.

MIBG scanning

This guanethidine derivative is taken up by chromaffin tissue, and its uses in the diagnosis of phaeochromocytoma are discussed in Chapter 9. It is particularly useful for imaging non-adrenal tumours and metastases (Figure 11). However, a proportion of tumours do not take up the radionuclide, and a false negative rate of 10% has been recorded. The radionuclide ^{123}I-MIBG has also been used for the intraoperative localization of a catecholamine-secreting tumour which was detected on conventional MIBG scan, but with no mass detectable on CT scan (Lehnert et al, 1988).

MANAGEMENT OF PHAEOCHROMOCYTOMA

Surgical extirpation of the tumour is the only curative therapy, but should only be carried out as an elective procedure after the most careful pre-operative preparation. If the diagnosis is strongly suspected on clinical or biochemical grounds, treatment should be commenced forthwith starting with the mixed α_1/α_2 non-competitive antagonist phenoxybenzamine. The starting dose is 10 mg every 12 h building up to a dose of 10 mg every 6 h. After the first few doses of α-adrenoceptor antagonist, the β_1/β_2-antagonist propranolol is given orally in a dose of 40 mg t.d.s. The fall in intravascular tone may cause substantial postural hypotension, and it is not unusual to witness a fall in haematocrit under such circumstances. Prior to surgery, it may be necessary to transfuse the patient up to an adequate haemoglobin. The side-effects of phenoxybenzamine include postural hypotension, nasal stuffiness, nausea, sedation, weakness and pedal oedema.

The pure α-blocking drug prazosin is not recommended. First it is a competitive antagonist and if the ambient catecholamine level is greatly raised, it will be displaced from its receptor. Second, α_2-receptors, a large proportion of which are vascular and extrasynaptic, are not blocked by this drug, and therefore it may not give adequate protection from the catecholamine surges characteristic of phaeochromocytoma. Third, the drug has a short half-life.

Theoretically, the mixed competitive α- and β-adrenoceptor blocking drug labetalol might be useful in the peroperative management of phaeochromocytoma. However, both its α- and β-blocking actions are weak. Furthermore, labetalol interferes indirectly in the HPLC-ECD estimation of both plasma and urinary adrenaline (Figure 4). We know of one case where a laparotomy was performed for suspected phaeochromocytoma due to labetalol interference in adrenaline estimation.

Prior to surgery, Ross et al (1967) has suggested a regimen whereby phenoxybenzamine is given by intravenous infusion for three consecutive days at a dose of 0.5 mg/kg over 4 h. This ensures that as many α-adrenoceptors as possible are irreversibly blocked before surgery. In our experience this regimen is safe and has been effective in attenuating potentially disastrous pressor crises during induction and tumour manipulation. Even so, given the large number of vasoconstrictor peptides that may be released by phaeochromocytomas (e.g. neuropeptide Y, endothelin), it is not surprising that the pressor episodes cannot be fully blocked by adrenoceptor blockade alone. Intraoperative continuous intra-arterial blood pressure recording, central venous pressure monitoring and continuous electrocardiographic recordings are recommended, and unexpected surges of blood pressure should be treated with intravenous infusions of sodium nitroprusside or phentolamine. Intravenous propranolol may be given intravenously to counteract sudden tachycardias, and lignocaine (lidocaine *USP*) must be available to counter more serious rhythm disturbances. With removal of the tumour, blood pressure may fall significantly; this is less likely to occur if attention has been paid to intravenous volume repletion prior to surgery. However, volume expanders such as dextran, albumin or blood must be available to correct this haemodynamic parameter should the need arise. Rarely blood pressure collapse necessitates the use of intravenous noradrenaline. However, since α-adrenoceptors may be grossly downregulated as well as residual adrenoceptors being blocked by α-antagonists, patients will tend to respond poorly to pressor amine administration. In patients with myocardial dysfunction, optimal fluid administration is best given with haemodynamic information obtained through a Swan–Ganz catheter. Similarly, a urinary catheter is recommended to obtain optimal information about fluid balance.

Premedication

Both diazepam and barbiturates may be used safely as sedatives (Hull, 1986), whereas droperidol and phenothiazine-related compounds, which may provoke a pressor crisis, should be avoided (Yusa et al, 1973). Morphine should be avoided since it may cause histamine release, which may in turn provoke a pressor crisis. Similarly, atropine should be avoided because it has a vagolytic effect, causing tachycardia.

Induction and intubation

Thiopentone has been widely used and is safe. Fentanyl and alfentanil are safe alternative agents. Sodium etomidate causes minimal cardiovascular disturbance and has been used safely (Hull, 1986). Endotracheal intubation should be performed under direct vision with the liberal use of topical anaesthesia.

Muscle relaxation

Vecuronium appears to be the muscle relaxant of choice, being devoid of autonomic effects and not provoking catecholamine release through histamine release (Gencarelli et al, 1981; Hull, 1986). Suxamethonium (succinylcholine *USP*) should be avoided due to stimulation of sympathetic ganglia. Tubocurarine and atracurium provoke histamine release, whereas pancuronium, which may release stored catecholamines through its indirectly acting amine properties, is not recommended (Jones and Hill, 1981).

Inhalation anaesthesia

Hypoxia must be avoided, since it sensitizes the myocardium to catecholamine-induced arrhythmias. Halothane may also sensitize the myocardium (Etsen and Shimosato, 1965). Isoflurane and enflurane, which are less arrhythmogenic, are preferred.

Postoperative management

Attention should be paid to volume status and the avoidance of hypovolaemia. Regulation of the circulating volume may take days to become normal; this is partly caused by the insensitivity of adrenergically innervated vasculature to relatively normal levels of catecholamines because of the downregulation of adrenoceptors during the time of tumour-induced hypercatecholaminaemia.

Plasma and urinary catecholamines may take days to weeks to fully normalize following successful tumour extirpation. There are two possible reasons for this. One is that catecholamine stores at the nerve endings are replete and it may take several days for these levels to normalize. Concurrent with this, because of downregulation, sympathetic activity may have to be increased in order to achieve the same pressor responses. As alpha adrenoceptors are gradually replaced, and sensitivity restored, so plasma and urinary catecholamines will gradually return to normal.

Results of surgery and follow-up

With complete surgical removal of the tumour, the majority of hypertensive patients are rendered normotensive. Residual hypertension is present in 30% of patients, presumably reflecting either underlying essential hypertension or end-organ damage. Life-long biochemical (by urinary catecholamine measurement) and clinical follow-up is recommended. This is because it is difficult to predict malignant behaviour in these tumours, and multiple primaries are present in up to 10% of patients (Modlin et al, 1979; Scott and Halter, 1982). Metastatic disease has a propensity for bone, and bone pain is an important symptom.

Management of malignant phaeochromocytoma

Patients with inoperable or only partially resectable lesions, as well as those with frankly metastatic disease, may survive many years with a good quality of life. The overall mortality at 5 years is about 44% (Scott and Halter, 1982; Averbuch et al, 1988). The quality of life may be improved by several modalities of treatment.

Pharmacological blockade

Phenoxybenzamine may be given orally in a dose sufficient to fully control symptoms, although side-effects frequently limit the dose given. Doses of up to 120 mg t.d.s. have occasionally been used. α-Methylparatyrosine is a useful adjunct and may have a dose-sparing effect on the α-blockers (Engelman et al, 1968; Robinson et al, 1977; Ram et al, 1985). β-Blockade is also administered.

Cytotoxic chemotherapy

Several authors have documented the effects of cytotoxic drugs in the management of phaeochromocytoma (Keiser et al, 1985; Averbuch et al, 1988). Cyclophosphamide, vincristine and dacarbazine have been given in repeated 21-day cycles in one report, a regimen associated with an 80% response in childhood neuroblastoma. In the largest chemotherapy report to date, this regimen has been associated with tumour shrinkage in 57% and biochemical response in 80% (Keiser et al, 1985). The treatment was given concurrently with α-adrenoceptor blockade.

External beam irradiation

Local therapy with 3000–5000 cGy provides useful palliation in cases of skeletal deposits, but less so if the deposits are in soft tissue (Scott and Halter, 1982).

MIBG therapy

This is discussed extensively in Chapter 11. Our experience of treating a small number of patients suggests that several hundred millicuries of MIBG labelled with iodine-131 are required. The response tends to be slow, but plasma catecholamines have fallen gradually over a period of years.

Tumour embolization

There have been a number of reports of the treatment of inoperable primary tumours and metastatic lesions with embolization using Gelfoam and finely divided lyophilized human dura to occlude the blood supply (Timmis et al, 1981). The feasibility of this approach is operator dependent, and the vascular supply of the tumour must be readily accessible. Patients must be fully α- and β-blockaded prior to this procedure.

Laparoscopic adrenalectomy for phaeochromocytoma

Recently, laparoscopic surgery has been used to remove a right adrenal phaeochromocytoma (Gagnier et al, 1992) after volume expansion and pharmacological blockade with prazosin. The patient, a 60-year-old man with a 3.5 cm phaeochromocytoma, maintained a stable blood pressure during the 2-h procedure, and no transfusion was required. The patient resumed eating the next day and was discharged on the fourth postoperative day. It is evident that this potentially hazardous procedure should only be performed by the most experienced surgeons.

SPECIAL PHAEOCHROMOCYTOMAS

Pregnancy

Phaeochromocytomas in pregnancy carry a high risk of morbidity and mortality to both mother and fetus (Schenker and Chowers, 1971; Schenker and Granat, 1982), with the vasoconstrictive effects of noradrenaline on uterine/placental blood flow accounting for fetal morbidity (Griffith et al, 1974). The differential diagnosis from severe pre-eclampsia may pose

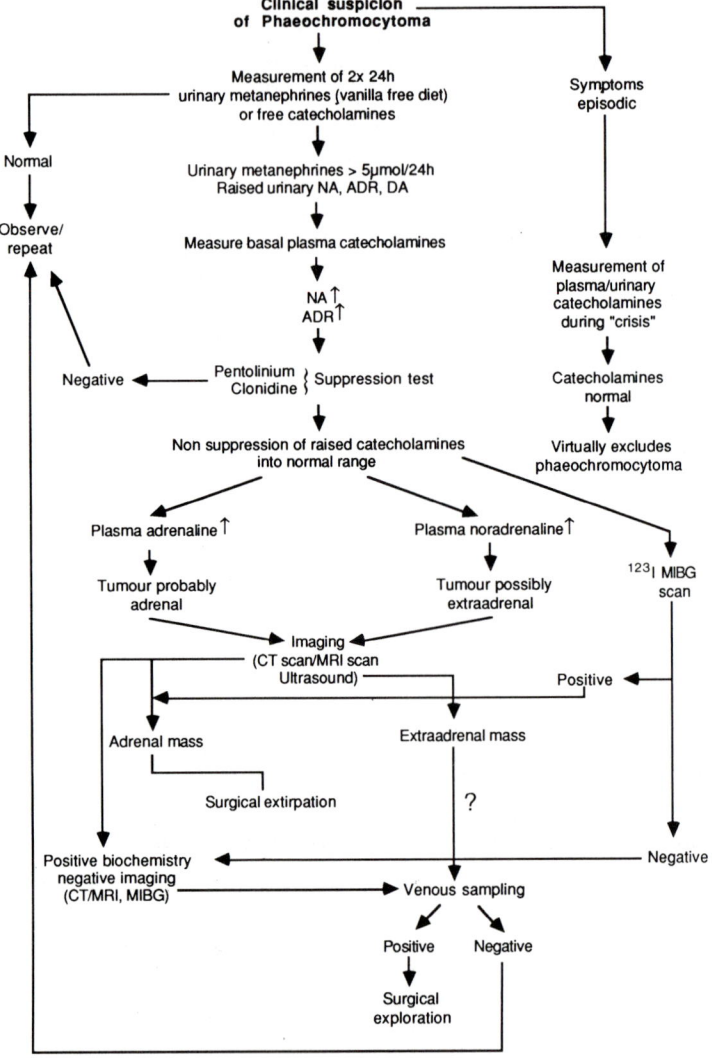

Figure 12. Strategy for the diagnosis of phaeochromocytoma.

problems, but remains biochemical. As soon as the diagnosis is confirmed, phenoxybenzamine in increasing doses should be commenced to lower the blood pressure, failing which methyltyrosine should be employed. In early pregnancy, termination is justified under α- and β-blockade. As pregnancy advances there is a risk that the enlarging uterus may compress the tumour, leading to increasing symptoms, and surgical extirpation may be attempted during the second trimester (Schenker and Granat, 1982). Tumour localization should preferably be with MRI. Since labour may be associated with pressor crises, an elective caesarean section should be performed via a vertical lower abdominal incision under α- and β-blockade. The incision may then be extended and the abdomen explored prior to tumour extirpation. In later pregnancy, if symptoms cannot be controlled, termination by hysterotomy may be required. This should be followed by immediate tumour resection.

Cardiac phaeochromocytomas

These may be difficult to diagnose, and patients often present with a long history of paroxysmal hypertension and cardiac arrhythmias. Conventional imaging may be unhelpful, and venous sampling may miss the site of origin of the tumour unless a coronary sinus sample is specifically taken. MRI is currently the best imaging technique for diagnosis (Figure 10), the lesions giving a bright appearance on the T2 weighted images.

SUMMARY

Use of current analytical techniques should lead to the successful diagnosis of most catecholamine-secreting tumours, and the experience and confidence which has evolved with the use of HPLC-ECD for plasma and urinary catecholamine estimation, as well as their greater diagnostic sensitivity and specificity, should soon render the older urinary assays based on catecholamine metabolites obsolete. Until then urinary metanephrine estimation will remain the diagnostic metabolite of choice. The diagnosis of small lesions and early recurrences will, however, continue to pose a great analytical challenge, and may call for the use of suppressive tests such as the pentolinium suppression test, venous catheterization, and MIBG scanning. The flow chart used for phaeochromocytoma diagnosis in our department is illustrated in Figure 12; and provides a strategy for the effective diagnosis of all but the most difficult lesions.

REFERENCES

Alezais A & Peyron S (1908) Un nouveau groupe de tumeurs epithéliale: les parangliomes. *C.R. Séances de la Société Biologique* **65:** 745–747.
Allison DJ, Brown MJ, Jones DH & Timmis JB (1983) Role of venous sampling in locating a phaeochromocytoma. *British Medical Journal* **286:** 1122–1124.

Averbuch SD, Steakley CS, Young RC et al (1988) Malignant phaeochromocytoma: Effective treatment with a combination of cyclophosphamide, vincristine and dacarbazine. *Annals of Internal Medicine* **109**: 267.

Bauer J & Belt E (1947) Paroxysmal hypertension with concomitant swelling of the thyroid due to phaeochromocytoma of the right adrenal gland. Cure by removal of the phaeochromocytoma. *Journal of Clinical Endocrinology and Metabolism* **7**: 30–46.

Beard CM, Sheps SG, Kurland LT, Carney JA & Lie JT (1983) Occurrence of phaeochromocytoma in Rochester Minnesota, 1950 through 1979. *Mayo Clinic Proceedings* **58**: 802–804.

Bittar DA (1982) Unsuspected phaeochromocytoma. *Canadian Anaesthetists' Society Journal* **29**: 183–184.

Bouloux PMG, Perrett D & Besser GM (1985) Methodological considerations in the determination of plasma catecholamines by high performance liquid chromatography coupled to electrochemical detection. *Annals of Clinical Biochemistry* **22**: 194–203.

Bouloux PMG, Grossmann AB & Besser GM (1986) Naloxone provokes catecholamine release in phaeochromocytomas and paragangliomas. *Clinical Endocrinology* **24**: 319–325.

Bravenboer B & Erkelens DW (1989) Acute hypertension mimicking phaeochromocytoma as main presenting feature of acute intermittent porphyria. *Lancet* **ii**: 928.

Bravo EL & Gifford RW Jr (1984) Phaeochromocytoma: diagnosis, localization and management. *New England Journal of Medicine* **301**: 682–686.

Brown MJ (1984) Simultaneous assay of noradrenaline and its deaminated metabolite dihydroxyphenylglycol in plasma: a simplified approach to the exclusion of phaeochromocytoma in patients with borderline elevation of noradrenaline concentration. *European Journal of Clinical Investigation* **14**: 67–72.

Brown MJ, Allison DJ, Lewis PJ et al (1981) Increased sensitivity and accuracy of phaeochromocytoma diagnosis achieved by plasma adrenaline estimation and a pentolinium estimation. *Lancet* **i**: 174–177.

Brunjes S, Johns VJ & Crane MG (1960) Phaeochromocytoma. Postoperative shock and blood volume. *New England Journal of Medicine* **262**: 393–395.

Buckels JAC, Webb AMC & Rhodes A (1983) Is paroxysmal thyroid swelling due to phaeochromocytoma a forgotten physical sign? *British Medical Journal* **287**: 1206–1207.

Canale MP & Bravo EL (1992) Serum chromogranin A in the differential diagnosis of suspected phaeochromocytoma. *Ninth International Congress of Endocrinology*, Nice, August 1992, abstract P-03.31.027.

Casola G, Nocolet V, Van Sonnenberg E et al (1986) Unsuspected phaeochromocytoma: risk of blood pressure alterations during percutaneous adrenal biopsy. *Radiology* **59**: 733–735.

Devoe LD, O'Dell BE, Castillo RA, Hadi HA & Searle N (1986) Metastatic phaeochromocytoma in pregnancy and fetal biophysical assessment after maternal administration of alpha-adrenergic, beta-adrenergic, and dopamine antagonists. *Obstetrics and Gynecology* **68**: 155–185.

Duncan MW, Compton P, Lazarus L & Smythe GA (1988) Measurement of norepinephrine and 3,4-dihydroxyphenylglycol in urine and plasma for the diagnosis of phaeochromocytoma. *New England Journal of Medicine* **319(3)**: 136–142.

Elliott WJ & Murphy MB (1988) Reduced specificity of the clonidine suppression test in patients with normal plasma catecholamines. *American Journal of Medicine* **84**: 419–424.

Elliott WJ, Murphy MB, Straus FH & Jabarak J (1989) Improved safety of glucagon testing for phaeochromocytoma by prior alpha receptor blockade. *Archives of Internal Medicine* **149**: 214–216.

Engelman K, Horwitz D, Jequier E et al (1968) Biochemical and pharmacological effects of alpha-methyltyrosine in man. *Journal of Clinical Investigation* **47**: 577.

Etsen BE & Shimosato S (1965) Halothane anesthesia and catecholamine levels in a patient with pheochromocytoma. *Anesthesiology* **26**: 688–691.

Eusebi V & Massarelli G (1971) Phaeochromocytoma of the spermatic cord: Report of case. *Journal of Pathology* **105**: 283–284.

Farquhar JW (1958) Phaeochromocytoma in childhood; case report and a brief review of 56 others recorded in the literature. *Journal of the Royal College of Surgeons of Edinburgh* **3**: 300–310.

Frankel F (1886) Ein Fall von doppelseitigen, vollig latent verlaufen Nebennierentumour und gleichzeitiger Nephritis mit Veranderungen am Circulationsapparat und Retinitis. *Virchows Archiv Pathology, Anatomy and Physiology* **103**: 244–263.

Fukumoto S, Matsumoto T, Harada SI, Fujiski J, Kawano M & Ogata G (1991) Phaeochromo-cytoma with pyrexia, marked inflammatory signs: A paraneoplastic syndrome with possible relation to IL6 production. *Journal of Clinical Endocrinology and Metabolism* **73:** 877–881.

Gagnier M, Lacroix A & Bolte E (1992) Laparoscopic adrenalectomy in Cushing's syndrome and phaeochromocytoma. *New England Journal of Medicine* **327:** 1033.

Gelato MC & Vassaloti G (1990) Insulin like growth factor II. Possible local growth factor in phaeochromocytoma. *Journal of Clinical Endocrinology and Metabolism* **71:** 1168–1174.

Gencarelli PJ, Roizen MF, Miller RD et al (1981) Org NC45 (Norcuron) and pheochromo-cytoma. Report of 3 cases. *Anesthesiology* **55:** 690.

Gifford RW, Kvale WF, Maher FT, Roth GM & Priestley R (1964) Clinical features, diagnosis and treatment of pheochromocytoma; a review of 76 cases. *Mayo Clinic Proceedings* **39:** 281–302.

Griffith MI, Felts JH, James FM et al (1974) Successful control of phaeochromocytoma in pregnancy. *Journal of the American Medical Association* **229:** 437–439.

Grouzmann O, Gicquel C, Plouin PF, Schlumberger M, Comoy E & Bohnon C (1990) Neuropeptide Y and neuron specific enolase levels in benign and malignant phaeochromo-cytomas. *Cancer* **66:** 1833–1835.

Helman LJ, Cohen PS, Averbuch SD, Cooper MJ, Keiser HR & Israel MA (1989) Neuro-peptide Y expression distinguishes malignant from benign phaeochromocytoma. *Journal of Clinical Oncology* **7:** 1720–1725.

Hervonen A (1971) Development of catecholamine storage cells in human fetal paraganglia and adrenal medulla: A histochemical and electron microscopic study. *Acta Physiologica Scandinavica Supplement* **368:** 94.

Hicks RJ, Wood B, Kalff V, Anderson ST & Kelly MJ (1991) Normalization of left ventricular function following resection of a phaeochromocytoma in a patient with a dilated cardio-myopathy. *Clinical Nuclear Medicine* **16(6):** 413–416.

Horton WA, Wong V & Eldridge R (1976) Von Hippel Lindau disease: clinical and patho-logical manifestations in 9 families with 50 affected members. *Archives of Internal Medicine* **136:** 769–777.

Hosaka Y, Rainwater LM, Grant CS, Farrow GM, van Heerden JA & Lieber MM (1986) Phaeochromocytoma: nuclear deoxyribonucleic patterns studied by flow cytometry. *Surgery* **100:** 1003–1010.

Hubschmann OR, Vijaynathan T & Countee RW (1981) Von Hippel Lindau disease with multiple manifestations: diagnosis and management. *Neurosurgery* **8:** 92–95.

Hull CJ (1986) Phaeochromocytoma. *British Journal of Anaesthesia* **58:** 1453–1468.

Humble RM (1967) Phaeochromocytoma, neurofibromatosis and pregnancy. *Anaesthesia* **22:** 296–303.

Hume DM (1960) Phaeochromocytoma in the adult and in the child. *American Journal of Surgery* **99:** 458–496.

Hyman A & Mencher D (1943) Phaeochromocytoma of the adrenal gland. *Journal of Urology* **49:** 755–771.

Jones DH, Reid JI, Hamilton CA et al (1980) The biochemical diagnosis, localization and follow-up of phaeochromocytoma: the role of plasma and urinary catecholamine measure-ments. *Quarterly Journal of Medicine* **195:** 341–361.

Jones RM & Hill AB (1981) Severe hypertension associated with pancuronium in a patient with a phaeochromocytoma. *Canadian Anethesthet. Society Journal* **28:** 394.

Keiser HR, Goldstein DS, Wade JL et al (1985) Treatment of malignant phaeochromocytoma with combination chemotherapy. *Hypertension* **7(supplement 1):** 1–18.

Kvale WF, Roth GM, Manger WM & Priestly JT (1956) Phaeochromocytoma. *Circulation* **14:** 622–630.

Kuchel O (1985) Pseudophaeochromocytoma. *Hypertension* **7:** 151–158.

Landsberg L & Young JB (1985) Catecholamines and the adrenal medulla. In Foster DW & Wilson JD (eds) *Williams Textbook of Endocrinology*, pp 891–965. Philadelphia: WB Saunders.

Langman J (1969) *Medical Embryology*, 2nd edn, p 389. Baltimore: Williams & Wilkins.

Lehnert H, Weber P, Nagele-Wohrle B et al (1988) Intraoperative localization of malignant phaeochromocytoma by [123]IMIBG single probe measurement. *Klinische Wochenschrift* **66:** 61–64.

MacDougall K, Isles CG, Stewart H et al (1988) Overnight clonidine suppression test in the diagnosis and exclusion of phaeochromocytoma. *American Journal of Medicine* **84:** 993–1000.

Manasse P (1896) Zur Histologie und Histogenese der primaren Nierengeschwulste. *Virchows Archiv Patholog, Anatomy & Physiology* **145:** 113–157.

Manger WM & Gifford RW Jr (1977) *Phaeochromocytoma.* New York: Springer-Verlag.

Manger WM, Gifford RW & Hoffmann BB (1985) Phaeochromocytoma; a clinical and experimental overview. *Current Problems in Cancer* **9:** 1–12.

Manu P & Runge LA (1984) Biochemical screening for phaeochromocytoma: superiority of urinary metanephrine measurements. *American Journal of Epidemiology* **120:** 788–790.

Margulies KB (1988) Carney's triad: guidelines for management. *Mayo Clinic Proceedings* **63:** 496–502.

Mathew CGP, Chin KS, Easton DF et al (1987a) A linked genetic marker for multiple endocrine neoplasia type 2A on chromosome 10. *Nature* **328:** 527–528.

Mathew CGP, Smith BA, Thorpe K, Royle NJ, Jeffrey AJ & Ponder BAJ (1987b) Deletion of genes on chromosome 1 in multiple endocrine neoplasia. *Nature* **328:** 524–526.

Mathew CGP, Easton DF, Nakamura Y, Ponder BAJ & MEN2A International Collaborative Group (1991) Presymptomatic screening for multiple endocrine neoplasia type 2A with linked DNA markers. *Lancet* **337:** 7–11.

Medeiros LJ, Wolf BC, Balogh K & Federman M (1985) Adrenal phaeochromocytoma: A clinicopathologic review of 60 cases. *Human Pathology* **16:** 580–589.

Modlin IM, Farndon JR, Shepherd A et al (1979) Phaeochromocytoma in 72 patients; clinical and diagnostic features, treatment and long term results. *British Journal of Surgery* **66:** 456–465.

Moley JF, Brother MB, Wells SA, Spengler BA, Biedler JL & Brodeur GM (1991) Low frequency of ras gene mutations in neuroblastoma, pheochromocytomas and medullary thyroid cancers. *Cancer Research* **51**(6): 1596–1599.

Northfield TC (1967) Cardiac complications of phaeochromocytoma. *British Heart Journal* **29:** 588–593.

O'Connor DT & Bernstein KN (1984) Radioimmunoassay of chromogranin A in plasma as a measure of exocytotic sympathoadrenal activity in normal subjects and patients with phaeochromocytoma. *New England Journal of Medicine* **311:** 764–770.

Padfield PL & Stewart MJ (1991) Ambulatory blood pressure monitoring in secondary hypertension. *Journal of Hypertension* **9**(suppl 8): S69–S71.

Page LB, Raker JW & Berberich FR (1969) Phaeochromocytoma with predominant epinephrine secretion. *American Journal of Medicine* **47:** 648–652.

Pearse AGE & Polak JM (1974) Endocrine tumours of neural crest origin. Neurolymphomas, apudomas and the APUD concept. *Medical Biology* **52:** 3.

Pinaud M, Desjars P, Tasseau F et al (1985) Preoperative acute volume loading in patients with phaeochromocytoma. *Critical Care Medicine* **13:** 460.

Proye C, Rossati P, Fontaine P et al (1986) Dopamine secreting phaeochromocytoma: an unrecognized entity? Classification of phaeochromocytomas according to their type of secretion. *Surgery* **100:** 1154–1161.

Quinn N (1988) False positive diagnosis of phaeochromocytoma in a patient with Parkinson's disease receiving levodopa. *Journal of Neurology, Neurosurgery and Psychiatry* **51:** 728–729.

Radtke WE, Kazmier FJ, Rutherford BD & Sheps SG (1975) Cardiovascular complications of phaeochromocytoma crisis. *American Journal of Cardiology* **35:** 701–705.

Ram CVS, Meese R & Hill SC (1985) Failure of alphamethyltyrosine to prevent hypertensive crises in phaeochromocytoma. *Archives of Internal Medicine* **145:** 2114.

Reubi JC, Waser B, Khosla S et al (1991) In vitro and in vivo detection of somatostatin receptors in phaeochromocytomas and paragangliomas. *Journal of Clinical Endocrinology and Metabolism* **74:** 1082–1089.

Robinson RG, DeQuattro V, Grushkin CM et al (1977) Childhood pheochromocytoma; treatment with alphamethyltyrosine for persistent hypertension. *Journal of Pediatrics* **91:** 143.

Ross EJ & Griffith DNW (1989) The clinical presentation of phaeochromocytoma. *Quarterly Journal of Medicine* **266:** 485–496.

Ross EJ, Prichard BN, Kaufman L, Robertson AI & Harries BJ (1967) Preoperative and operative management of patients with phaeochromocytoma. *British Medical Journal* **28:** 191–198.

Sackel SG, Manson JE, Harawi SJ & Burakoff R (1985) Watery diarrhoea syndrome due to an adrenal phaeochromocytoma secreting vasoactive intestinal peptide. *Digestive Diseases and Sciences* **30:** 1201–1207.

Samaan NA & Hickley RC (1987) Phaeochromocytoma. *Seminars in Oncology* **14:** 297–305.

Sardesai SH, Mourant AJ, Sivathandon T, Farrow R & Gibbons DO (1990) Phaeochromocytoma and catecholamine induced cardiomyopathy presenting as heart failure. *British Heart Journal* **63:** 234–237.

Schenker JG & Chowers I (1971) Phaeochromocytoma and pregnancy. *Obstetrical and Gynecological Survey* **26:** 739–747.

Schenker JG & Granat M (1982) Phaeochromocytoma and pregnancy—an updated appraisal. *Australian and New Zealand Journal of Obstetrics and Gynaecology* **22:** 1–10.

Schmedtje JF Jr, Sax S, Pool JL, Goldfarb RA & Nelson EB (1987) Localization of ectopic phaeochromocytomas by magnetic resonance imaging. *American Journal of Medicine* **83:** 770–772.

Scott HW Jr & Halter SA (1982) Oncologic aspects of phaeochromocytoma: the importance of follow-up. *Surgery* **96:** 1061–1066.

Scott I, Parkes R & Cameron DP (1988) Phaeochromocytoma and cardiomyopathy. *Medical Journal of Australia* **148:** 94–96.

Shapiro B, Sisson JC, Lloyd R, Najako M, Satterlee W & Beierwaltes WH (1984) Malignant phaeochromocytoma. Clinical, biochemical and scintigraphic characterization. *Clinical Endocrinology* **20:** 189–203.

Sheps SG, Jiang NS & Klee GG (1988) Diagnostic evaluation of phaeochromocytoma. *Endocrinology and Metabolism Clinics of North America* **17(2):** 397–414.

Sheps SG, Jiang NS, Klee GG & van Heerden JA (1990) Recent developments in the diagnosis and treatment of phaeochromocytoma. *Mayo Clinic Proceedings* **65:** 88–95.

Shermin D, Cohn PS & Zipin SB (1990) Phaeochromocytoma presenting as rhabdomyolysis and acute myoglobinuric renal failure. *Archives of Internal Medicine* **150:** 2384–2385.

Shulkin BL, Shapiro B & Sisson JC (1987) Phaeochromocytoma, polycythaemia and venous thrombosis. *American Journal of Medicine* **83:** 773–776.

Simpson NE, Kidd KK & Goodfelow PJ (1987) Assignment of multiple endocrine neoplasia type 2a on chromosome 10 by linkage. *Nature* **328:** 528–530.

Smits M & Huizinga J (1961) Familial occurrence of phaeochromocytoma. *Acta Genetica Statistics Medicine* **11:** 137–153.

Sode J, Getzen LC & Osborne DP (1967) Cardiac arrhythmias and cardiomyopathy associated with phaeochromocytoma: report of three cases. *American Journal of Surgery* **114:** 927–931.

Stackpole RH, Melicow MM & Uson AC (1963) Phaeochromocytoma in children. *Journal of Pediatrics* **63:** 315–330.

Stewart AF, Burtis WJ, Wu T et al (1987) Two forms of parathyroid like adenylate cyclase stimulating protein derived from tumours associated with humeral hypercalcaemia of malignancy. *Journal of Bone and Mineral Research* **2:** 587–593.

Suzuki K, Miyashita A, Inouc Y ct al (1991) Interleukin 6 producing phaeochromocytoma *Acta Haematologica* **85(4):** 217–219.

Tevetoglu F & Lee CH (1956) Adrenal phaeochromocytoma simulating diabetes insipidus. Report of a case and review of the other pediatric cases. *American Journal of Diseases of Children* **91:** 365–379.

Thomas JE, Rooke JD & Kvale WF (1966) The neurologist's experience with pheochromocytoma. A review of 100 cases. *Journal of the American Medical Association* **197:** 754–758.

Timmis JB, Brown MJ & Allison DJ (1981) Therapeutic embolization of phaeochromocytoma. *British Journal of Radiology* **54:** 420.

Tippett PA, McEwan AJ & Ackery DM (1986) A re-evaluation of dopamine excretion in phaeochromocytoma. *Clinical Endocrinology* **25:** 401–410.

Turner CE (1983) Gastrointestinal pseudo-obstruction due to phaeochromocytoma. *American Journal of Gastroenterology* **78:** 214–217.

van Heerden JA, Sheps SG, Hamberger B et al (1982) Phaeochromocytoma; current status and changing trends. *Surgery* **91:** 367.

White PD, Lishman WA & Wyke MA (1986) Phaeochromocytoma as a cause of reversible dementia. *Journal of Neurology, Neurosurgery and Psychiatry* **49:** 1449–1451.

Yusa T, Hashimoto Y & Shima T (1973) Droperidol and phaeochromocytoma. *Japanese Journal of Anaesthesiology* **22:** 474.

Zweifler AJ & Julius S (1982) Increased platelet catecholamine content in phaeochromocytoma: a diagnostic test in patients with elevated catecholamines. *New England Journal of Medicine* **306:** 890.

Index

Note: Page numbers of article titles are in **bold** type.

545